# The Glycaemic Index

## A Physiological Classification of Dietary Carbohydrate

# The Glycaemic Index

## A Physiological Classification of Dietary Carbohydrate

**Thomas M.S. Wolever**

*Department of Nutritional Sciences*
*University of Toronto*
*Ontario*
*Canada*

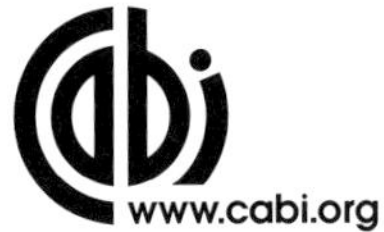

**CABI is a trading name of CAB International**

CABI Head Office
Nosworthy Way
Wallingford
Oxfordshire OX10 8DE
UK

Tel: +44 (0)1491 832111
Fax: +44 (0)1491 833508
E-mail: cabi@cabi.org
Web site: www.cabi.org

CABI North American Office
875 Massachusetts Avenue
7th Floor
Cambridge, MA 02139
USA

Tel: +1 617 395 4056
Fax: +1 617 354 6875
E-mail: cabi-nao@cabi.org



A catalogue record for this book is available from the British Library, London, UK.

A catalogue record for this book is available from the Library of Congress, Washington, DC.

ISBN-10: 1-84593-051-7
ISBN-13: 978-1-84593-051-6

Typeset by SPi, Pondicherry, India
Printed and bound in the UK by Biddles Ltd, King's Lynn.

# Contents

# Preface

The term 'glycaemic index' (GI) first appeared in the literature in 1981. Initially, the concept was applied to the treatment of diabetes and there was vigorous debate and large differences of opinion about its role in this respect. The American Diabetes Association concluded that the GI had no clinical utility and it was not recommended in the management of diabetes. By contrast, Diabetes Australia was so strongly supportive it felt that GI was essential information for everyone with diabetes; the result was the world's first food labelling programme, the GI Symbol Program, operated by Glycemic Index Ltd, a non-profit corporation whose members are the University of Sydney, Diabetes Australia and the Juvenile Diabetes Research foundation. Nevertheless, for about 15 years after the initial publication, scientific interest in the GI was only moderate because it was considered relevant only to diabetes and did not have support from the American Diabetes Association.

However, public and scientific interest in the GI has exploded over the past 10 years as it became evident that GI-influenced human health and performance in many ways. Of particular interest has been the role of GI in the management of body weight, and more and more popular diet books make reference to it. Unfortunately, along with increased interest in the GI has come widespread promulgation of over-simplified, misleading and faulty information about it. Scientists, health professionals and lay people use the term 'glycaemic index' inappropriately. Foods are given incorrect GI values in popular books and peer-reviewed scientific publications. Incorrect methods are used to measure the GI of foods. The clinical utility of the GI is, more often than not, presented in an unbalanced fashion, with it either being praised with exaggerated benefits far beyond what is justified by any research, or being unjustifiably condemned as having no clinical utility. The results of clinical trials of low-GI diets are inappropriately extrapolated by some to apply to diets containing novel carbohydrates which reduce glycaemic responses by a different mechanism. Recommendations about how to use GI information are sometimes not consistent either with sound nutritional principles or with the way the GI was used in the clinical trials demonstrating benefits.

All this inappropriate information about GI is not helpful – at best it is confusing – at worst it could destroy the GI concept altogether. Either way, such misunderstanding reduces our ability to learn more about the role of the GI in health and disease and to determine how best to use the GI to help those who could derive benefit from it. Therefore, I offer this book in the hope that it will help students, scientists and health professionals to understand the current state of knowledge about GI, to evaluate properly studies and other information about the GI and to use the most appropriate and up-to-date methods in their research, clinical work, product development or health education programs. In addition, I hope it will stimulate critical and creative thinking about the GI! It is not my intent to insist that my opinions about the GI are correct simply because that is the way it has always been done. I hope that the views presented in this book are based on the results of sound research and sound reasoning; I also hope that I am willing to be proven wrong.

# 1
# Historical Introduction

Over 150 years ago, Claude Bernard introduced the concept that the *milieu interieur*, the internal environment of the body, was controlled by homeostatic mechanisms. He was profoundly interested in carbohydrate metabolism, and considered that both the gut and the liver were central in the control of the blood glucose concentration. He suggested that carbohydrate was fed into the liver from the intestine and stored there (Bernard, 1848, 1855) and released (La Coudraie and Malloizel, 1881) as necessary to conserve the constancy of the *milieu interieur*. After his death, the liver continued to be considered central in the control of carbohydrate metabolism, a role later emphasized by the fact that individuals with liver disease may have episodes of hyperglycaemia (Johnston *et al.*, 1977) and hypoglycaemia (Sherlock, 1975). In addition, in individuals with diabetes who have normal liver function, there is a close relationship between hepatic glucose output and the fasting blood glucose (FBG) concentration (DeFronzo, 1988). With the discovery of the endocrine function of the pancreas, and later insulin itself, the role of the gastrointestinal tract in the regulation of carbohydrate metabolism was minimized. However, the small intestine is now known to be the largest endocrine organ in the body, and by virtue of the gut hormones, once again, has been implicated in the control of carbohydrate metabolism (Bloom and Polack, 1981; Drucker, 1998). This role was further enhanced by the discovery that modification of intraluminal events within the upper gastrointestinal tract by dietary fibre may profoundly affect the blood glucose and endocrine responses elicited by carbohydrate foods.

## 1.1 The Dietary Fibre Hypothesis

Interest in dietary fibre arose from the observations of Dennis Burkitt and Hugh Trowell, medical missionaries who noted, during their years of medical service in Africa, that many of the diseases common in developed countries were virtually unknown among rural Ugandans living on their traditional diets (Burkitt and Trowell, 1975). It is recognized that many factors have a role in the development of non-infectious diseases, including the effects of physical activity and obesity. The role of diet is less clear and much more controversial. Nevertheless, Burkitt and Trowell suggested that there was an association between a lack of fibre in the diet and many 'Western' diseases including coronary heart disease (CHD) (Trowell, 1972), diabetes (Trowell, 1973, 1974) and colon cancer (Burkitt, 1971). These observations have been confirmed by many subsequent epidemiological studies, and the role of dietary fibre in reducing the risk of heart disease (Lupton and Turner, 2003), diabetes (Salmerón *et al.*, 1997a,b; Wolever *et al.*, 1997a) and colon cancer (Bingham *et al.*, 2003; Peters *et al.*, 2003) is now well established.

Since it is not absorbed, dietary fibre influences disease risk by influencing events within the lumen of the gastrointestinal tract. In the 1970s, this was a novel concept, and the mechanisms discovered for dietary fibre led not only to the glycaemic index (GI), but also to the development of novel pharmacological (e.g. α-glucosidase inhibitors) and nutritional approaches (e.g. fructo-oligosaccharides) to prevent and treat various disorders. The mechanisms of action suggested for dietary fibre included: dilution of the energy density of the diet, resulting in reduced food intake and obesity; altered rates of gastric emptying; reduced rate and/or extent of the absorption of carbohydrate, fatty acids and cholesterol; the passage of fibre into the colon, leading to stool bulking and reduced transit times; and colonic fermentation leading to the production of short-chain fatty acids (SCFA) which influence local and systemic metabolism. For example, SCFA reduce the pH of the colonic contents, which in turn, alters intraluminal metabolism and absorption of sterol and nitrogen compounds. SCFA provide fuel for colonic mucosa and are absorbed and influence systemic metabolism. More recently, it has been shown that unabsorbed carbohydrates alter the populations of specific colonic bacterial species. This alteration, in turn, influences local and systemic immune function. These concepts will be discussed in more detail later in this book. Of most relevant to the development of the GI, however, was work on the effect of dietary fibre on postprandial glucose and insulin responses.

Early on it was suggested (Heaton, 1973), and later demonstrated both *in vitro* and *in vivo* (Elsenhaus *et al.*, 1980; Jenkins and Wolever, 1981; Blackburn *et al.*, 1984), that certain forms of dietary fibre, notably the viscous gelling agents such as guar gum, a galactomannan extracted from the cluster bean, *Cyampopsis tetragonoloba*, were able to reduce the rate of uptake of carbohydrate from the small intestine (Blackburn *et al.*, 1984) and reduce the excursions of blood glucose and insulin following the ingestion of fibre-containing test meals (Jenkins *et al.*, 1976). We showed that incorporation of guar into the diets of subjects with diabetes resulted in improved glycaemic control, as judged by reduced urinary glucose output (Jenkins *et al.*, 1977). In order to see if guar could have any practical use in the management of diabetes, an effective method of administration was required. If guar worked by trapping the food within an intraluminal gel and reducing the rate of digestion, it would have to be hydrated and intimately mixed with the food in order to reduce postprandial glucose responses; if guar were sprinkled on food, or taken between meals it was not effective in this respect (Wolever *et al.*, 1978). Although mixing guar with foods such as bread, instant potato, soups and cereals prior to eating was effective in reducing glucose and insulin responses, it made them highly viscous and unpalatable (Wolever *et al.*, 1979). Guar crispbread turned out to be one palatable solution to this problem (Jenkins *et al.*, 1978a) and patients with diabetes were able to use guar crispbread for periods of up to 1 year with some success (Jenkins *et al.*, 1980c).

Unfortunately, we were unable to develop the use of guar as a practical tool in the management of diabetes for several reasons. The manufacturer of guar crispbread was unable to continue to support the research programme, and we were unable to find any other industrial backing. Manufacturers felt that there was no future in guar-enriched foods (products which would now be known as 'functional foods'). In addition, we had to rely on the crude measure of urinary glucose output as an assessment of postprandial glucose levels. At this time, there was no way of measuring blood glucose concentrations throughout the day in patients with diabetes outside of a metabolic ward situation. Glycated haemoglobin had not yet been discovered, and portable glucose monitors had not yet been developed. Indeed, lancet devices using a fine needle had only just been developed and our colleagues in the diabetes clinic were assessing procedures for home glucose monitoring such as having patients place a drop of blood on a filter paper and mailing to the laboratory a small disc of blood-soaked paper punched out with a hole punch. The difficulty in assessing glycaemic control made it difficult to know whether dietary fibre supplements had any benefits. Therefore, we decided to turn our attention to studying the glycaemic responses elicited by high-fibre foods; work which lead directly to the development of the GI. Before describing this, however, it is important to review studies on the glycaemic impact of foods originating from other laboratories prior to the appearance of the GI.

## 1.2 Early Studies on the Glycaemic Effects of Carbohydrates

Clinicians were interested in the glycaemic effects of foods at a very early stage, even before blood glucose could be measured easily. Because of methodological limitations, the results of some of the early papers are often difficult to interpret or do not agree (but are not necessarily inconsistent) with our current understanding about the glycaemic effects of carbohydrates. However, results can be found from over 80 years ago which are completely consistent with modern results. The following is not a complete review of the early literature, but a sampling of those cited by later workers in the area and which therefore appear to have been influential in shaping understanding about the glycaemic effects of carbohydrates prior to the development of the GI.

### 1.2.1 Studies before 1970

Before 1970, it was almost universally held that available carbohydrates should be categorized as being 'simple' (i.e. mono- and disaccharides) or 'complex' (i.e. starch). The idea that simple carbohydrates elicit higher glycaemic responses than complex carbohydrates originated from the work of Allen prior to the 1920s in dogs; in these studies blood glucose was not even measured. Allen's objective was to determine the appropriate management of diabetes at a time when insulin and oral hypoglycaemic drugs were not available and diet was the only known treatment. Partially depancreatized dogs were fed various different diets with urinary glucose excretion being the measure of glycaemic control and rate of progression of diabetes. Allen found that feeding dogs glucose caused diabetes to progress more rapidly than starch, but that there was no difference between the effects of different starches such as bread, oatmeal, rice, potato or pearled barley (Allen, 1920). Allen attributed the difference between 'sugar' and starch to the rate of absorption, and concluded that: '. . . a rapid flood of carbohydrate is more injurious to the pancreatic function than a slow absorption'.

In the early 1920s, carbohydrate tolerance was studied by measuring glucose excretion in the urine or glucose concentration in the blood. Indeed, an experimental issue which interested many investigators at this time was to determine the renal threshold for glucose, since it was not known if people without diabetes ever had 'sugar' in their urine (Folin and Berglund, 1922). We now know that the chemical methods used to measure urinary glucose at that time reacted with substances other than glucose; thus, the results of these early papers are probably unreliable because of false positives.

During this early period, blood glucose responses elicited by various nutrients and foods were sometimes measured, but the results are often difficult to interpret or unreliable for a number of reasons such as the use of a very small number of subjects (often only one); non-standardized fasting times, starting times, blood sampling intervals and doses of nutrients fed; and a lack of description of the composition of the test meals. Some of these problems are illustrated by the results Folin and Berglund (1922) (Fig. 1.1). The glycaemic response elicited by 200 g glucose was determined in six subjects – the carbohydrate tolerance of the six subjects differed markedly and the blood sampling interval and time over which blood samples were taken also varied from subject to subject (Fig. 1.1, top). The responses elicited by various carbohydrates including maltose, starch, fructose, galactose and lactose were studied in one subject. None of them elicited an appreciable rise in blood glucose (Fig. 1.1). Unfortunately, these results cannot reliably be compared with those elicited by glucose because the subject's blood glucose concentration after oral glucose was not measured until 1.5 h after the glucose load. By this time, blood glucose was only moderately above the fasting concentration and most of the glycaemic response elicited by oral glucose had, presumably, been missed. To be fair to the authors, however, the major purpose of the study was to determine the relationship between 'blood sugar' and 'urine sugar' in an attempt to gain some understanding about the metabolism of different sugars. Thus, the timing,of the blood samples was probably related to when the subjects could pass urine rather than a desire to comparing the glycaemic responses elicited by the different test meals.

Gray (1923) was concerned about how to diagnose diabetes and felt that measuring blood sugar was better than measuring urine sugar. However, there was concern at the time that feeding subjects large doses of glucose might be harmful because of Allen's conclusion (Allen, 1920) that glucose was more damaging to the pancreas than starch. Therefore, Gray (1923) reviewed the blood glucose responses elicited by various doses of glucose and other carbohydrates with a view to establishing normal ranges. The results presented in this paper are difficult to interpret for several reasons. The different test meals were tested in different groups of subjects

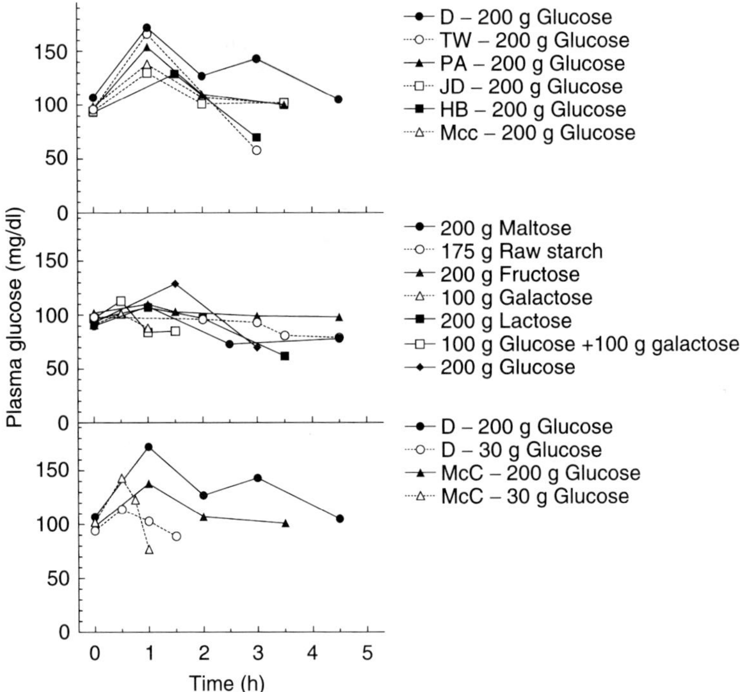


**Fig. 1.1.** Plasma glucose response curves published by Folin and Berglund (1922). Each curve is the response of a single individual. Top: six individuals' responses to 200 g glucose. Middle: one individual's (subject HB) response to various different carbohydrates. Bottom: two subjects' responses to 30 and 200 g glucose.

varying in size from $n = 4$ to 300. The doses of carbohydrates were not consistent, and the results of different doses were often combined in ranges. Also, curiously, the tables giving the mean blood glucose responses elicited by the different carbohydrates do not include the fasting value, and thus, one has to use the overall mean value for fasting glucose for all the subjects. This may not necessarily represent the fasting glucose for the group of subjects testing each test meal. The results from Gray (1923) suggest that glycaemic responses generally increase with the dose of glucose consumed, but 50 g glucose elicited a higher response in 21 subjects than 70–100 g glucose in 300 subjects (Fig. 1.2, left). These data do not fit the expected dose–response relationship derived from recent data (Fig. 1.2, right). By contrast, MacLean reported glycaemic responses elicited by 5, 10, 20 and 50 g glucose in the one subject (Fig. 1.2, centre) and these results fit the expected non-linear dose–response relationship very well (Fig. 1.2, right).

Another result from Gray (1923), which is not consistent with current concepts, is that sucrose and fructose elicited higher glycaemic responses than glucose (Fig. 1.3, top). On the other hand, MacLean (1922) showed that 50 g fructose elicited only about 15% of the glycaemic response elicited by 50 g glucose. Gray also shows that the responses elicited by starch and a mixed meal were similar to those elicited by glucose (Fig. 1.3, bottom), however, the nature of the starch and the composition of the mixed meal were not indicated.

Rowe and Rogers (1927) compared the glycaemic response elicited by 100 g glucose with that elicited by two shredded wheat biscuits and 3 oz milk, because the latter was being considered as a possible diagnostic test for diabetes. Twenty subjects consumed both test meals with blood glucose being measured at fasting and at 30, 90 and 150 min. These methods are suitable for comparing the glycaemic impact of the two test meals. I calculated the incremental areas under

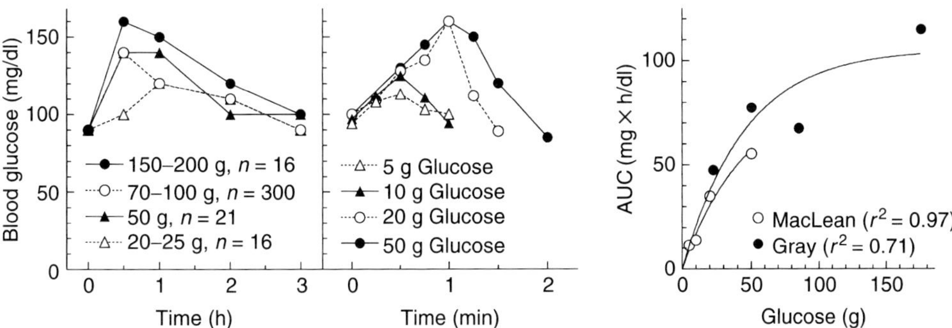


**Fig. 1.2.** Early dose–response curves: glycaemic responses elicited by different doses of glucose in normal subjects. Left, redrawn from Gray (1923). Centre, redrawn from MacLean (1922). Right, non-linear regression of incremental area under the curve (AUC) on dose of glucose; solid lines represent regression lines with the equation AUC $= K \times (1 - e^{-0.0222g})$ where $K$ is a constant and g is the grams of glucose (the rate constant is the same as that derived in Fig. 4.1 using data from my laboratory).

the mean glucose response curves shown in the Chart 2 of Rowe and Roberts (1927), and found that the glycaemic response elicited by shredded wheat, 659 mg × min/dl, was 38% of that elicited by 100 g glucose, 1736 mg × min/dl. To see whether this result is similar to what would be expected based on our current knowledge, one needs to know the amount of available carbohydrate and GI of the test meals. Rowe and Rogers (1927) did not indicate the nutrient composition of the shredded wheat test meal, but according to current food tables it would contain 37 g of available carbohydrate and have a GI of 70 (48 g of shredded wheat = 33 g available carbohydrate with GI of 75 (Foster-Powell *et al.*, 2002) and 92 g milk = 4 g available carbohydrate with a GI of 32). Using the formula shown in Fig. 4.1, the expected relative response of the shredded wheat meal (37 g available carbohydrate, GI = 70) is 44% of that for 100 g glucose (100 g

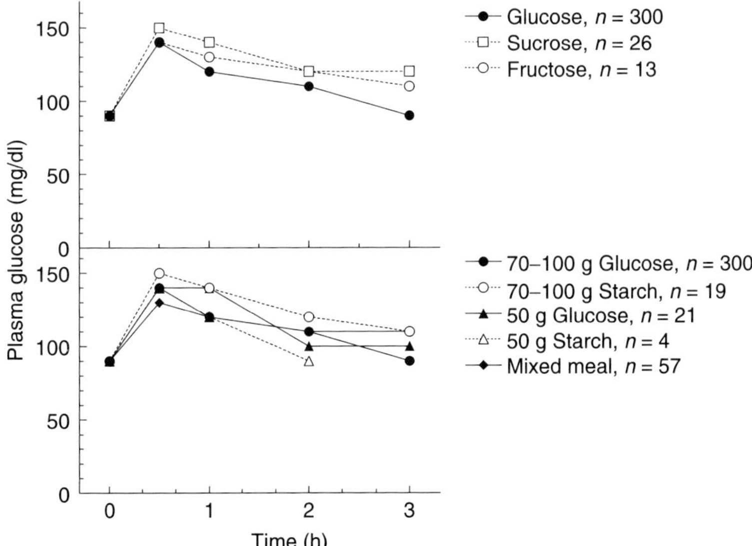


**Fig. 1.3.** Comparison of glycaemic responses elicited by different sugars (top) and glucose, starch and mixed meals (bottom) redrawn from Gray (1923).

available carbohydrate, GI = 100); a value very similar to the observed value of 38%.

During this period of time, it was generally felt that there were no significant differences in the assimilation of different starches (Allen, 1920), and there was evidence that there was little difference between cooked starches and glucose (Gray, 1923). Indeed, on this point, Allen (1920) concluded: 'Whenever permanent diabetes is present... starch brings on glycosuria more slowly than sugar, but just as surely.... The clinical lesson from such experiments is that even if a patient becomes free from glycosuria on withdrawal of sugar only, nevertheless other foods should also be limited'. The idea that different starchy foods have the same glycaemic impact was also put forward by MacLean (1922) based on a comparison of the glycaemic responses elicited by 250 g potatoes vs 100 g oatmeal (Fig. 1.4), probably based on studies in one subject. (Note also the different schedule of blood sampling for the different tests.) MacLean (1922) states that 'The ordinary starchy foods, such as potatoes, rice, corn-flour, and oatmeal, behave almost exactly like glucose when given in proportionate amounts'.

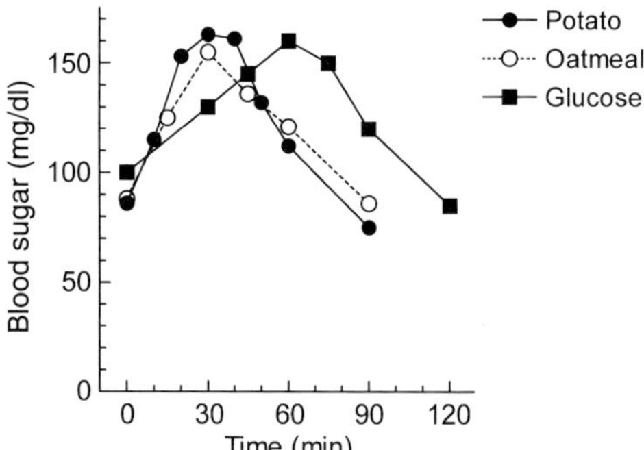


**Fig. 1.4.** Glycaemic responses elicited by 50 g glucose, 250 g potatoes and 100 g oatmeal. Redrawn from MacLean (1922).

Although it was felt that all cooked starches elicited large glycaemic responses, it was known in the 1920s that raw starches had virtually no glycaemic effect in humans (Rosenthal and Ziegler, 1929) (Fig. 1.5). It was known at this time that raw starches were virtually completely digested during passage through the human alimentary tract (Langworthy and Deuel, 1922), but there was controversy as to the extent to which digestion and absorption occurred in the small intestine, as opposed to breakdown by bacterial fermentation in the colon (Rosenthal and Ziegler, 1929). Those of us working in the carbohydrate field today tend to think that the significance of colonic fermentation in humans only began to be appreciated about 25 years ago; in fact, the discussion of Rosenthal and Ziegler (1929) reads like it was written recently and clearly shows that the importance of colonic fermentation was appreciated over 75 years ago.

Conn and Newburgh (1936) were mainly interested in comparing the effects of carbohydrate and protein on glycaemic responses, but as part of these studies they observed that portions of apple and bread containing 53 g available carbohydrate elicited lower glycaemic responses than 53 g glucose in patients with diabetes. Calculation of the area under the curve (AUC) from the

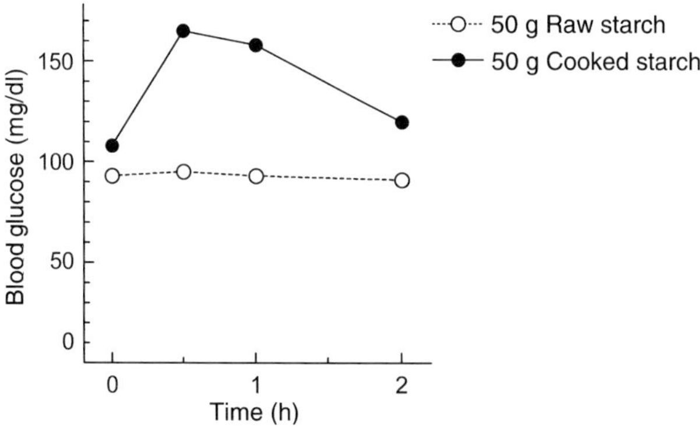


**Fig. 1.5.** Glycaemic response elicited by 50 g raw starch and 50 g cooked starch (250 g potato). Redrawn from Rosenthal and Ziegler (1929).

graphs of the data shown in this paper indicate that apple and bread elicited glycaemic responses 52% and 76% of that elicited by glucose, consistent with the GI values of these two foods, 38 and 71, respectively (Foster-Powell *et al.*, 2002).

### 1.2.2 Studies after 1970

After about 1970, authors began to be specifically interested in comparing the glycaemic responses elicited by different carbohydrates. Thus, study designs were more appropriate for this purpose, with groups of 8 to 20 subjects being studied with each subject testing each test meal. However, important details about the nature of the test foods and cooking methods used are sometimes lacking. In addition, the methods used to quantify glycaemic responses were evolving during this time and one can begin to see how differences in data analysis could influence markedly the interpretation of the results obtained.

Lütjens *et al.* (1975) compared the glycaemic responses elicited by 50 g carbohydrate portions of glucose, sucrose, bread and starch, in the form of potato. The way the potato starch was cooked and served is not indicated. The authors compared glucose and insulin concentrations at each point in time. They concluded that since neither the glucose nor insulin values showed any significant differences after the various carbohydrates, it was not important what type of carbohydrate is administered. However, the statistical analysis presented is not consistent with this conclusion because it shows that blood glucose concentrations at some time points differed significantly (Fig. 1.6). The authors did not calculate the areas under the blood glucose response curves (AUC), but doing so using the data presented indicates that sucrose, bread and potato, respectively, elicited glycaemic responses 76%, 71% and 53% that of glucose.

Crapo *et al.* (1977) published a series of papers in which the glucose and insulin responses elicited by 50 g carbohydrate portions of glucose, baked potato, rice, white bread and maize were determined in normal subjects, subjects with impaired glucose tolerance (IGT) (Crapo *et al.*, 1980) and subjects with type 2 diabetes (Crapo *et al.*, 1981). Although the same protocol was used in these papers, the method of data analysis differed. In the normal subjects, Crapo *et al.* (1977) found that the different carbohydrates elicited virtually identical total AUC values. Nevertheless, they concluded that different carbohydrate sources elicited different glycaemic responses on the basis of significantly different glucose concentrations between 30 and 60 min. For the studies in subjects with IGT and diabetes, Crapo *et al.* (1980, 1981) calculated incremental AUC (IAUC) values. In the paper with IGT subjects, there was no statistical comparison of the AUC values, but the authors noted that the responses elicited by bread, rice and maize were 25% to 36% lower than those elicited by glucose and potato. In the paper in subjects with diabetes, Crapo *et al.* (1981) found significant differences in AUC between the different carbohydrate sources, with bread, rice and maize eliciting glucose responses 11–41% lower than potato and glucose. When comparing the results of these studies, the authors did not compare the relative glycaemic responses (RGR), but pointed out that the difference in glycaemic response between foods in subjects with IGT or diabetes were two to three times greater than those in normal subjects (Crapo *et al.*, 1980, 1981).

Figure 1.7 shows my recalculation of the results of the studies by Crapo *et al.* (1977, 1980,

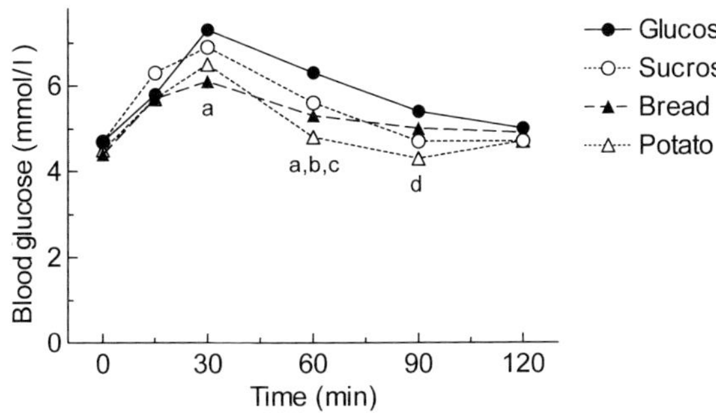


**Fig. 1.6.** Mean blood glucose responses elicited by 50 g carbohydrate from glucose, sucrose, bread or potato in nine normal subjects. Statistically significant differences ($P < 0.05$): a, glucose vs bread; b, glucose vs potato; c, sucrose vs potato; and d, sucrose vs bread. Redrawn from Lütjens *et al.* (1975).

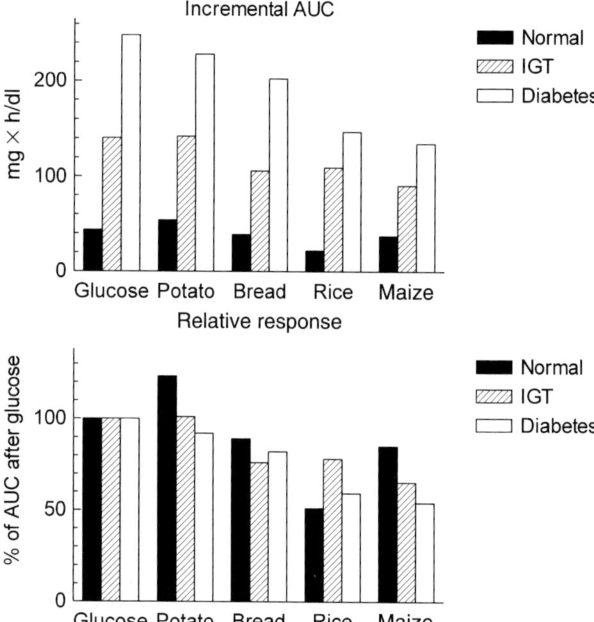


**Fig. 1.7.** Mean incremental areas under the curve (top) and relative responses (bottom) elicited by 50 g carbohydrate portions of glucose, baked potato, bread, rice and maize in normal subjects, and subjects with IGT and type 2 diabetes. Recalculated from Crapo *et al.* (1977, 1980, 1981).

1981). The top of Fig. 1.7 shows the IAUC values calculated from the mean glucose concentrations; it can be seen that subjects with IGT and diabetes have AUC values which are three- and fivefold greater than normal subjects, and that the differences in AUC between foods is larger in subjects with diabetes and IGT than without. However, when expressed relative to the AUC after glucose, the glycaemic responses elicited by potato, bread, rice and maize were similar in the different groups of subjects (Fig. 1.7, bottom). Indeed, using the SD of the relative responses of potato, rice, maize and bread as the measure of differences in glycaemic response between foods, the difference in relative response between foods is smaller in subjects with diabetes (SD = 18) and IGT (SD = 15) than in normal subjects (SD = 29).

Vaaler *et al.* (1980) measured the plasma glucose and insulin responses elicited by 300 kcal portions of glucose, potato, rice, white bread and brown bread. Since the test meals contained equal amounts of energy, their content of carbohydrate varied from 58 to 75. The authors did not calculate the AUC, but doing so from the mean glucose concentrations given, results in mean IAUC values of 111, 70, 77, 49 and 64 mg × h/dl, respectively, for glucose, potato, rice, white bread and brown bread. Thus, the responses of potato, rice, white bread and brown bread, expressed as a percentage of that for glucose, were 62%, 70%, 44% and 58%, respectively. However, these values cannot be considered approximations of the GI because the test meals contained different amounts of carbohydrate. After adjusting for this, using the regression equation shown in Fig. 4.1, the approximate 'GI' values of these four foods becomes 64, 72, 50 and 64, respectively.

The largest number of foods tested for glycaemic response prior to the GI was reported by Otto's group who expressed the glucose AUC elicited by 25 g carbohydrate portions of different foods in subjects with diabetes as a percentage of that elicited by 25 g glucose. This is nearly the same methodology as used for GI. However, at the time we published the first paper on GI (Jenkins *et al.*, 1981a) we were unaware of this work because, apart from a few abstracts (Schauberger *et al.*, 1977), only one paper was ever published by the group (Spaethe *et al.*, 1972). In addition, Otto used the information differently than we conceived; we envisaged the GI as being used as an aid to selecting carbohydrate foods to enable a high carbohydrate intake to be maintained with minimal glycaemic impact. By contrast, Otto's concept was to adjust the amounts of different carbohydrate foods consumed so as to maintain a constant glycaemic impact (Spaethe *et al.*, 1972). The mean of the RGR for 13 foods published by Otto's group (Spaethe *et al.*, 1972; Schauberger *et al.*, 1977), 46.5%, is similar to the mean of the GI values for the same 13 foods summarized by Foster-Powell *et al.* (2002), 48.2 (ns) and the correlation between the values is excellent ($r = 0.886$, $P < 0.001$, Fig. 1.8).

## 1.3 The Inception of the GI

Two technological advances which occurred in the late 1970s were invaluable in allowing us to study the glycaemic responses of foods: the development of the Autolet® lancet device (Owen Mumford Ltd., Woodstock, UK) which allowed subjects to obtain their own blood samples, and the development of an automatic glucose analyser (Yellow Springs Instruments, Yellow Springs, WI) which could measure glucose accurately, easily and rapidly using a 25 μl sample of whole blood. Prior to this, assessing glucose responses was a labour-intensive process, which required a trained individual to obtain venous blood samples. Since one phlebotomist can take venous blood sample from only one subject at a time, a limited number of subjects could be studied on any one occasion. Once subjects could obtain their own finger-prick capillary blood samples, a large number of subjects could be studied simultaneously.

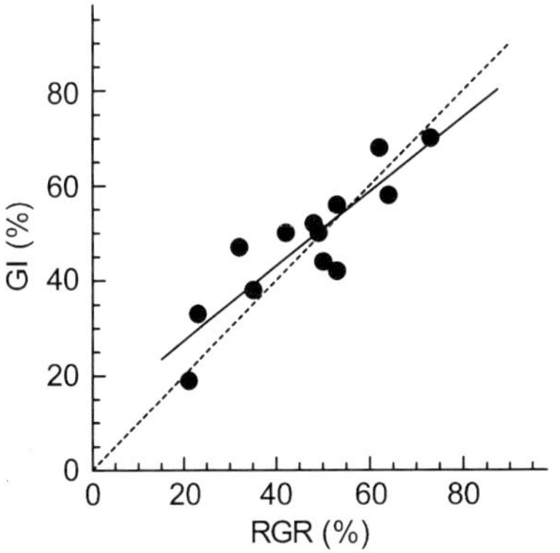


**Fig. 1.8.** Correlation between relative glycaemic responses (RGR) of 13 foods published by Otto's group (Spaethe *et al.*, 1972; Schauberger *et al.*, 1977) and the mean GI values for the same foods from the International GI Tables (Foster-Powell *et al.*, 2002). The following are the foods shown, with the value in brackets being the food ID number from the International GI Tables; fructose (580), dried peas (467, 469, 474), carrots (599), apple (388), whole grain rye bread (84), banana (397), potato (605), pasta (533), rice (277), orange (415), sucrose (589), oatmeal porridge (209) and wheat bread (101).

Since we had found that the ability of dietary fibre to reduce glycaemic responses was related to its viscosity, we began by comparing the glycaemic responses of foods containing what we considered to be viscous and non-viscous fibres. Since guar was obtained from a legume, we studied legumes as sources of viscous fibre, and found them to elicit lower glycaemic responses than other starchy carbohydrate foods (Jenkins *et al.*, 1980d). The low glycaemic responses elicited by lentils and soybeans *in vivo* were associated with much slower rates of digestion of the foods *in vitro* (Jenkins *et al.*, 1980a). We went on to compare the responses of different whole or fibre-depleted cereal products, bread, rice and spaghetti, and found that while the presence of cereal fibre had no effect, there was a difference between bread, rice and spaghetti (Jenkins *et al.*, 1981c). These results were so surprising that we wanted to compare the glycaemic responses elicited by a large number of foods. The result was the GI (Jenkins *et al.*, 1981a).

We faced a number of problems in planning this study. One was how to control for the fact that we could not test all the foods in the same group of subjects. Since glycaemic responses vary in different people, we decided to control for between-subject variation by giving everyone 50 g glucose and express the results of each subject relative to his or her own response to glucose. We also realized that it would take a long time to test a large number of foods and it was possible that subjects' carbohydrate tolerance might change over time. Thus, the glycaemic response elicited by 50 g glucose was tested repeatedly in each subject. Finally, we needed to be able to express the glycaemic response using a single number. Since we wanted to know how much the food raised blood glucose, we thought the best way to express this would be the IAUC, ignoring area beneath the fasting level. But we did not know how to measure it!

We knew that AUC could be calculated using the trapezoid rule, but the problem was how to determine the AUC between two time points when blood glucose was greater than fasting at one but less than fasting at the other. As an example, let us take the situation where, at time $T_1$ glucose is $A$ above fasting, and at time $T_2$ glucose is $B$ below fasting. We needed to find the area of the triangle whose height is $A$ and whose base is $t$ (the difference between $T_1$ and the time that the straight line between $A$ and $B$ crosses the fasting level). The area of this triangle will be $At/2$, but the problem is finding $t$ – at what exact time did the blood glucose cut the baseline? I remember discussing various options with David Jenkins, including plotting the glycaemic response curve on graph paper, cutting it out, and weighing it! It seemed to me there had to be an easier way. I suddenly realized that this could be worked out mathematically; there were two nested triangles, one had a height of $A$ and base of $t$, and the other had a height of $(A + B)$ and a base of $T$.

$$\text{Since, } t/T = A/(A+B),$$

$$\text{therefore, } t = TA/(A+B),$$

$$\text{thus, AUC} = At/2 = TA^2/[(A+B) \times 2].$$

We were fortunate that the decisions made to address these three methodological issues turned out to be good ones. We did not really understand the importance of these issues, or even feel the need to test whether the assumptions made were correct. It was only later that, prompted by criticisms of the GI, we began to consider these issues and found that the GI actually does control for between-subject variation (Wolever, 1992), that taking the average of several responses of the reference food is necessary to normalize the results (Wolever *et al.*, 1991a) and that the method of AUC calculation we used may be more valid and precise than other methods commonly used (Wolever, 2004a). In addition, we were unaware of much of the previous work showing that different foods elicited different glycaemic responses.

## 1.4 The Development of the GI

After the publication of the first GI paper, there was growing interest in the GI. Groups in France (Bornet *et al.*, 1987, 1989), Italy (Parillo *et al.*, 1985), Scandinavia (Hermansen *et al.*, 1987), Israel (Indar-Brown *et al.*, 1992) and Australia (Colagiuri *et al.*, 1986; Chew *et al.*, 1988) confirmed that different starchy foods elicited different glycaemic responses in normal and diabetic subjects and found that these differences were maintained in the context of mixed meals. A number of these groups showed that reducing the GI of the diet improved glycaemic control in diabetes (Fontvieille *et al.*, 1988, 1992; Brand *et al.*, 1991; Frost *et al.*, 1994). In addition, these and other groups were elucidating the mechansisms responsible for the different glycaemic responses (Brand *et al.*, 1985; Holm *et al.*, 1988, 1989; Liljeberg *et al.*, 1992; Liljeberg and Björck, 1996, 1998). This work contributed much towards the scientific validation of the GI concept.

Until about the middle of the 1990s, the only clinical application of the GI was considered to be in the treatment of diabetes. In this respect the GI was not accepted in North America, despite the positive results of ourselves and others, because studies from the USA consistently concluded that the GI had no clinical utility (Coulston *et al.*, 1984a,b, 1987; Hollenbeck *et al.*, 1986, 1988; Laine *et al.*, 1987); consequently the American Diabetes Association (1994) did not recommend it.

However, things began to change with the application of the GI to dietary data collected by Dr Walter Willett's group at Harvard University in the Nurses' Health and Male Health Professionals Studies, prospective studies involving well over 100,000 participants. The first papers from Willett's group using the GI appeared in 1997 and showed that a low diet GI reduced the risk of developing diabetes (Salmerón *et al.*, 1997a,b). This stimulated other work not only from Harvard group but also from others around the world examining the effect of GI on the risk of diabetes, metabolic syndrome, cardiovascular disease, cardiovascular disease risk factors and cancer; these papers are reviewed in Chapter 8. Another important factor which raised the profile of the GI in North America was the work from Dr David Ludwig's group at Harvard suggesting that GI has an important role to play in the regulation of body weight (Ludwig *et al.*, 1999a,b; Ludwig, 2000; Pawlak *et al.*, 2004). This work was important because it expanded the potential clinical utility of the GI from the treatment of diabetes to the treatment and prevention of a wide range of disorders and showed how GI could be relevant to the normal population.

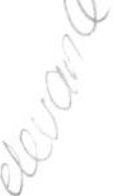

An indication of the extent to which scientific interest in the GI is increasing can be obtained by considering the number of publications in the

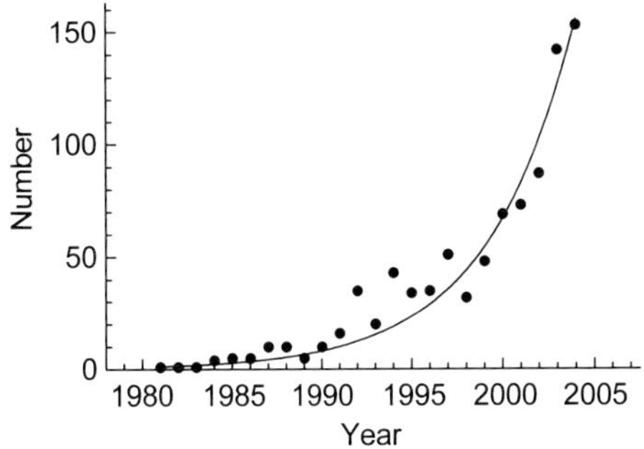


**Fig. 1.9.** Growth in the number of scientific publications on glycaemic index per year.

scientific literature appearing on the topic. Figure 1.9 shows the number of papers published in the scientific literature per year from 1981 to 2004 based on a search of the ISI Web of Knowledge(TM) database (http://isi6.isiknowledge.com/portal.cgi/WOS) for the term 'glycaemic index' in the title, abstract or keywords. The number increases nearly exponentially, with the slope increasing markedly after 1997, when the first papers from the Health Professionals Studies appeared.

## 1.5 Summary

There has been interest in measuring the glycaemic impact of foods for nearly 100 years. Early attempts were limited by the difficulty in measuring blood glucose concentrations and by other methodological issues. Recent interest in measuring the glycaemic impact of foods arose from the dietary fibre hypothesis and was focused primarily on the treatment of diabetes. The term 'glycaemic index' was coined in 1981 by Jenkins *et al.* (1981a). Since the late 1990s interest in the GI has exploded because it has been found to be relevant in many areas of human health and performance.

# 2

# Determining the GI of Foods – Methodological Considerations

To be practically useful, the definition of the term 'glycaemic index' and the methods used to determine the GI of foods must be standardized so that the values obtained are not only reproducible but also mean the same thing in different countries. Unfortunately, the definition of certain nutrients differs in different countries. Most unfortunately for the GI, dietary carbohydrates fall into this category, with long-standing disagreements about the terminology used to describe the term 'carbohydrate' and its components from a regulatory point of view. In North America, the amount of 'carbohydrate' on the food label includes total carbohydrate measured by difference, whereas in Europe, 'carbohydrate' on the food label includes available carbohydrates measured directly. Similar problems occur with the term 'dietary fibre' and 'starch'. I believe these disagreements have contributed to misunderstanding and confusion about the GI, and are certainly the source of differences in methodology used to determine the GI of foods.

The method used to determine the GI of foods is deceptively complex with numerous issues to be considered. The importance of some issues, such as how AUC is calculated, or how 'carbohydrate' is defined, is sometimes not appreciated, and the method used not described in some papers on GI. In these cases, it is difficult to compare the results with other data in the literature. On the other hand, some investigators go to great lengths to control and describe factors, such as careful selection of subjects without personal or family history of diabetes, which actually have little or no impact on the GI values obtained. In addition, there are a number of important issues about methods which have not been resolved, and there are many questions for which no data exist. What follows in this chapter is a description of the recommended method for determining the GI of foods, and a detailed justification as to why things are done that way, and, where data exist, the consequences of using different methods.

## 2.1 Definition of the 'Glycaemic Index'

The GI is defined as the incremental area under the blood glucose response curve elicited by a 50 g available carbohydrate portion of a food expressed as a percentage of the response after 50 g anhydrous glucose taken by the same subject.

This definition raises many questions such as: What is 'incremental area under the curve?' How is 'blood glucose' measured? What is 'available carbohydrate?' What kind of subjects should be studied? Does it have to be a 50 g carbohydrate portion? Does the reference food have to be glucose? Before addressing these issues, it is important to consider questions of a more philosophical nature, the answers to which must take into account the purpose of the GI, and what distinguishes GI from information about food composition which can be obtained from chemical analysis. These issues relate to the 'meaning' of the GI rather than its definition.

### 2.1.1 Meaning of 'glycaemic index'

The GI was originally meant to be an index of the blood glucose raising potential of the available carbohydrate in foods. Monro (2002) has shown that GI does not indicate the glycaemic impact of a food. He rightly points out that GI is a property of the carbohydrates in foods, not a property of foods, and also that GI is a value which is independent of the portion size of the food or the amount of carbohydrate consumed. He believes, therefore, that GI is '. . . not suitable for dietary management of postprandial glycaemia. . . . ', and should be redefined (Monro, 2003). However, I believe current evidence suggests that the original meaning of GI should be retained because it provides a unique and useful measure of the biological quality of the available carbohydrate in foods. I will review this evidence in Chapter 9. However, here it is important to point out a number of principles that follow from this meaning.

#### *2.1.1.1 Glycaemic index is not the same as glycaemic response*

The term 'glycaemic index' is often used incorrectly to mean 'glycaemic response' in a variety of situations including: mixed meals, foods containing unavailable carbohydrate and differences between subjects. In the context of mixed meals, for example, it has been stated that: 'Adding fat to bread reduces its glycaemic index'. In this case, the correct terminology would be: 'Adding fat to bread reduces the glycaemic response'. Also, investigators sometimes determine the glycaemic responses of mixed meals and calculate a 'GI' of the meals by expressing the glycaemic responses as a percentage of the response of the same subjects to bread or glucose. This is inappropriate because the GI is a property of individual carbohydrate foods tested by themselves with nothing added. It is known that fat and protein affect glycaemic responses, but these effects have nothing to do with the glycaemic response of the carbohydrate. In addition, the effects of added fat and protein on glycaemic responses differ in normal subjects, subjects with type 1 diabetes and subjects with type 2 diabetes (discussed in Chapter 5, this volume). On the other hand, the GI of individual carbohydrate foods is the same in all of these different types of subjects. Thus, the GI of mixed meals should be calculated from the GI values of the individual foods whereas the 'glycaemic responses' of mixed meals should be measured *in vivo*. The relative differences between the observed glycaemic responses should be predicted by the relative differences in calculated meal GI.

Some investigators persist in using the term 'glycaemic index' to describe the fact that foods containing low amounts of available carbohydrate, such as vegetables, have low glycaemic responses (Tremblay *et al.*, 2002). This is inappropriate because it is possible to tell from the food label that a food has little or no carbohydrate, and thus will not raise blood glucose. We can also know from the food label how much unavailable carbohydrate (non-starch polysaccharides (NSP), inulin, etc.) a food contains and since, by definition, unavailable carbohydrate is not available to the body as glucose, it does not raise blood glucose. A food in which some of the available carbohydrate has been replaced by unavailable carbohydrate (e.g. resistant starch (RS)) will elicit a lower glycaemic response than the normal food fed at the same level of total carbohydrate, but this could be known from the label, because the amount of available carbohydrate is less. It is not correct to equate this with a low-GI food because the long-term effects of reducing available carbohydrate intake are not the same as reducing the GI (Chapter 9, this volume).

The terms 'glycaemic index' and 'glycaemic response' should also not be confused because these entities have different mathematical and statistical properties (Wolever, 1992). Theoretically, the GI adjusts glycaemic response areas to each individual's response to a reference food, thus correcting for between-subject variation. In order to test this hypothesis, we determined the glycaemic responses of bread, rice and spaghetti in 12 subjects with diabetes with each subject repeating each food four times (Wolever *et al.*, 1990). The results showed that the glycaemic responses (i.e. incremental AUC values) differed significantly for the different foods and also differed significantly in the different subjects. Indeed, 62% of the total variance was accounted for by variation between subjects (Fig. 2.1). The exact magnitude of between-subject variation of glycaemic responses depends on the homogeneity of the subjects chosen, and in this case was large because subjects were chosen to be dissimilar by including subjects with both type 1 and type 2 diabetes on a variety of different treatments. However, when the AUC values were expressed as a percentage of each subject's average AUC after white bread (i.e. the GI), the difference between subjects was no

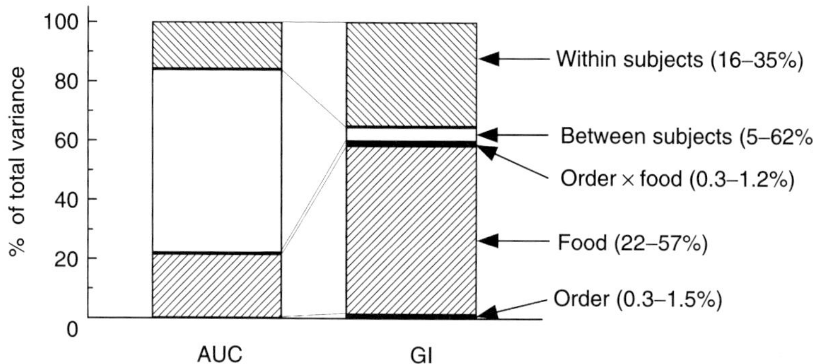


**Fig. 2.1.** Partitioning of variance of incremental areas under the glycaemic response curve (AUC) and glycaemic index values (GI) from tests in 12 subjects with diabetes whose glycaemic responses were measured after consuming bread, rice and spaghetti with each subject repeating each food four times (Wolever *et al.*, 1990).

longer significant, with between-subject variation accounting for only 5% of the total variance (Fig. 2.1). The proportion of total variance explained by variation within-subjects and variation between foods increased by more than twofold when results were expressed as GI. However, this is because the reduction in between-subject variation reduces total variation; when expressed as coefficient of variation (CV = 100 × SD/mean), expressing results as GI reduces between-subject variation without changing variation between foods or variation within subjects (Table 2.1).

### *2.1.1.2 Low-carbohydrate foods*

Foods containing no carbohydrate, such as bacon or eggs, do not have a GI. The GI is not an index of how much the food raises blood glucose, it is an index of the extent to which the available carbohydrate in the food raises the blood glucose.

It was originally intended that the GI should apply to 'high' carbohydrate foods such as grains, breads, cereals, etc. A problem arises when one considers manufactured food products which contain a considerable amount of their energy as fat and protein, such as meal replacement bars, or certain natural foods such as dairy products and nuts. It is known that fat and protein may affect glycaemic responses, as will be discussed in Chapter 5. Thus, the glycaemic response elicited by foods containing large amounts of fat and protein may be low because of the effects of fat and protein on insulin secretion or gastric emptying, rather than because of the intrinsic nature of the carbohydrate.

For example, let us consider a food bar such as Ironman PR Bar (PR Nutrition, San Diego, California) containing about 40% energy as carbohydrate, 30% fat and 30% protein, the main carbohydrate ingredients of which are high-fructose corn syrup (HFCS) and sucrose (University of Arizona, accessed 12 January, 2005). A 50 g available carbohydrate portion of this bar contains about 17 g fat and 35 g protein,

**Table 2.1.** Sources of variation of incremental area under the glycaemic response curve (AUC) and glycaemic index values (GI) expressed as standard deviations (SD) and coefficient of variation (CV).[a]

| | AUC values | | GI values | |
|---|---|---|---|---|
| Source of variance | SD | CV (%) | SD | CV (%) |
| Food | 262 | 31 | 22.9 | 30 |
| Within subjects | 210 | 25 | 15.9 | 21 |
| Between subjects | 408 | 49 | 5.8 | 8 |

[a]Data from Wolever *et al.* (1990) and Wolever (1992).

and elicits a mean glycaemic response about 55% that of a 50 g carbohydrate portion of white bread (Hertzler, 2000). Thus, the approximate GI of the bar is 55 × 0.71 = 39, a value 35% less than the GI of its carbohydrate ingredients (taken to be sucrose, GI = 60). However, it must be noted that my estimate of the GI of the carbohydrate ingredients assumes the HFCS in the Ironman PR bar is a 50:50 mixture of glucose and fructose; if the HFCS contained predominantly fructose, then the expected GI would be lower, but if the HFCS was predominantly glucose, then the expected GI would be higher (Chapter 5, this volume describes how to calculate the GI of a mixture of carbohydrate foods).

Tests on other types of food bars and candy bars suggest that, in the context of a food bar, protein may have more impact on the glycaemic response than fat. Hertzler (2000) showed that a 50 g available carbohydrate portion of PowerBar (Powerfood, Berkeley, California), containing 2 g fat and 12 g protein, elicited a mean glycaemic response 75% that of bread. PowerBar contains 40–45% of carbohydrate as glucose and fructose (mean GI = 60) and 50–55% as maltodextrin (GI = 100), brown rice (GI = 90) and oat bran (GI = 56) (PowerBar Sport When To Use/FAQ), thus (assuming oat bran to be a relatively minor ingredient) the GI of its carbohydrate ingredients is likely between 70 and 80, compared to the observed approximate GI of 75 × 0.71 = 53. On the other hand, 50 g available carbohydrate portions of Snickers candy bar (M&M Mars, Hackettstown, New Jersey) and Mars candy bar contain only 2–4 g protein but 14–21 g fat. The major carbohydrates in these candy bars are sugar (GI = 60) and corn syrup (GI = 100) so, assuming somewhat more sugar than corn syrup, the GI value of the carbohydrate mixture is likely between 70 and 80. Snickers elicited a mean glycaemic response 97% that of bread (GI ≈ 69) (Hertzler, 2000), and we found Mars bar to have a GI of 68 (Jenkins *et al.*, 1981a).

Thus, although the presence of some protein and fat do not necessarily have a major effect on the glycaemic response to carbohydrate, it is likely that high amounts do. This is an important issue, because if, as I believe it should be, the GI is a measure of the biological effect of the available carbohydrate in foods on glycaemic responses, independent of the effects of fat and protein on gastric emptying and insulin secretion, then it is not appropriate to determine GI on foods high in protein and fat. However, systematic dose–response studies have not been done on the effect on glycaemic responses of adding protein and fat alone and in combination to carbohydrate. Thus, it is difficult to determine a threshold for protein and fat contents of moderate and low-carbohydrate foods above which it might be considered inappropriate to determine GI.

#### 2.1.1.3 GI is measured for single foods and calculated for mixed meals

The GI has been criticized because it is a property of single foods which may not reflect the glycaemic effects of foods when they are consumed in a mixed meal due to the effects of added fat and protein (Hollenbeck *et al.*, 1986; American Diabetes Association, 1994, 2002; Franz *et al.*, 1994, 2002). To this end, some investigators are now measuring GI values of mixed meals by expressing the glycaemic response of a mixed meal containing 50 g carbohydrate as a percentage of the response after 50 g glucose or 50 g carbohydrate from bread. This approach is problematic because the magnitude of the difference in glycaemic response between the reference food and the mixed meal is not only due to differences in the carbohydrate, but also to the added fat and protein. The RGR of foods are the same in different groups regardless of their glucose tolerance status (see Section 2.2.4.1). However, this is not so for fat and protein. The effects of fat and protein on glycaemic responses have not been systematically studied, but it is known that the effects are influenced by different sources of fat and protein, the habitual diet the subject is consuming, the way the fat and protein is incorporated into the meal, and most importantly, the glucose tolerance status of the subjects (these issues are reviewed in Chapter 4, this volume). The implication of this is that the glycaemic effect of a mixed meal containing fat and protein, relative to that elicited by a reference food without fat and protein, may not be the same in different subjects. Therefore, the results of studies where the GI of mixed meals is measured are likely to be only applicable to the specific meal and in the specific group of subjects studied.

However, the GI values measured in individual foods can be applied to gain an insight into the relative glycaemic effects of mixed meals containing fat and protein in both normal and diabetic subjects. To do this, the GI of the mixed meal is mathematically *calculated* from the GI values and carbohydrate contents of the individual foods present in the mixed meal. This calculation ignores the effects of added fat and protein. The way this is done, and the validity of the approach is reviewed in Chapter 4. If done using the appropriate methods, the calculated GI of mixed meals is usually very closely related to the observed glycaemic responses elicited by the meals. Even if this were not so, the approach of determining the glycaemic effects of foods individually before combining them into a mixed meal is useful for helping to understand what determines the glycaemic responses of mixed meals.

The point being made here is that the GI is *measured* in individual foods and *calculated* for mixed meals. Thus, the criticism that the GI is not useful because it is only measured in single foods is way off the mark. Far from being a weakness, the fact that the GI is measured only in single foods is a major strength of the concept and is precisely what allows the GI to be useful.

#### *2.1.1.4 Exclusion of non-glycaemic carbohydrates*

The GI is intended to be a measure of how much the available carbohydrate in a high-carbohydrate food raises blood glucose. Therefore, unavailable, or non-glycaemic, carbohydrates should be excluded from the 50 g carbohydrate portion because, by definition, these carbohydrates do not raise blood glucose. When the GI was first developed, this was a fairly simple concept to apply in practice, because the only 'unavailable' carbohydrate for which analytic data were available was 'dietary fibre'. However, unavailable or partially available carbohydrates now include RS, unavailable oligosaccharides (e.g. inulin and fructo-oligosaccharides), modified starches, polydextrose and sugar alcohols, and these compounds are appearing more and more in the food supply. It is now appreciated that it is difficult, if not impossible, to measure the amount of carbohydrate in foods which is actually absorbed from the human small intestine. A method for measuring RS, which is accepted by the Association of Official Analytical Chemists, has been developed (McCleary and Monaghan, 2002). However, measured RS may overestimate the amount of carbohydrate entering the colon after consumption of starchy foods (Englyst and Cummings, 1986, 1987; Danjo *et al.*, 2003), particularly for amounts of RS over 1 g (Fig. 2.2). Most polyols are partly absorbed, and it is not only difficult to determine exactly how much is absorbed, but it is known that the proportion of the amount consumed which is absorbed probably varies in different individuals and also varies depending on whether they are consumed alone or with other foods (Beaugerie *et al.*, 1990). In addition, a proportion of some sugar alcohols which are absorbed are not metabolized, but excreted intact in the urine. Livesey (2003) reviewed the metabolism of polyols recently, and provided a useful table showing the approximate absorption and urinary excretion of different kinds of sugar alcohols which can be used to estimate available carbohydrate for GI determinations (Table 2.2).

Since it is difficult or impossible to actually measure the amount of 'available' carbohydrate in foods, it could be argued that most of the GI measurements in the literature have not properly excluded unavailable carbohydrate, and that the reductions in GI could be due to reductions in carbohydrate absorption. From this, it could be argued that unavailable carbohydrate should not be excluded from the 50 g carbohydrate load.

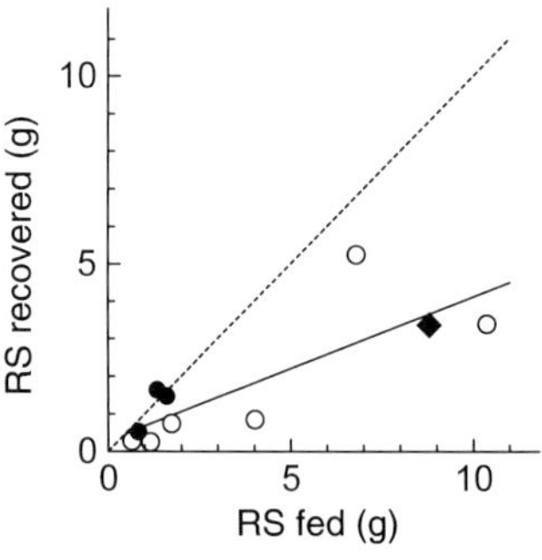


**Fig. 2.2.** Amount of resistant starch (RS) fed vs the amount recovered from the terminal ileum. (●) Mean recovery of RS in potatoes from groups of two to five subjects with an ileostomy (Englyst and Cummings, 1987); (○) recovery of RS in banana from individual subjects with an ileostomy (Englyst and Cummings, 1986); (◆) mean recovery of RS in high amylose maize starch from seven normal volunteers measured by intubation (Danjo *et al.*, 2003). Dotted line = line of identity; solid line = regression line.

**Table 2.2.** Approximate absorption and excretion of polyols.

| | Absorption (%) | Urinary excretion (%) | Available[a] (%) |
|---|---|---|---|
| Erythritol | 90 | 90 | 0 |
| Xylitol | 50 | <2 | 50 |
| Sorbitol | 25 | <2 | 25 |
| Mannitol | 25 | 25 | 25 |
| Isomalt | 10 | <2 | 10 |
| Lactitol | 2 | <2 | 0 |
| Maltitol | 40 | <2 | 40 |
| Maltitol syrup | 45 | <2 | 45 |
| Polyglycitol | 40 | <2 | 40 |

[a]Per cent (g/100 g) to be included as 'available carbohydrate' for GI determinations.
Adapted from Livesey (2003).

However, the latter would only follow if the former were true. I will show in the next chapter that there are differences in the amount of carbohydrate absorbed from different starchy foods, but that these are not nearly large enough to explain the differences observed in their GI values. Errors, which may exist in the literature due to not accounting for unavailable carbohydrate, are so small as to be virtually non-detectable without a huge increase in the number of subjects used to determine GI values, even for foods naturally containing large amounts of RS. Therefore, to retain the meaning of the GI, unavailable carbohydrates should be excluded.

## 2.1.2 Suggested protocol for determining the GI of foods

### *2.1.2.1 Subjects*

Male or non-pregnant and non-lactating female subjects aged 18–75 years can be included. For most purposes, healthy subjects with normal glucose tolerance are used, but subjects with IGT or diabetes may be included. The inclusion of pregnant or lactating females or subjects with unstable diabetes mellitus is not recommended because the carbohydrate tolerance status of such subjects is changing rapidly with time, and therefore the subject may not be in the same state when the glycaemic responses of the test and reference foods are determined. The number of subjects included depends on the magnitude of the confidence interval (CI) desired. For most purposes, use of ten subjects is recommended.

### *2.1.2.2 Procedures*

Subjects are studied in the morning (between 7:00 and 9:30 am) after an overnight fast of 10–14 h. On each test occasion the subject is weighed, and a fasting blood sample is obtained by finger-prick. Then the subject starts to consume a test meal. When the subject takes the first bite of the test meal, a timer is started and additional blood samples are taken by finger-prick at 15, 30, 45, 60, 90 and 120 min after starting to eat. After the last blood sample, the subject is offered tea or coffee and a snack and is free to leave. During the 2 h of the test, subjects remain seated quietly. Whole blood or plasma glucose is measured using any recognized reference method.

The test meals consist of portions of the test food containing 50 g available carbohydrate. If this results in a portion size, which is too large to consume by the subjects, the amount of available carbohydrate can be reduced. GI values based on 25 g available carbohydrate portion sizes have been published. The effect of reducing the amount of carbohydrate in the portion will be discussed below. Ideally available carbohydrate is based on direct measurement and does not include RS or other unavailable carbohydrates. If the food contains carbohydrates which are partly absorbed and/or not metabolized (e.g. sugar alcohols), the unabsorbed and/or non-metabolized portion should not be included in the 50 g available carbohydrate load (Table 2.2). In North America, methods for determining carbohydrate differ, and it is acceptable to define available carbohydrate as total carbohydrate minus dietary fibre measured by the AOAC method, minus any unavailable carbohydrate ingredients not included in dietary fibre. In the absence of definitive data, the proportions of carbohydrates absorbed and metabolized may have to be estimated from the available literature.

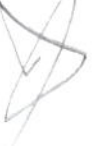

Subjects should have a drink with the test meal, and can choose to have one or two cups of water, tea or coffee with or without 2% milk and artificial sweetener; the volume and type of drink the subject chooses should remain the same for all tests done by that subject. Test meals are consumed within 10 min.

Subjects are studied for a series of tests including a certain number of test foods and at least three tests of the reference food (anhydrous glucose or white bread are commonly used). Generally, the reference food tests are done at the beginning, middle and end of a series with the order of the other foods randomized. If more than 12 foods are tested at one time, one reference standard generally should be included for every 3 months, or for every five to six test foods (whichever is sooner) to ensure that the subjects' carbohydrate tolerance is not changing with time.

The incremental area under the curve (IAUC) under each blood glucose response curve is calculated as follows:

For times $t_0, t_1, \ldots, t_n$, the blood glucose concentrations are $G_0, G_1, \ldots, G_n$, respectively. IAUC $= \sum_{n}^{x=1} A_x$ where $A_x =$ the IAUC for the $x$th time interval (i.e. between $t_{x-1}$ and $t_x$).

For the first time interval (i.e. $x = 1$): if $G_1 > G_0$, $A_1 = (G_1 - G_0) \times (t_1 - t_0)/2$
otherwise, $A_1 = 0$

For the other time intervals (i.e. $x > 1$)
if $G_x \geq G_0$ and $G_{x-1} \geq G_0$, $A_x = \{[(G_x - G_0)/2] + [(G_{x-1} - G_0)/2]\} \times (t_x - t_{x-1})$
if $G_x > G_0$ and $G_{x-1} < G_0$, $A_x = [(G_x - G_0)^2/(G_x - G_{x-1})] \times (t_x - t_{x-1})/2$
if $G_x < G_0$ and $G_{x-1} > G_0$, $A_x = [(G_{x-1} - G_0)^2/(G_{x-1} - G_x)] \times (t_x - t_{x-1})/2$
if $G_x \leq G_0$ and $G_{x-1} \leq G_0$, $A_x = 0$

The individual IAUC values for each test food in each subject are expressed as a percentage of the mean IAUC value for the repeated reference food tests taken by the same subject. The mean of the resulting values for each food is the GI value for that food.

### 2.1.3 Performance of method

An interlaboratory study was conducted recently in which seven centres experienced in GI methodology participated (Toronto, Canada; Sydney, Australia; Dunedin, New Zealand; Potchefstroom, South Africa; Milan, Italy; Lund, Sweden; and Trinidad and Tobago). Each laboratory determined the GI of four centrally provided foods and locally obtained white bread, using centrally provided anhydrous glucose. Two centres collected venous blood and five collected capillary blood by finger-prick. The variation of the results was greater for the two centres which collected venous plasma, which probably reflects a real difference between venous and capillary blood sampling, as will be discussed below. The average SD of the centre mean GI values for the five foods was 9 (Wolever *et al.*, 2003a).

## 2.2 Effects of Variation in Methods

### 2.2.1 Calculation of AUC

There are many ways of calculating the AUC. Major differences in results or interpretation of the results may be obtained from the same data depending on how the AUC is calculated (Wolever and Jenkins, 1986; Ha *et al.*, 1992). One consideration is whether the trapezoid rule can be used to calculate the AUC, or whether a more sophisticated and complex model should be used. The other consideration is the area which is included in the AUC.

The AUC is estimated based on measures of blood glucose concentration obtained at various instants in time. Ideally, AUC should be based on blood glucose concentrations measured continuously. This is at present impossible to achieve and even indwelling devices to measure blood glucose 'continuously' actually produce measurements at intervals of approximately 30–60 s. Usually, glucose is measured at 15–30 min intervals, and to determine AUC one has to estimate what is happening to blood glucose between the times when it is measured. The simplest method is to draw a straight line between each point, and this is the basis of the trapezoid rule. This is not physiological. A more physiological approach would be to connect the points when glucose is measured with a smooth curve (Fig. 2.3). The problem with this is that it is difficult to know what should be the shape of this curve. In addition, the calculations involved are complex. When the trapezoid method was compared with polynomial interpolation of third and fourth degree, Simpson's integration and cubic interpolatory splines, the different methods produced slightly different results, but the variation was no more than 2%, and the estimates were highly correlated with each

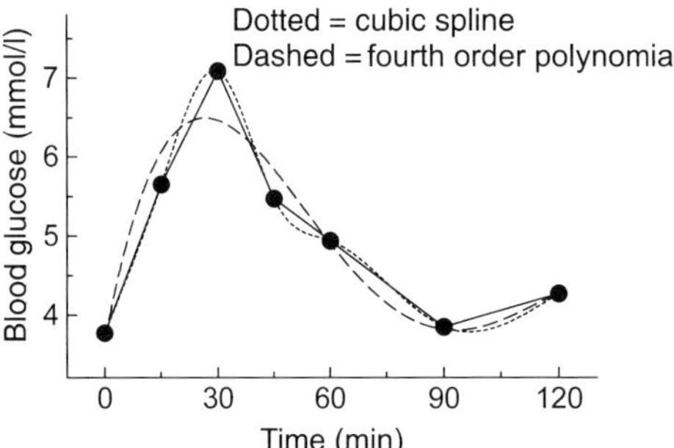


**Fig. 2.3.** Examples of models to generate a smooth glycaemic response curve from data points (•) compared with straight lines connecting the points.

other ($r > 0.998$) (Le Floch *et al.*, 1990). Thus, it appears that the trapezoid method is suitable for calculating AUC. The next question is what area should be included.

Different ways of calculating the AUC are shown in Fig. 2.4. The GI is based on the IAUC, defined as the area beneath the curve above the fasting level only; area beneath the fasting level is ignored. Thus, IAUC cannot have a value < 0. It was initially used because it indicates the amount to which the food raises blood glucose above the fasting concentration. Net incremental AUC (netAUC) (Gannon *et al.*, 1989) includes all area below the curve, including area below the fasting concentration. Since it is calculated by applying the trapezoid rule to both positive and negative blood glucose increments, the effect is to subtract area below the fasting level from that above. Thus, netAUC can have a value < 0. AUCcut (Ha *et al.*, 1992) is calculated in the same way as IAUC, but only includes area before the blood glucose concentration drops below (cuts) the baseline (fasting concentration); area after the glucose concentration cuts the baseline is not included. IAUC above the lowest blood glucose concentration attained (AUCmin) (Vorster *et al.*, 1990) is calculated by subtracting the lowest blood glucose concentration attained during the test period from each of the other blood glucose concentrations, and calculating the AUC by applying the trapezoid rule to the resulting increments. Total AUC (TAUC) is the area under the blood glucose response curve above a blood glucose concentration of zero.

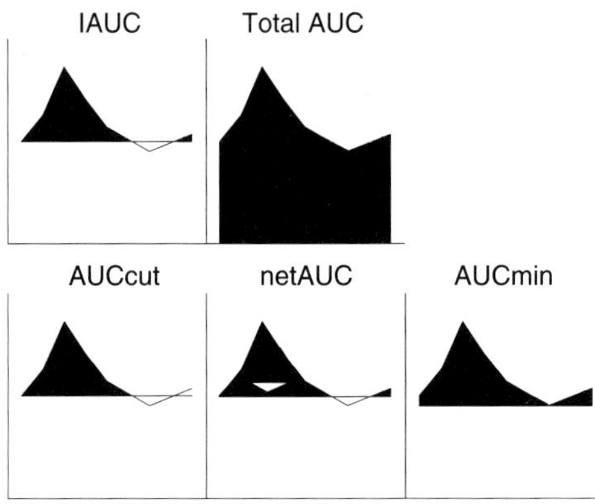


**Fig. 2.4.** Area subtended by different methods used to calculate area under the curve.

TAUC of blood glucose always has a value much greater than that for the incremental methods, because much of the TAUC is determined by the concentration of fasting glucose. In subjects with diabetes, about 80% of the variance in TAUC is determined by the basal or fasting glucose concentration (Le Floch *et al.*, 1990). The different methods of calculating IAUC will all have the same value if the postprandial blood glucose concentrations obtained are all greater than the fasting level. The different methods produce different results if blood glucose drops below the fasting level. This is illustrated in Table 2.3 which shows the results of sample calculations on two sample blood glucose profiles using different methods of calculating AUC. Table 2.3 also shows that the different methods of calculating AUC can result in markedly different values when the AUC for the food is expressed as a percentage of that after glucose.

There is no 'right' or 'wrong' way of calculating AUC; indeed, different methods may be most appropriate depending on the purpose of the analysis. Unfortunately, in some of the literature, the method of calculating AUC is not indicated, and it can, therefore, be difficult to know if the magnitudes of the relative effects of different test meals found in one study are comparable to those found in another. For the GI to be a valid and useful property of foods, and for valid comparisons of experimental results with published GI values, a standardized method of calculating AUC must be used.

TAUC is useful for comparing the effects of different treatments on average blood glucose concentrations, but it is an insensitive method

**Table 2.3.** Example of different methods of calculating AUC.

| | Blood glucose concentrations (mmol/l) at time (min) | | | | | | | | | | | |
|---|---|---|---|---|---|---|---|---|---|---|---|---|
| | 0 | 15 | 30 | 45 | 60 | 90 | 120 | IAUC | netAUC | AUCcut | AUCmin | TAUC |
| Glucose | 3.67 | 6.11 | 6.06 | 4.44 | 3.17 | 3.61 | 4.00 | 85.9 | 75.9 | 81.7 | 135.9 | 516 |
| Food | 3.94 | 5.00 | 5.11 | 3.44 | 3.50 | 3.83 | 4.33 | 35.4 | 18.6 | 30.8 | 78.6 | 491 |
| | | Food AUC expressed as % of glucose AUC: | | | | | | 41 | 25 | 38 | 58 | 95 |

for detecting differences in response between foods, since most of the TAUC is determined by the fasting glucose concentration, which is not affected by the test meal about to be consumed. We have shown that using netAUC and AUCmin result in GI values which are more variable (less precise) than IAUC. AUCcut performs similarly to IAUC, but is more difficult to calculate than IAUC, and in a study involving five foods, resulted in the SD of GI value of each of five foods being slightly higher (by 0.2–1.2) than those based on IAUC. Thus, IAUC appears to be the best method to calculate GI values (Wolever, 2004a).

### 2.2.2 Amount of 'available carbohydrate' in the portion tested

#### *2.2.2.1 Definition of 'available carbohydrate'*

The term 'available carbohydrate' is somewhat ambiguous; it originally meant a carbohydrate that provided glucose for metabolism, but it could also mean a carbohydrate that provides energy to the body. Energy can be provided either by the monosaccharides absorbed in the small intestine, or from the SCFA produced during the fermentation of unabsorbed carbohydrates in the colon. For this reason, the FAO carbohydrate report (1998) recommended using the term 'glycaemic carbohydrate' to mean carbohydrates, which provide glucose for metabolism. According to this definition, glycaemic carbohydrates are those which are absorbed in the human small intestine and metabolized in the body rather than excreted in the urine. However, the term 'glycaemic carbohydrate' is not ideal, because glycaemic carbohydrates do not necessarily produce glucose during metabolism, for example, fructose, which is clearly an available or glycaemic carbohydrate, does not necessarily yield glucose, but can be oxidized directly for energy. Thus, in this book, I will continue to use the term 'available carbohydrate' to mean carbohydrates which are absorbed from the small intestine and metabolized in the body via pathways which can, at least potentially, yield glucose.

As has been indicated above, and will be discussed in more detail later, it is difficult, if not impossible, to determine precisely the physiologically available carbohydrate in foods. Therefore, we need to rely on methods which define available carbohydrate from a chemical point of view. Ideally, methods for analysing carbohydrates directly, including sugars, total and resistant starch and NSP (McCleary and Monaghan, 2002; Champ *et al.*, 2003) should be used to determine the available carbohydrate. Unfortunately, these are not used for regulatory purposes in many parts of the world, particularly the USA, in which carbohydrates are analysed by difference and dietary fibre by gravimetric methods, both of which can include non-carbohydrate components. However, the amount of RS contained in most natural foods, and not included in the measurement of dietary fibre is relatively small, and accounting for it by feeding a larger portion size is unlikely to have any significant impact on the glycaemic response obtained. For example, in a recent interlaboratory study (Wolever *et al.*, 2003a), one of the test foods was pearled barley, a food which contains more RS than most other foods. The portion size fed in the study, 79.6 g, was based on analysis of total carbohydrate by difference and total dietary fibre. One of the centres involved in the study, experienced in measuring RS, found that 15.2% of the starch in the barley was RS, and thus, the 79.6 g portion size actually contained 44.2 g glycaemic starch. Increasing carbohydrate intake from 44.2 to 50 g would be expected to increase the glycaemic response by about 8% (Wolever and Bolognesi, 1996a). When the portion size of barley was increased to 93.9 to adjust for its RS content, this resulted in a non-significant increase in the GI from 39.3 ± 13.1 to 44.4 ± 13.1 (mean ± SD, $n = 10$). Although the 13% higher GI value found for the higher portion size of barley was similar to the expected difference, over 300 subjects would be required for an 80% chance of detecting a difference of 8% at $P < 0.05$.

However, large amounts of RS or other unavailable carbohydrates can be added to foods in the manufacturing process. Since these are added, they can be accurately measured, and accounting for them in determining the portion size to feed is critical to the interpretation of the results. For example, foods enriched with RS elicit lower glycaemic responses than portions of control products containing an equal amount of total carbohydrate (Hoebler *et al.*, 1999). However, Jenkins *et al.* (1998) found that 50 g available carbohydrate (not including RS) portions of muffins or cereal containing about 33% and 45% of total starch as RS elicited the same glycaemic response as 50 g available carbohydrate portions of control muffins and cereals. This suggests that at least some types of RS added to foods may not slow the rate of absorption of the available starch and reduce blood glucose and insulin responses simply by displacing available carbohydrate. The long-term effects of this on blood glucose, insulin and lipids may not be the same as that of slowing carbohydrate absorption. The issue of reduced carbohydrate intake vs reduced GI is addressed in Chapter 9.

Determining the GI of foods containing polyols, and other partly absorbed carbohydrates, presents a special problem because it is difficult to measure their absorption and metabolism, few data exist, and the different polyols vary in the degree to which they are absorbed and metabolized. Nevertheless, enough data exist to estimate the proportion of carbohydrate which is absorbed and metabolized (Table 2.2), and, in the absence of definitive information, such estimates are, in my view, better than not making any correction. Indeed, errors as high as 20% have only a small effect on the GI value obtained, especially for carbohydrates which do not raise blood glucose appreciably.

### *2.2.2.2 Use of portion sizes containing less than 50 g available carbohydrate*

If a portion size less than 50 g available carbohydrate is to be used, then the amount of available carbohydrate in the reference food has to be reduced to be the same as that in the test food. The effect of using portions of foods containing less than 50 g available carbohydrate on the GI values obtained has not been studied. One question is whether the RGR of carbohydrates are the same at any level of carbohydrate intake. Another question is whether the variability of glycaemic responses is the same at different levels of carbohydrate intake.

Figure 2.5 shows the glycaemic responses elicited by 25, 50 and 100 g available carbohydrate doses of barley, spaghetti, instant potato, sucrose and glucose relative to a dose of white bread containing the same amount of available carbohydrate. These relative responses are calculated as $F/B$ where $F$ is the mean AUC elicited by the food in a group of subjects and $B$ is the mean AUC elicted by bread; the values are not termed GI because they are not calculated using correct GI methods. Nevertheless, the mean relative responses of the five foods tested at all three levels of carbohydrate vary by less than 5%, being 91 at 25 g carbohydrate, 92 at 50 g carbohydrate and 88 at 100 g carbohydrate. This suggests that the relative responses of foods are the same at different levels of available carbohydrate intake (at least between 25 and 100 g).

The within-subject variation of glycaemic responses and its effect on the resulting GI values is discussed in detail below. In brief, increased variation of glycaemic responses not only increases the variation of the resulting GI values,

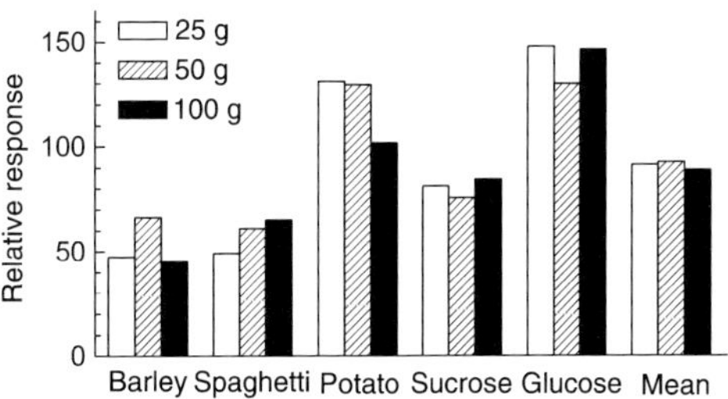


**Fig. 2.5.** Mean incremental AUC of blood glucose in a group of normal subjects elicited by 25, 50 and 100 g available carbohydrate doses of barley, spaghetti, instant potato, sucrose and glucose expressed as a percentage of that elicited by a dose of white bread containing the same amount of available carbohydrate. Data from Wolever and Bolognesi (1996a) and Lee and Wolever (1998).

but also skews the distribution and increases the mean of the resulting GI values. Thus, if within-subject variation of glycaemic responses, expressed as CV, increased as the portion of available carbohydrate decreased, this would have a deleterious effect on the accuracy and precision of the GI values obtained. We found recently that within-subject variation of glycaemic responses of normal subjects decreased from 98% to 28% as the dose of available carbohydrate from white bread increased from 0 to 20 g, but decreased only marginally more to 26% as the dose of available carbohydrate increased to 50 g (Table 2.4). This suggests that 20 g is the minimum amount of available carbohydrate which should be used for determining GI.

### 2.2.3 Method of blood sampling and glucose measurement

Capillary blood sampling was used initially for convenience and to minimize expense. Subjects can either take their own capillary blood, or samples can be taken more quickly and less invasively compared to taking blood from a forearm vein either by needle or indwelling catheter. Initially, there were concerns that measuring glucose in capillary blood may not be as precise as measuring it in venous plasma, because of the variable need to 'milk' the finger which may dilute the blood with interstitial fluid. This would be a problem if the concentration of glucose in interstitial fluid differed from that in the blood, but this is difficult to assess in practice (see Section 2.2.3.1). Regardless of this concern, there are a number of theoretical considerations, and experimental results, which suggest that measuring glucose in capillary blood is preferable to measuring it in venous plasma.

The concentration of glucose in venous plasma is less than that in arterial plasma because the tissues take up glucose from the blood as it passes from the arteries, through the capillaries to the veins (Jackson *et al.*, 1973; Coppack *et al.*,1990). The amount of glucose taken up depends on a number of factors such as the concentration of insulin, the concentration of glucose and the subject's insulin sensitivity. The difference in concentration between arterial and venous plasma glucose concentrations (A–V difference) depends not only on the rate of uptake of glucose by tissues, but also on blood flow. For example, at a given rate of glucose uptake, reduced blood flow will result in a larger A–V difference. Venous blood is typically sampled from a forearm vein, and flow through these vessels is markedly affected by ambient temperature. Thus, it has been shown that the venous plasma glucose response to a standard meal is less at an ambient temperature of 23°C than 33°C, with blood flow being over four times greater at the higher temperature (Frayn *et al.*, 1989). Such variation in venous plasma glucose can be minimized by warming the hand in dry air at 65°C. By increasing peripheral blood flow and reducing the A–V glucose difference, this has the effect of arterializing the venous blood. Since capillary blood glucose concentration is closer to arterial, it presumably is less affected by variation in ambient temperature.

Another feature influencing venous plasma glucose differently from arterial glucose may be the fact that insulin is secreted from the normal

**Table 2.4.** Within-subject variation of glycaemic responses in normal subjects who took 0, 5, 10, 20, 25 or 50 g available carbohydrate portions of white bread on repeated occasions.

| Dose (g) | Number of subjects | Number of repeats | Mean AUC (mmol × min/l) | Within-subject SD (mmol × min/l) | Within-subject CV (%) |
|---|---|---|---|---|---|
| 0 | 18 | 4.4 ± 0.3 | 10.0 ± 2.4 | 8.3 ± 2.4 | 99 ± 11 |
| 5 | 18 | 4.1 ± 0.2 | 32.5 ± 4.4 | 18.8 ± 3.0 | 60 ± 4 |
| 10 | 18 | 4.6 ± 0.3 | 57.4 ± 6.3 | 18.9 ± 1.8 | 37 ± 4 |
| 20 | 18 | 4.4 ± 0.3 | 102.8 ± 10.6 | 27.4 ± 1.8 | 28 ± 3 |
| 25 | 24 | 4.0 ± 0.3 | 105.1 ± 8.0 | 28.1 ± 3.9 | 27 ± 3 |
| 50 | 105 | 7.1 ± 0.6 | 182.7 ± 7.1 | 44.8 ± 2.2 | 26 ± 1 |

Values are mean ± SEM.

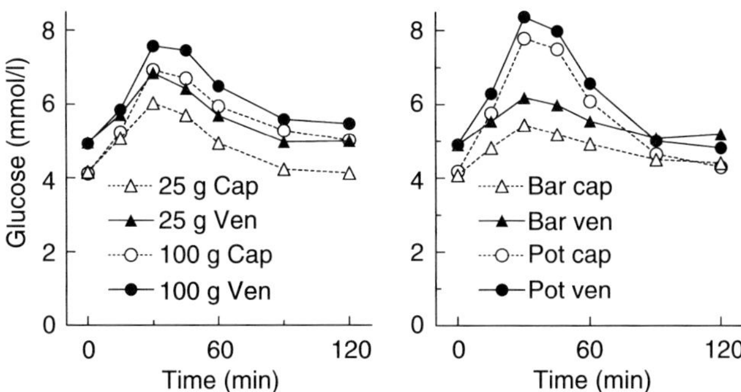


**Fig. 2.6.** Glucose responses in simultaneously obtained venous plasma (●,▲) and finger-prick capillary whole blood (○,△) after 25(△,▲) or 100 g (○,●) available carbohydrate from white bread (left) or 50 g available carbohydrate from pearled barley (△,▲) or instant mashed potato (○,●; right). Data from Wolever and Bolognesi (1996a).

pancreas in pulses (Matthews *et al.*, 1983) occurring at a frequency of one for every 2–3 min. Venous plasma glucose concentrations also vary up and down with a similar frequency to those of plasma insulin (Abdallah *et al.*, 1997). Presumably, therefore, the variations in plasma glucose are due to variation in tissue uptake elicited by the variable insulin concentrations. However, the glucose concentration in arterial blood would presumably vary less on a minute by minute basis than the glucose concentration in venous blood because it has not yet reached the insulin-sensitive tissues.

The glucose concentration in plasma is greater than that in whole blood because the water content of plasma is higher than that of red cells (93% vs 73%) with the glucose concentration in the water in these two compartments being identical (Burrin and Alberti, 1990). When glucose responses after different test meals were measured in simultaneously obtained venous plasma and capillary whole blood, fasting and postprandial capillary whole blood glucose concentrations were less than those in venous plasma glucose (Wolever and Bolognesi, 1996a). The difference between venous plasma and capillary whole blood glucose concentrations appears to be smaller 2 h after 100 g carbohydrate loads than after 25 or 50 g loads, but this is not the case for foods with different GI values (Fig. 2.6). The IAUC of capillary whole blood glucose was larger than that of venous plasma, and the difference appeared to vary more with amount of carbohydrate than with GI (Fig. 2.7). The random error associated with measurements of glucose in capillary whole blood was less than that associated with measurement of glucose in venous plasma for test meals consisting of single foods or mixed

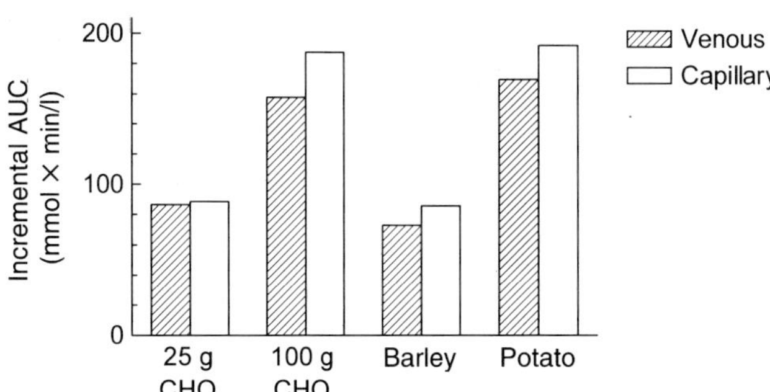


**Fig. 2.7.** Comparison of incremental areas under the glucose response curve measured in venous plasma or finger-prick capillary whole blood (tests shown in Fig. 2.4).

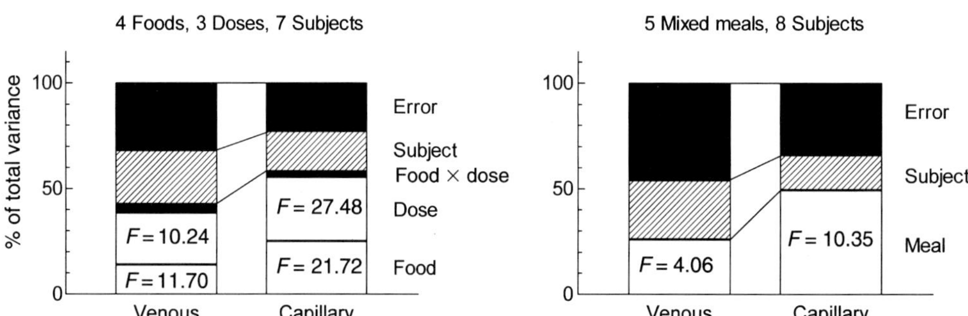


**Fig. 2.8.** Comparison of partitioning of variance from glucose measurements in simultaneously obtained venous plasma or capillary whole blood for individual foods (left) or mixed test meals (right). Data from Wolever and Bolognesi (1996a,b).

meals (Wolever and Bolognesi, 1996a,b) (Fig. 2.8). Therefore, differences in glycaemic response are more readily detected with capillary than venous blood sampling (Granfeldt *et al.*, 1995).

Data from an interlaboratory study also suggest that measuring glucose responses in venous plasma results in greater within-subject variation of plasma glucose responses and greater variation of GI values than measuring glucose in capillary blood (Wolever *et al.*, 2003a). In this study, five centres collected capillary blood and two collected venous blood. Each subject repeated the 50 g oral glucose trial three times, and the coefficient of variation (CV = 100 × SD/mean) of the three IAUC values after the glucose trials were calculated for each subject. The mean CV for the 47 subjects from capillary blood centres, 23.4 ± 2.1%, was significantly less than that for the 21 subjects from venous plasma centres, 56.8 ± 4.4%. The AUC values for subjects tended to be smaller from venous plasma centres, and, although the mean GI values did not differ, the variation of the GI values was much greater for the venous plasma centres (Fig. 2.9).

The site from which capillary blood is taken may affect the results. Finger-tip capillary blood responds more rapidly to changes in blood glucose than other sites. Thus, when glucose concentrations are rising rapidly after a meal, finger-prick capillary glucose concentrations are higher than capillary blood obtained from forearm, thigh or abdomen (Ellison *et al.*, 2002; Jungheim and Koschinsky, 2002; van der Valk *et al.*, 2002), whereas, when glucose concentrations are falling, finger-prick capillary glucose is lower. It is not known how blood sampling from sites other than

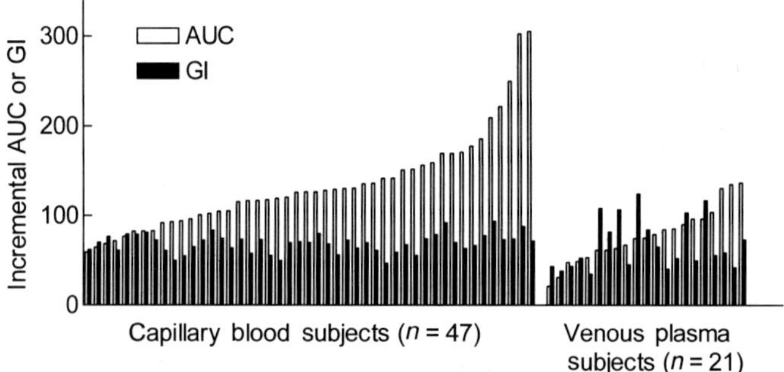


**Fig. 2.9.** Incremental areas under the blood glucose response curves (AUC) and mean GI values for 68 subjects who tested the GI of five different foods. Each AUC value is the mean AUC for all test foods and glucose taken by each subject, and each GI value is the mean GI of the five test foods taken by that subject. Data from Wolever *et al.* (2003a).

the finger-tip affects the IAUC and GI values of foods.

#### 2.2.3.1 *Interstitial vs blood glucose*

Interstitial fluid is the water compartment which is both outside of cells and outside of the blood stream. Hormonal signals and nutrients which are carried in blood reach the target tissues only by diffusing through the interstitial fluid. Thus, the concentration of glucose in interstitial fluid, at least theoretically and in a steady-state situation, would be expected to be similar to that in the blood in nearby capillaries, but rapid changes in blood glucose are followed more slowly by interstitial glucose (Fischer *et al.*, 1987). Measurement of glucose in interstitial fluid is difficult, with microdialysis (Lonnoth *et al.*, 1987), filtration (Schmidt *et al.*, 1993) or wick (Fischer *et al.*, 1987) methods being used. Interstitial glucose concentrations have sometimes been reported to be the same as those in blood (Fischer *et al.*, 1987; Lonnoth *et al.*, 1987) and sometimes 25–50% less (Schmidt *et al.*, 1993; Sternberg *et al.*, 1995). Some of the discrepancy may be explained by the fact that insertion of the probe injures the tissue and disrupts blood flow, with low initial recoveries of glucose eventually recovering after several days (Wientjes *et al.*, 1998). Recent appreciation of the differences in capillary glucose concentrations in different sites of the body (Ellison *et al.*, 2002; Jungheim and Koschinsky, 2002; van der Valk *et al.*, 2002) may also explain some of the discrepancies, because subcutaneous interstitial glucose in abdominal adipose tissue is usually compared with plasma glucose obtained from a forearm vein.

#### 2.2.3.2 *Handling of blood samples*

Red blood cells metabolize glucose, and continue to do so when blood is withdrawn from the body. Thus, if a whole blood sample is left in a tube on a bench at room temperature, the blood glucose concentration falls linearly with time. This is a potential source of measurement error, especially if tubes are left out for variable lengths of time. The fall in blood glucose can be stopped by removing the plasma or serum from contact with the cells. If one centrifuges the blood without anticoagulant, one has to wait for about 30–60 min for the blood to clot (during which time the blood glucose will fall) or else the serum removed will clot. If one wants to remove the plasma rapidly from the cells, an anticoagulant must be present in the blood collection tubes to prevent the plasma from clotting. Blood collection tubes containing a glycolytic inhibitor (such as fluoro-oxalate) are commonly used, but studies show that if such tubes are left at room temperature, glucose concentration falls for about 1 h before the inhibitor takes effect. The most reliable way to inhibit glycolysis and prevent the glucose concentration from falling is to place the sample in a refrigerator or on wet ice as soon as it has been obtained. This immediately arrests the fall in blood glucose.

#### 2.2.3.3 *Method of measuring glucose*

Glucose can be measured in whole blood or plasma using various different methods. The CV of analytical variation for measuring glucose is <3% for typical clinical laboratories (Burrin and Alberti, 1990; Widjaja *et al.*, 1999). In our hands, the CV of repeated determinations of fasting glucose ($n = 100$ each measured 3 times, range 3.54–5.35 mmol/l) by YSI was 1.26% (Velangi *et al.*, 2005). In a recent interlaboratory study, three different methods of measuring glucose were used amongst the five laboratories which collected capillary blood, including: whole capillary blood glucose by glucose oxidase after mixing 1 ml 0.025 M NaOH and 50 μl 0.3 M $ZnSO_4$ solution with 50 μl whole blood, measurement of glucose in capillary plasma by hexokinase, and whole capillary blood glucose using an automatic analyser (YSI Stat 2300, Yellow Springs Instruments, OH, USA). There was no significant effect of the method of blood sampling on either the mean of variation of the GI values obtained. This suggests that any recognized and well-standardized reference method of measuring glucose is suitable for determining the GI of foods.

However, the reproducibility of dry chemistry analysers such as portable glucose metres is not as good as reference methods, with the CV of analytical variation being typically <8% (Burrin and Alberti, 1990; Widjaja *et al.*, 1999). The CV of analytical variation for various portable glucose metres ranged from 1.5% to 8.0% (Engel *et al.*, 1998; Solnica *et al.*, 2003). This degree of precision is considered adequate for the purposes of self-monitoring of blood glucose in diabetes. However, it may not be adequate for GI testing. For reference methods of measuring glucose (CV < 3%), a glucose concentration of 5.0 mmol/l would be expected to lie between 4.7 and 5.3 mmol/l ( ± 6%); however, for dry methods of measuring glucose (CV < 8%), the concentration would lie between 4.2 and 5.8 mmol/l ( ± 16%). Since variances are additive, the variation of the incremental AUC, which is calculated from many individual glucose concentrations, would be expected to be considerably higher than the variation of each glucose measure. We recently evaluated the performance of a portable glucose meter for measuring GI of seven types of potato, and found that GI values determined by the meter were more variable than and did not agree well with those determined by YSI (Velangi *et al.*, 2005). By YSI, GI values varied from 56 ± 5 to 88 ± 8 ($P = 0.004$), but by the meter, although the range of GI values was similar (57 ± 10–81 ± 12) the means for the seven foods did not differ significantly ($P = 0.11$). This suggests that a reference method for measuring glucose should be used for determining the GI values of foods.

## 2.2.4 Type of subjects studied

Generally 'normal' subjects are studied, although GI values for many foods in the literature are based on tests in people with diabetes. It is generally accepted that GI values from these groups of subjects are comparable, and can be used interchangeably. However, different subjects have different degrees of within-subject variation of glycaemic responses, which influences the precision and may affect the mean of the results obtained. The implication of this is that between-subject variation of glycaemic responses does not need to be controlled when selecting subjects for determining the GI of foods, but the degree of within-subject variation may be important to consider. In an attempt to obtain a homogeneous group of subjects, investigators may tend to select young, fit subjects with no family history of diabetes for glycaemic response studies. Ironically, this type of subject may not be ideal for determining GI values because they will tend to be insulin-sensitive with low glycaemic responses, and day-to-day variation in response which is relatively high in relation to the mean.

### *2.2.4.1 Mean GI values in different subjects*

For most foods and most subjects, mean GI values are the same in subjects with different degrees of carbohydrate intolerance. This is based on the results of studies such as those shown in Fig. 2.10 which show strong correlations between GI values determined in normal subjects and subjects with diabetes (Fig. 2.10A), subjects with type 2 diabetes and subjects with type 1 diabetes (Fig. 2.10B) and European and African subjects (Fig. 2.10C). In addition, the mean of the GI values for the 21 foods determined in normal subjects, 78 ± 6, was not significantly different from that in subjects with diabetes, 74 ± 6, and the mean of the GI values in the European subjects, 54 ± 5, was the same as that in the African subjects,

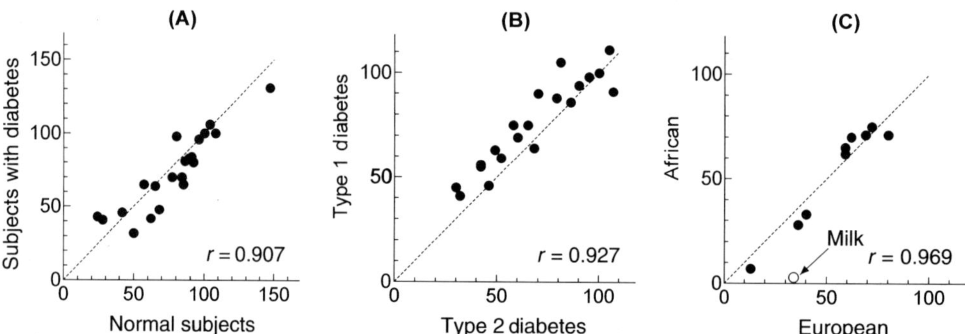


**Fig. 2.10.** Correlations between GI values for the same foods measured in normal and diabetic subjects (A), subjects with type 2 diabetes and subjects with type 1 diabetes (B) and normal European and normal African subjects (C). Dotted lines = lines of identity. Data from Jenkins *et al.* (1981a, 1983), Wolever *et al.* (1987) and Walker and Walker (1984).

54 ± 5, with the exception of milk. Milk had a lower GI in Africans than in Europeans, and the mean of the GI values for 20 foods tested in subjects with type 1 diabetes, 76 ± 5, was significantly greater than that for the same foods tested in subjects with type 2 diabetes, 68 ± 5 ($P$ = 0.001). The example of milk illustrates the only situation where major differences in GI between subjects may occur, that is, when the efficiency of absorption of the test food is relatively different than that of the reference food. Africans and Europeans absorb glucose and starch to the same extent, but Africans have a much higher prevalence of low intestinal lactase activity than Europeans, so the Africans would absorb the lactose in milk to a lesser extent than the Europeans. The small difference in GI between subjects with type 1 and type 2 diabetes can be explained by the fact that within-subject variation differs in these subject groups.

#### *2.2.4.2 Day-to-day variation of glycaemic responses in different subjects*

Day-to-day (or within-subject) variation of glycaemic responses differs markedly in different groups of subjects. Within-subject variation is assessed by having the subject repeat exactly the same test meal (usually the reference test meal) on different days. Early on we assessed the day-to-day variation of glycaemic responses in subjects who were normal, or who had type 2 diabetes treated with diet or oral agents, type 2 diabetes treated with insulin, or type 1 diabetes (Wolever *et al.*, 1985) (Table 2.5). This showed that the average within-subject CV (CV = 100 × SD/mean) in subjects with type 2 diabetes, 15%, was significantly less than that in subjects with type 1 diabetes, 29%, and normal subjects having an intermediate value. Rasmussen *et al.* (1992) determined the variation of plasma glucose and insulin responses in ten subjects with type 2 diabetes who repeated trials of white bread three times each. They obtained a mean CV for plasma glucose within subjects of 19%, similar to our value of 15%, but a much higher CV for plasma insulin, 41%. More recently, we determined the reproducibility of plasma glucose and insulin responses in lean and obese normal subjects, subjects with IGT and subjects with type 2 diabetes after 75 g oral glucose and a solid mixed test meal 'bar' (Wolever *et al.*, 1998a,b). Reproducibility after glucose was similar to that after the bar (Table 2.6). This study confirmed that subjects with IGT and type 2 diabetes tended to have lower within-subject variation than normal subjects, significantly so after glucose (12% in subjects with diabetes vs 39% in lean normal subjects). However, in contrast to Rasmussen *et al.* (1992), the CV values for insulin (19–29%) were similar to those for glucose (12–39%) and did not differ between different subject groups (Table 2.6).

Differences in within-subject variation are important, because, as shown above (Fig. 2.1), most of the variation of GI values is due to within-subject variation. Because the GI is a ratio of two independently variable glycaemic response AUC values, not only is the variation of GI

**Table 2.5.** Between- and within-subject variation in glycaemic responses in different groups of subjects who took 50 g glucose (normal subjects) or 50 g available carbohydrate portions of white bread (subjects with diabetes) on repeated occasions.

| Subject group | *n* (range) | Mean (mmol × min/l) | $CV_{between}$ (%) | SD (mmol × min/l) | $CV_{within}$ (%) |
|---|---|---|---|---|---|
| Normal (*n* = 11) | 8.3 (4–15) | 208 ± 55[a] (129–290) | 26.4 | 57 ± 40[a] (14–136) | 25.0 ± 12.0[ab] (9.0–46.9) |
| Type 2 not on insulin (*n* = 10) | 7.8 (5–11) | 658 ± 222[b] (291–1045) | 33.7 | 96 ± 38[a] (50–167) | 15.9 ± 7.1[ab] (5.6–27.1) |
| Type 2 on insulin (*n* = 12) | 10.6 (6–27) | 968 ± 224[c] (611–1373) | 23.1 | 139 ± 41[a] (89–205) | 14.8 ± 4.4[a] (8.6–22.1) |
| Type 1DM (*n* = 14) | 9.4 (5–35) | 1066 ± 358[c] (555–1658) | 33.6 | 268 ± 134[b] (78–640) | 29.1 ± 19.8[b] (7.1–71.3) |

[abc]Means in a column with different letter superscripts differ significantly, $P < 0.05$. Values are mean ± SD with the range in brackets.
Data from Wolever *et al.* (1985).

**Table 2.6.** Mean and within-subject variation of incremental areas under the plasma glucose and insulin response curves in different groups of subjects who took 75 g glucose 4 times and 50 g available carbohydrate from a mixed solid test meal wafer four times.

| | Mean (mmol × min/l) | | CV (%) | |
|---|---|---|---|---|
| | GTT | BAR | GTT | BAR |
| *Plasma glucose* | | | | |
| Normal lean ($n = 10$) | 215 ± 44[a] | 108 ± 24[a] | 38.7 ± 6.1[a] | 30.6 ± 6.3 |
| Normal obese ($n = 9$) | 268 ± 36[a] | 106 ± 13[a] | 26.0 ± 5.9[ab] | 32.5 ± 4.6 |
| IGT ($n = 9$) | 537 ± 26[b] | 276 ± 19[b] | 18.9 ± 2.7[ab] | 16.5 ± 3.7 |
| Type 2 diabetes ($n = 8$) | 803 ± 59[c] | 435 ± 43[c] | 11.6 ± 1.8[b] | 18.1 ± 1.6 |
| *Plasma insulin* | | | | |
| Normal lean ($n = 10$) | 15.2 ± 2.0 | 9.4 ± 1.4 | 20.6 ± 2.4 | 19.7 ± 3.4 |
| Normal obese ($n = 9$) | 24.2 ± 4.6 | 11.2 ± 1.7 | 29.0 ± 5.0 | 21.2 ± 2.6 |
| IGT ($n = 9$) | 35.6 ± 7.4 | 23.2 ± 4.6 | 19.5 ± 3.1 | 23.7 ± 4.0 |
| Type 2 diabetes ($n = 8$) | 20.6 ± 5.6 | 16.1 ± 3.7 | 18.8 ± 4.0 | 20.2 ± 4.1 |

Values are mean ± SD with the range in brackets.
[abc]Means in a column with different letter superscripts differ significantly, $P < 0.05$.
Data from Wolever *et al.* (1988a,b).

values greater than the within-subject variation of the glycaemic responses, but also increasing within-individual variation of glycaemic responses skews the distribution of the GI values and increases the mean (Wolever *et al.*, 1991a).

Absolute glycaemic responses of normal subjects are not normally distributed because of differences in response between subjects (left side of Fig. 2.11). However, within subjects, the responses are normally distributed as illustrated in the right side of Fig. 2.11. The data shown here represent 720 individual tests of 50 g available carbohydrate portions of white bread taken by 98 subjects each of whom tested bread at least three times (range 3–35, median 5). The left side of Fig. 2.11 shows that the normalized AUC values (each AUC was expressed as a *Z* score, i.e. the number of SDs from the mean of the same subject) are normally distributed. The same is true for subjects with diabetes (Wolever, 1990b). Thus, mathematical

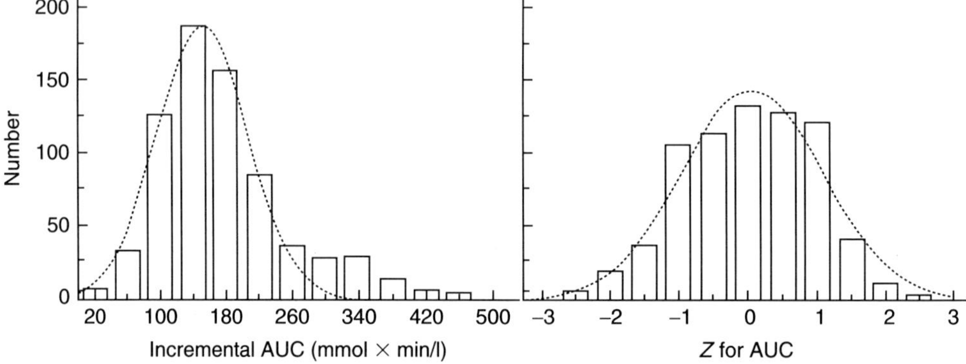


**Fig. 2.11.** Distribution of glycaemic response (incremental area under the curve) elicited by 50 g available carbohydrate portions of white bread. Data represent 720 individual tests of bread taken by 98 normal subjects with each subject doing at least three tests (range 3–35). Bars represent numbers of subjects with the value being the centre of the bin. Dotted lines represent the normal distribution with the same mean and SD. Left: distribution of AUC values is significantly skewed. Right: distribution of *Z* scores is not significantly different from the normal distribution.

modelling using the normal distribution can be used to illustrate the effects of altering the variation of glycaemic responses on the GI values obtained. Table 2.7 shows examples of GI calculations with within-subject CV of glycaemic responses being either 30% (representing subjects with type 1 diabetes) or 15% (representing subjects with type 2 diabetes). In addition the effect of using the average of three trials of the reference food to calculate the GI is illustrated. If $C$ equals the within-subject CV of glycaemic response AUCs elicited by the reference food, then $C/\sqrt{3}$ equals the CV of the average of three trials of the reference food. Thus, in Table 2.7, the CVs of the reference food have been reduced by a factor of $\sqrt{3} = 1.73$. Assuming a normal distribution,

**Table 2.7.** Model of effect of altering day-to-day variation of glycaemic responses on GI values.

a. CV = 30%; one trial of reference food.

| | | −2SD (−60%) | −1SD (−30%) | Test mean | +1SD (+30%) | +2SD (+60%) |
|---|---|---|---|---|---|---|
| Deviation | Area | 360 | 630 | 900 | 1170 | 1440 |
| −2SD (−60%) | 480 | 75 | 131 | 188 | 244 | 300 |
| −1SD (−30%) | 840 | 43 | 75 | 107 | 139 | 171 |
| Reference mean | 1200 | 30 | 53 | 75 | 98 | 120 |
| +1SD (+30%) | 1560 | 23 | 40 | 58 | 75 | 92 |
| +2SD (+60%) | 1920 | 19 | 33 | 47 | 61 | 75 |

b. CV = 30%; average of three trials of reference food.

| | | −2SD (−30%) | −1SD (−15%) | Test mean | +1SD (+15%) | +2SD (+30%) |
|---|---|---|---|---|---|---|
| Deviation | Area | 360 | 630 | 900 | 1170 | 1440 |
| −2SD (−34.6%) | 784 | 46 | 80 | 115 | 149 | 184 |
| −1SD (−17.3%) | 992 | 36 | 64 | 91 | 118 | 145 |
| Reference mean | 1200 | 30 | 53 | 75 | 98 | 120 |
| +1SD (+17.3%) | 1408 | 26 | 45 | 64 | 83 | 102 |
| +2SD (+34.6%) | 1616 | 22 | 39 | 56 | 72 | 89 |

c. CV = 15%; one trial of reference food.

| | | −2SD (−30%) | −1SD (−15%) | Test mean | +1SD (+15%) | +2SD (+30%) |
|---|---|---|---|---|---|---|
| Deviation | Area | 630 | 765 | 900 | 1035 | 1170 |
| −2SD (−30%) | 840 | 75 | 91 | 107 | 123 | 139 |
| −1SD (−15%) | 1020 | 62 | 75 | 88 | 102 | 115 |
| Reference mean | 1200 | 53 | 64 | 75 | 86 | 98 |
| +1SD (+15%) | 1380 | 46 | 55 | 65 | 75 | 85 |
| +2SD (+30%) | 1560 | 40 | 49 | 58 | 66 | 75 |

d. CV = 15%; average of three trials of reference food.

| | | −2SD (−30%) | −1SD (−15%) | Test mean | +1SD (+15%) | +2SD (+30%) |
|---|---|---|---|---|---|---|
| Deviation | Area | 630 | 765 | 900 | 1035 | 1170 |
| −2SD (−17.3%) | 992 | 64 | 77 | 91 | 104 | 118 |
| −1SD (−8.7%) | 1096 | 58 | 70 | 82 | 94 | 107 |
| Reference mean | 1200 | 53 | 64 | 75 | 86 | 98 |
| +1SD (+8.7%) | 1304 | 48 | 59 | 69 | 79 | 90 |
| +2SD (+17.3%) | 1408 | 45 | 54 | 64 | 74 | 83 |

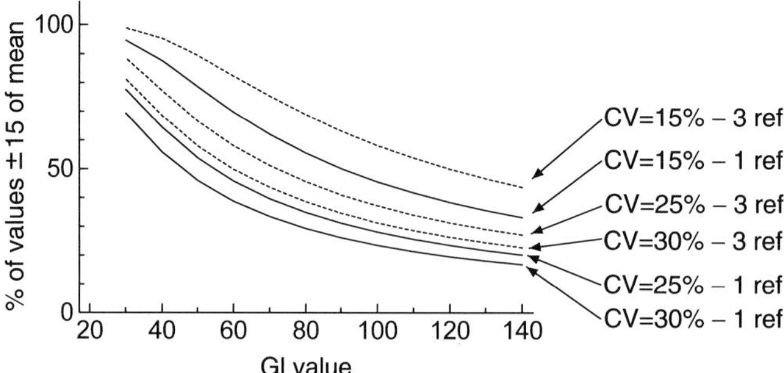


**Fig. 2.12.** Estimated percentage of subjects whose individual GI values will lie within a range of ± 15 from the true GI for different values of GI, for different degrees of within-subject variation of AUC values (CV = coefficient of variation, 30% represents subjects with type 1 diabetes, 25% represents normal subjects and 15% represents subjects with type 2 diabetes), and for GI values calculated using either one repeat of the reference food (1 ref) or three repeats (3 ref). Data derived from mathematical modelling (see text).

approximately 47% of all GI values fall within the range of the nine GI values outlined by the bold lines (AUC for both reference and test foods within ± 1 SD of mean). Approximately 44% of all GI values fall between the inner 9 and outer 16 GI values (AUC for either reference or test food more >1 SD but <2 SD from the mean). Approximately 9% of all GI values fall outside the range of all 25 GI values on each table (AUC for either reference or test food >2 SD from the mean). The range of GI values in the example representing type 1 diabetes with only one test of the reference food goes from 19 to 300, which is 25–400% of the true value. Using the mean of three reference tests reduces the range of GI values obtained from 29% to 245% of the true value. Using a CV of 15%, representing subjects with type 2 diabetes, and the mean of three trials of the reference food, yields a range of GI values from 60% to 157% of the true value.

A grid similar to that shown in Table 2.7 was created, but with deviations going from −3 to +3 SDs in steps of 0.5 SDs. Assuming a normal distribution, the average GI value and the likelihood of obtaining a value in that cell was calculated. This allows one to estimate the theoretical effect of changing the mean and CV of AUC values for the reference and test foods on the distribution and mean GI of the values obtained. Figure 2.12 shows the estimated % of subjects whose individual GI values will lie within a range of ± 15 from the true GI for different values of GI (mean AUC for theoretical test food expressed as a percentage of the mean AUC for the theoretical reference food) and for different degrees of within-subject variation of AUC values. The percentage of GI values within ± 15 from the true mean increases as the within-subject CV is reduced and also as the GI value is reduced. Figure 2.13 shows the observed proportion ( ± 95% CI) of 47 normal subjects with a GI value ± 15 from the mean for five foods with GI ranging from 35 to 91 (Wolever *et al.*, 2003a), plotted against the expected proportion from Fig. 2.12. The relatively good correlation suggests that the type of mathematical modelling illustrated in Table 2.7 and Fig. 2.12 is valid.

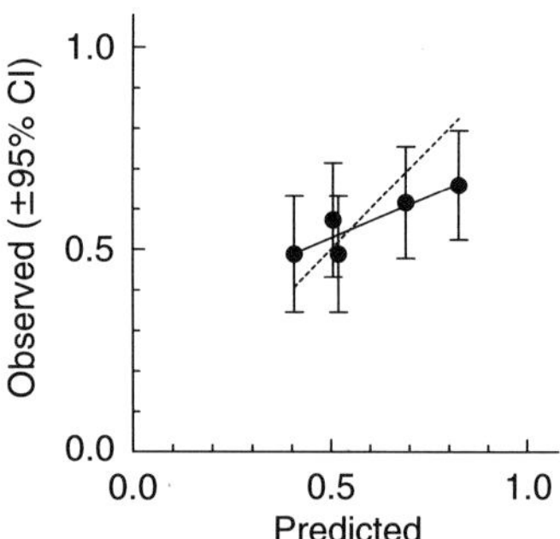


**Fig. 2.13.** Observed (with 95% confidence interval, CI) vs predicted proportion of 47 subjects with an individual GI value within ± 15 of the mean for five foods with GI ranging from 35 to 91. Predicted proportion derived from Fig. 2.12, observed proportion derived from Wolever *et al.* (2003a). Dotted line = line of identity; solid line = regression line.

Theoretical consideration of the effects of increased random variation of glycaemic responses on GI values also suggests that as the variation increases, the mean GI increases. The magnitude of the effect predicted by the model discussed above is shown in Fig. 2.14, which shows how the difference in GI (theoretical observed minus true) increases both as day-to-day variation of glycaemic responses increases and as the GI itself increases. Thus, it would be predicted that subjects with high within-subject variation, such as those with type 1 diabetes, would have somewhat higher GI values than subjects with low within-subject variation, such as those with type 2 diabetes. Figure 2.10B shows that GI values determined in subjects with type 1 diabetes are slightly, but significantly, higher than GI values determined in subjects with type 2 diabetes. The magnitude of the observed difference, 7.7, is greater than that expected by the model shown in Fig. 2.14, but this may be explained by the fact that the model calculations include the entire population of subjects; whereas the real data are drawn from a sample of the real population which reduces the precision of the observed means.

#### 2.2.4.3 *Effect of preprandial glucose on postprandial glycaemic response*

Early on, we noted that the incremental area under the blood glucose response curve of subjects with type 1 diabetes was inversely related to their FBG concentration immediately preceding the test meal (Jenkins *et al.*, 1984); that is the higher FBG, the lower the incremental area under the blood glucose response curve (AUC). Later we reported that the same phenomenon tended to occur in normal subjects and those with type 2 diabetes although the strength of the relationships were much less than in subjects with type 1 diabetes (Wolever *et al.*, 1985). Others have noted a similar phenomenon (Nielsen and Nielsen, 1989) but suggested that the correlation between FBG and AUC was apparent only when FBG >13 mmol/l. However, our data do not support this. Figure 2.15 shows data for 205 trials of reference white bread done by 18 subjects with type 1 diabetes, and 931 trials of reference white bread done by 54 subjects with type 2 diabetes. The solid dots represent trials for which fasting glucose was <13.0 mmol/l, and the open circles represent trials for which fasting glucose was ≥13.0 mmol/l. For subjects with type 1 diabetes, FBG was significantly related to AUC when FBG <13 mmol/l, $r = -0.318$ ($P < 0.001$); when FBG ≥13 mmol/l, there was a strong trend for a negative correlation, $r = -0.263$, which missed statistical significance ($P = 0.092$). Similarly, for subjects with type 2 diabetes, there was a weak correlation when FBG < 13 mmol/l, $r = -0.106$, which was statistically significant because of the large number of points ($P = 0.002$); with the correlation when FBG ≥ 13 mmol/l being stronger ($r = -0.163$), but not statistically significant ($P = 0.12$). The regression lines for AUC on FBG had almost identical slopes and *y*-intercepts in subjects with both type 1 and type 2 diabetes when FBG < 13 or ≥13 mmol/l (Fig. 2.15). These data suggest that the negative correlation between FBG and AUC is the same across the entire range of FBG, but is less strong (i.e. the

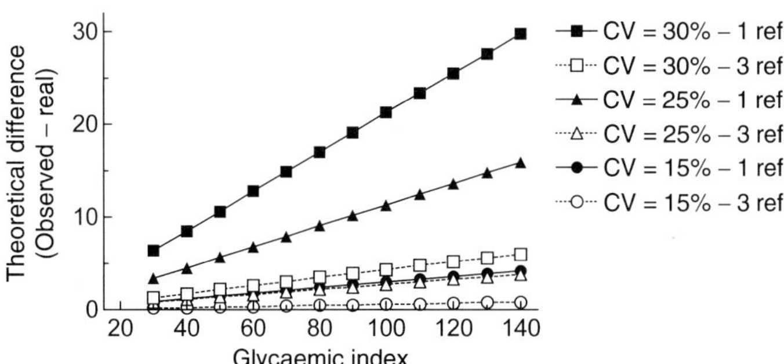


**Fig. 2.14.** Theoretical effect of increased day-to-day variation (CV) and number of reference foods used on the difference in GI (observed minus real) based on mathematical modelling.

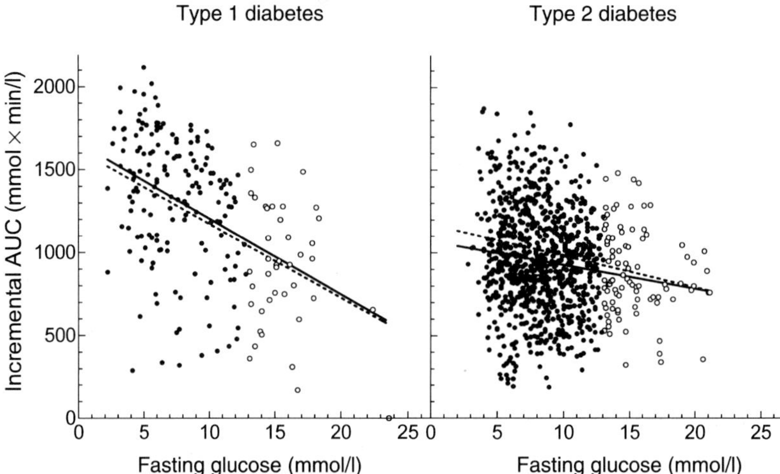


**Fig. 2.15.** Relationship between fasting glucose and incremental area under the curve for repeated tests of white bread taken by subjects with type 1 diabetes (left) and type 2 diabetes (right). Solid lines = regression lines for fasting glucose <13 mmol/l (filled circles); dotted lines = regression lines for fasting glucose >12.9 mmol/l (open circles). See text for further description.

slope is less) in people with type 2 diabetes than in those with type 1 diabetes.

Table 2.8 shows mean data for repeated trials of white bread to compare the relationships between FBG and AUC in 18 individual subjects with type 1 diabetes compared to 54 subjects with type 2 diabetes each of whom tested white bread at least three times. The subjects with type 1 diabetes did an average of 11 trials of bread each, compared to 17 for subjects with type 2 diabetes (ns). Although mean FBG did not differ significantly between type 1 and type 2 subjects, the variation of FBG in subjects with type 1 diabetes was more than twice that in subjects with type 2 diabetes ($P < 0.001$). Mean AUC was significantly higher in subjects with type 1 dia-

**Table 2.8.** Within-subject relationships between fasting glucose and incremental area under the curve elicited by test meals of white bread containing 50 g available carbohydrate taken repeatedly by subjects with type 1 and type 2 diabetes.

| | Type 1 | Type 2 | *P** |
|---|---|---|---|
| Number of subjects | 18 | 54 | – |
| Number of repeated trials per subject | 11.4 ± 3.0 | 17.2 ± 1.9 | ns |
| Fasting glucose (mmol/l) | 9.4 ± 0.6 | 8.9 ± 0.3 | ns |
| SD of fasting glucose (mmol/l)[a] | 3.9 ± 0.4 | 1.8 ± 0.1 | <0.001 |
| CV of fasting glucose (%)[a] | 43.5 ± 3.7 | 20.2 ± 1.4 | <0.001 |
| IAUC (mmol × min/l) | 1109 ± 81 | 876 ± 33 | 0.002 |
| SD of IAUC (mmol × min/l)[a] | 278 ± 27 | 155 ± 8 | <0.001 |
| CV of IAUC (%)[a] | 28.0 ± 4.0 | 18.3 ± 0.9 | <0.001 |
| Adjusted CV of IAUC (%)[b] | 19.2 ± 3.1 | 15.6 ± 0.9 | ns |
| Regression slope (min)[c] | –48.8 ± 6.5 | –17.2 ± 9.9 | 0.078 |
| Regression *y*-intercept (mmol × min/l)[c] | 1115 ± 80 | 877 ± 33 | 0.002 |
| Correlation coefficient (*r*)[c] | –0.634 ± 0.063 | –0.164 ± 0.060 | <0.001 |
| *n* (%) with significant *r*-value[c] | 8 (44%) | 7 (13%) | 0.004 |

Significance of difference between Type 1 and Type 2; ns=not significant.
[a]SD=standard deviation; CV=coefficient of variation (100 × SD/mean); IAUC=incremental area under the blood glucose response curve.
[b]CV of residuals; i.e. differences between individual IAUC values and estimates of IAUC at the same fasting glucose from the regression equation of IAUC on fasting glucose.
[c]Slope, y-intercept, correlation coefficient and significance of correlation coeffcient for regression of IAUC on fasting glucose.

betes by about 26%, but the variation in AUC in subjects with type 1 diabetes was almost twice that in subjects with type 2 diabetes ($P < 0.001$). The correlation coefficients and regression equations between FBG and AUC were calculated for each individual subject. Although the slope of the regression line in type 1 subjects was nearly three times that in type 2 subjects, because of high variation in the type 2 subjects, the difference did not reach statistical significance ($P = 0.078$). However, the mean correlation coefficient in type 1 subjects was nearly four times that in type 2 subjects (−0.634 vs −0.164, $P < 0.001$), and the correlation between FBG and AUC was significant in 44% of the type 1 subjects compared to only 13% of the type 2 subjects ($P = 0.004$). If the individual correlations between FBG and AUC are used to adjust the AUC values for the variation in FBG and the variability of the adjusted AUC values is calculated, one finds that the mean CV (CV = 100 × SD/mean) in type 1 subjects is reduced by nearly 50% to 19.2%, a value which is not longer significantly different from the mean CV of the adjusted AUC values in the type 2 subjects, 15.6% (Table 2.8).

Figure 2.16 shows the correlations between FBG and AUC in the eight subjects with the largest number of white bread trials. All the subjects whose data are shown in Fig. 2.16 had type 2 diabetes, except subject #2, who had type 1 diabetes. These data illustrate that the variation in FBG is less in most of the subjects with type 2 diabetes than the subject with type 1 diabetes, and that the slopes of the regression lines and degree of significance of the correlation coefficients are less in the subjects with type 2 than type 1 diabetes. Thus, part of the reason for the lack of correlation between FBG and AUC in type 2 diabetes is the smaller range of variation in FBG and AUC in type 2 subjects. However, this is not the whole story. Subject 1 (type 2 diabetes) has the same range in FBG as subject 2 (type 1 diabetes), but the correlation coefficient is much less. All of these facts shed some light as to why incremental AUC is reduced when FBG is high.

One potential reason why incremental AUC gets smaller as FBG increases is because of more and more glucose being lost in the urine as the blood glucose increases. However, if loss of glucose into the urine were the only reason, then the slope of the regression line for AUC on FBG should be the same in subjects with type 1 and type 2 diabetes, particularly those with a high range of variation of FBG, such as subjects #1 and #2. The fact that this is not so suggests that other factors must be playing a role, and a likely factor is what is termed 'glucose effectiveness', i.e. the ability of plasma glucose to stimulate its own removal. Glucose enters cells via different types of glucose transporters of which more than a dozen different types are known (Wood and Trayhurn, 2003). Factors which increase the transport activity of glucose transporters include glucose, insulin and exercise (Khayat *et al.*, 2002; Koistinen and Zierath, 2002). The most well-known transporters are the class I facilitative transporters GLUT1–4. GLUT1–3 transporters are not sensitive to insulin, that is, the rate at which they transport glucose is not affected by the insulin concentration. GLUT2 is primarily expressed in liver, pancreas, intestine and kidney and is believed to be part of the glucose sensing mechanism. GLUT3 is primarily expressed in brain. GLUT1 is expressed in all tissues, and particularly in brain and red blood cells, but also in muscle and fat. GLUT1, therefore, is a mechanism by which muscle can take up glucose in the absence of insulin at a rate which depends on the concentration of glucose in the blood. Insulin-stimulated glucose uptake is primarily mediated by GLUT4. A rise in plasma insulin increases glucose transport by causing GLUT4 transporters to be translocated from vesicles in the cytoplasm of cells to the surface of cells, and by increasing the intrinsic glucose transport activity of the transporters themselves (Furtado *et al.*, 2002).

### 2.2.5 Type of reference food

The 'reference food' is the carbohydrate source against which other foods are compared, and, by definition, has a GI of 100. The original reference food was glucose (Jenkins *et al.*, 1981a), but later, when we started doing tests mainly in subjects with diabetes, we used whole meal bread (Jenkins *et al.*, 1983). The rationale for switching was because bread was considered a more physiological carbohydrate source. It was felt that the high osmolarity of oral glucose solutions may delay gastric emptying and/or produce nausea in some individuals which, in turn, might make glycaemic responses more variable (Thompson *et al.*, 1982), as well as being unpleasant for the subjects. Since the whole meal bread produced the same glycaemic response as white bread, we began using white bread as the reference food. This raises

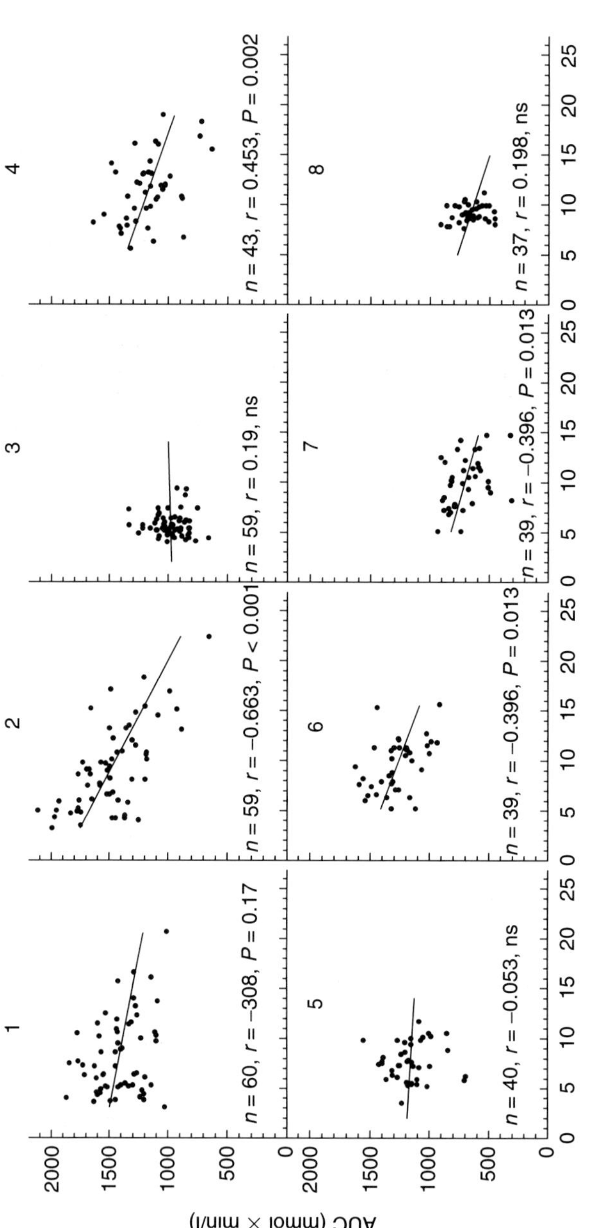


**Fig. 2.16.** Relationship between fasting blood glucose and incremental area under the blood glucose response curve elicited by 50 g available carbohydrate from white bread in eight individual subjects with diabetes. Subject 2 had type 1 diabetes, all the others had type 2 diabetes. Lines are regression lines.

two questions. Is bread better than glucose as a reference food for GI testing? Since GI values based on different reference foods differ; is it valid to convert GI values based on one reference food to those based on another?

Subjects may prefer eating bread rather than glucose, and this is one reason why bread may be preferred as a reference food. If glycaemic responses elicited by bread were less variable than those elicited by glucose, this would be a strong reason to use bread instead of glucose. However, there is no evidence that day-to-day variation of glycaemic responses when subjects take repeated tests of glucose differs from that for bread. Table 2.5 shows that, in 11 normal subjects, the mean ( ± SEM) CV within subjects for repeated tests of 50 g glucose was 25 ± 4% (Wolever *et al.*, 1985), and in 47 subjects who repeated trials of 50 g oral glucose two to three times in the interlaboratory GI study, mean CV was 23.4 ± 2.1% (Wolever *et al.*, 2003a). For bread, the mean within-subject CV was 27.7 ± 5.0% in ten subjects who repeated bread trials three times each (Wolever *et al.*, 2003a) and 20.4 ± 1.8% in 13 subjects who repeated bread trials four times each. The fact that the average CV for glucose, 24%, is virtually identical to that for bread, 24%, suggests that, at least from a technical point of view, either are equally good reference foods for determining the GI of foods.

GI values for foods based on bread as a reference ($GI_{wb}$) are higher than those based on glucose (GI). Therefore, when reading the literature on GI it is important to know what the reference food is. I showed in my PhD thesis that the $GI_{wb}$ values could be converted to GI values by simply dividing the $GI_{wb}$ values by $100/x$ where $x$ is the mean GI value of white bread. In my studies the mean GI of white bread was 75, and so $GI_{wb}$ values were adjusted by dividing by 1.333. The mean GI value of the 21 foods, 58.52 ± 4.52, was virtually identical to the mean of the adjusted $GI_{wb}$ values, 58.43 ± 4.65. The linear regression of the adjusted $GI_{wb}$ values on GI values produced a regression line which was virtually superimposed on the line of identity across the entire range of GI values (Fig. 2.17). This showed that it is valid to adjust GI values based on reference foods other than glucose. The adjustment factor from my PhD thesis, 1.333, was less than that recommended by Dr Jennie Brand-Miller, 1.4. But this is probably because I used 50 g dextrose in my PhD thesis. Dextrose is glu-

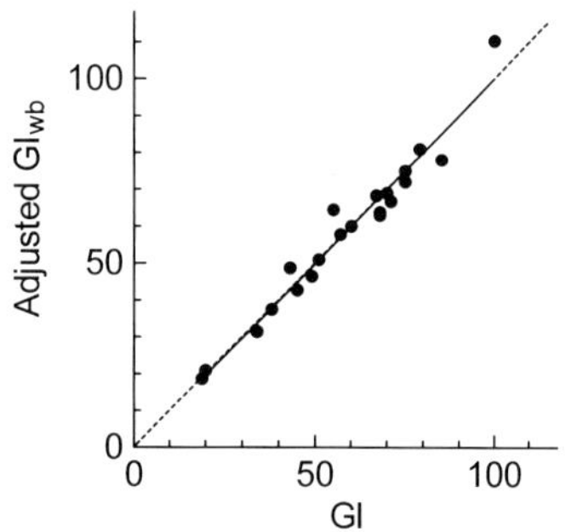


**Fig. 2.17.** Relationship between glycaemic index calculated using glucose as the reference food (GI) and glycaemic index calculated using white bread as the reference food ($GI_{wb}$) and adjusted by multiplying the $GI_{wb}$ values by $W/100$, where $W =$ the GI of white bread (glucose = 100). Data are from groups of normal subjects each of whom consumed both glucose and white bread. Dotted line = line of identity, solid line = regression line. Data from Wolever (1986).

cose monohydrate which has a molecular weight 10% more than that of anhydrous glucose. Thus, to obtain 50 g anhydrous glucose, 55 g of dextrose is required. Increasing my conversion factor of 1.333 by 5% yields a factor of exactly 1.4! In the interlaboratory GI study, 50 g anhydrous glucose was the reference food, and the mean GI of white bread tested in 47 subjects was 71.0, resulting in a conversion factor of 1.408.

It is not ideal to have two different sets of GI values in the literature. Therefore, it is recommended that GI values be expressed on the glucose scale. It is valid to use bread or some other food as the reference, but the results should be adjusted to the glucose scale. If a reference food other than glucose is to be used, then the GI value of the reference food relative to glucose should be well characterized and periodically checked to ensure that an accurate conversion factor is used.

### 2.2.6 Time of day tests are done

Blood glucose responses vary throughout the day depending on the time of day (Malherbe *et al.*, 1969; Genuth, 1973; Service *et al.*, 1983; Wolever and Bolognesi, 1996c), the nature of the meal consumed (Service *et al.*, 1983; Daly *et al.*, 1998), the nature of the previous meal consumed (Jenkins *et al.*, 1982b; Collier *et al.*, 1987; Wolever *et al.*, 1988a, 1995a; Nestler *et al.*, 1988; Liljeberg and

Björck, 2000) and intermeal spacing (Staub, 1921; Trougott, 1922). These studies suggest that absolute glycaemic responses may vary at different times of the day. However, it is generally assumed that the relative effects of meal components on glycaemic responses is the same; i.e. if a change in the nature of the test meal has a certain effect at breakfast, the relative effect will be the same at lunch or dinner.

Most glycaemic response tests are done in the morning after an overnight fast, but some have been done at lunch time after a standard breakfast and the results used to draw general conclusions about the validity of the GI (Coulston *et al.*, 1984a, 1987) or about the effects of varying meal size and composition (van Amelsvoort *et al.*, 1990a,b). There is evidence that treatments which influence blood glucose responses at breakfast and dinner may not have such large effects at lunch. For example, in a study of low-GI diets in healthy subjects, Jenkins *et al.* (1987a), glycaemic responses were lower after low-GI breakfast and dinner meals, but the expected difference at lunch was not seen. Similarly, in subjects with type 2 diabetes, there was no difference in blood glucose after a low-GI lunch, but the expected difference was seen after breakfast (Brand *et al.*, 1991). In addition, in subjects with IGT, the α-glucosidase inhibitor acarbose reduced glucose and insulin responses to a lesser extent after lunch than after dinner or breakfast, despite the same dose being taken (Chiasson *et al.*, 1996). On the other hand, this is not a universal effect, with the expected reductions in glucose and/or insulin being observed at lunch in some studies (Hollenbeck *et al.*, 1988; Järvi *et al.*, 1999).

One problem with interpreting these studies is that the test meals fed at breakfast, lunch and dinner were not the same. Thus, it is not really possible to know if the difference in relative effects seen at different times of the day was really due to diurnal variation or simply to differences in the meals. We did a study in eight normal subjects to see if the relative glycaemic effects of two breakfast cereals were the same when fed in the morning after an overnight fast, or at mid-day, exactly 4 h after starting to eat a standard breakfast consumed under supervision in the laboratory (Wolever and Bolognesi, 1996c). As expected, when consumed at breakfast after an overnight fast, the high-fibre, oat loop cereal (GI = 61) elicited a glycaemic response almost exactly 50% of that elicited by a portion of maize flakes (GI = 124) containing the same amount of available carbohydrate (Fig. 2.18), but there was no difference in glycaemic response between the cereals when consumed at mid-day, 4 h after a standard breakfast. It is not known if time of day affects the RGR in other groups of subjects, such as those with insulin resistance or diabetes. In addition, our results do not indicate whether the lack of difference at lunch was due to the time of day *per se*, or to the fact that a meal had been consumed 4 h previously. Nevertheless, the results suggest that time of day may need to be taken into account when interpreting the literature. In addition, they are the basis for my recommendation that studies done for the purpose of determining the GI of foods should be done in the morning after an overnight fast.

It is of interest that diurnal variation affects not only blood glucose and insulin responses, but also chylomicron–triglyceride responses. When a single fat-rich test meal is fed in the morning after an overnight fast, serum triglyceride concentrations peak about 3–5 h after the meal. However, when a second meal is consumed 4–6 h after the first one, there is more rapid appearance of chylomicrons into the circulation, with a peak in serum triglycerides about 1 h after the meal (Wolever, 1990a; Fielding *et al.*, 1996). It has been suggested that the early postprandial peak in chylomicrons is due to the fact that a propor-

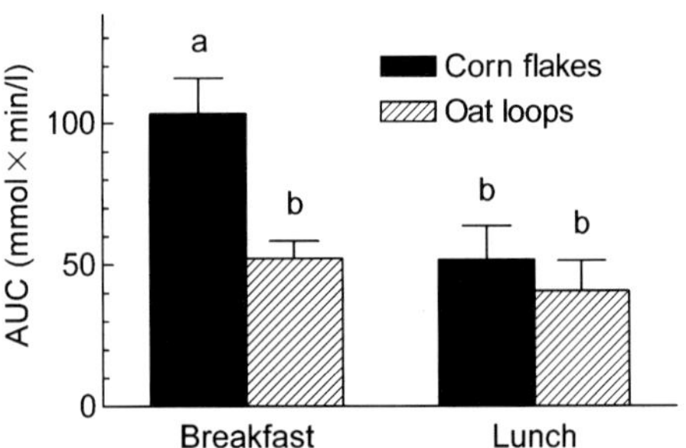


**Fig. 2.18.** Mean ± SEM incremental areas under the glycaemic response curve (AUC) of eight normal subjects after consuming equal-available carbohydrate portions of corn flakes or oat loops either in the morning after 10–14 h overnight fasts (breakfast) or 4 h after a standard breakfast (lunch). Means with different letter superscripts differ significantly ($P < 0.05$). Data from Wolever and Bolognesi (1996c).

tion of the fat in the first meal remains in the intestine or the enterocytes and enters the circulation with ingestion of the second meal (Fielding *et al.*, 1996). The early postprandial peak is similar whether the second meal is rich in fat or carbohydrate (Evans *et al.*, 1998). In contrast to the reduced difference in glycaemic response between carbohydrate foods fed at lunch, the difference in blood levels of different fatty acids appears to be maintained or even enhanced after the second meal (Jackson *et al.*, 2002).

### 2.2.7 Preparation of subjects before the test day

The glycaemic responses elicited by the reference test meal vary from day-to-day within subjects. Since most of the variation in GI values is due to within-individual variation (Fig. 2.1), the precision of GI results can be improved by procedures which reduce within-subject variation. The use of capillary as opposed to venous blood sampling is associated with reduced within-subject variation (Figs 2.8 and 2.9), as is the use of the mean AUC of three trials of the reference test in each subject (Table 2.7). Factors such as stress (Surwit *et al.*, 1992; Armario *et al.*, 1996), recent exercise (Mikines *et al.*, 1988; Langfort *et al.*, 1991; Borghouts and Keizer, 2000), cigarette smoking (Frati *et al.*, 1996), length of fasting time (Berkus *et al.*, 1990; Horton and Hill, 2001; Emberson *et al.*, 2002) and previous meal (Jenkins *et al.*, 1982b; Collier *et al.*, 1987; Nestler *et al.*, 1988; Wolever *et al.*, 1988a, 1995a; Liljeberg and Björck, 2000) have been shown to affect carbohydrate metabolism. Thus, variation in these factors may increase day-to-day variation in blood glucose responses. In an attempt to control some of these factors, some investigators provide subjects with a standard dinner to be consumed at a set time, the evening before a glycaemic response test, and ask them not to smoke or to do any vigorous physical activity for 24 h before the test (Wolf *et al.*, 2001a,b). These steps add cost to the study and make it more difficult for subjects to comply with the experimental protocol, and, at the time, it was not known whether this actually reduced day-to-day variation. Therefore, we did a study to see whether within-individual variation of glycaemic responses to a standard breakfast test meal could be reduced by controlling subjects' dinner, activities, stress and fasting time for 24 h prior to the test.

Thirteen healthy subjects performed four controlled and four uncontrolled trials using a randomized block design. During the controlled trials, subjects were asked not to smoke or do any vigorous exercise for 24 h, consume a standard dinner provided to them, and to fast for a set length of time ($\pm$ 15 min). During the uncontrolled trials, subjects were asked not to smoke on the morning of the test or to do any unusually vigorous physical activity for 24 h before the test. Subjects were allowed to do usual vigorous physical activity, and were asked to eat their normal dinner meal and to fast between 10 and 14 h. To reduce anxiety, subjects who were not familiar with finger-prick blood glucose response testing conducted a trial test to familiarize themselves with procedure before starting the study. The objective of the study was to see if the difference in subject preparation, controlled vs uncontrolled, influenced the within-individual variation of glycaemic responses expressed as CV (100 × SD/mean). To our surprise, mean CV for the controlled trials (CVc), 24.3 $\pm$ 3.0%, tended to be *greater* than that for the uncontrolled trials (CVu), 20.4 $\pm$ 1.8%, but the difference was not statistically significant. However, CVc was greater than CVu in 10 of the 13 individual subjects ($P = 0.046$) (Campbell *et al.*, 2003) (Fig. 2.19). The $P$-value is the chance CVc > CVu on 10 of 13 subjects, assuming that the probability of CVc > CVu is really 0.5. Based on this statistical analysis, we could not conclude that CVc was different from CVu, but we feel this is strong evidence that CVc is not less than CVu.

Thus, this study suggests that controlling subjects' diet and activities the day before a test by the methods we used does not improve the reproducibility of glycaemic response tests, and may actually make it worse. Providing a standard meal and documenting the compliance to the control measures increases the cost of doing studies. Not allowing subjects to do their regular exercise nor eat their regular diet and making them control the fasting time increases the inconvenience to subjects and may make some unwilling to participate in glycaemic response tests. Therefore, until there is evidence to the contrary, I recommend allowing subjects to undertake their usual physical activities and eat their normal diet on the day before doing a glycaemic response test.

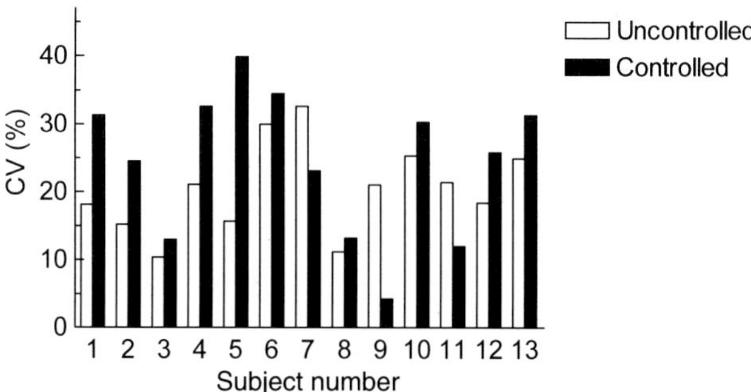


**Fig. 2.19.** Within-individual coefficients of variation (CV = 100 × SD/mean) of glycaemic responses elicited by 50 g available carbohydrate portions of white bread taken on four occasions after controlled diet and activities the day before or on four occasions after uncontrolled diet and activities in 13 normal subjects. Ten of the 13 subjects have higher CV after controlled diet and activities ($P$ = 0.046) (Campbell *et al.*, 2003).

### 2.2.8 Effect of volume and type of drink consumed with the test meal

Questions often asked about GI methodology is whether the volume of the test meal should be constant, and what type of drink, if any, can be used.

#### *2.2.8.1 Volume*

The volume of test meals influences the rate of gastric emptying (Hunt *et al.*, 1985), which, in turn, affects glycaemic responses (Thompson *et al.*, 1982; Torsdottir *et al.*, 1984, 1986; Mourot *et al.*, 1988; Thomsen *et al.*, 1994). The volume of a test meal can be increased in many ways, for example, by consuming more of the test meal (increased carbohydrate content), or by diluting the test meal with water (reduced osmolarity), or by adding dietary fibre, or even by adding air. The effects of these different manoeuvres on gastric emptying are probably different. However, when considering the volume of a drink consumed with the test meal, the major variables to consider would be the effects of the increased volume and the effects of the reduced osmolarity. Brouns *et al.* (1995) showed that, with a constant delivery of carbohydrate of about 1.2 g/min in various solutions containing 45–90 g/l carbohydrate with osmolarity of 243–374 mOsm/kg, the rate of gastric emptying was not affected by differences in osmolarity, but appeared to be triggered by the carbohydrate content of the drinks. However, the osmolarity of the solutions in this study are much lower than in many nutrition studies in which the effect of volume has been examined (Table 2.9).

In general, several-fold increases in the volume of test meals tend to have a modest effect to increase glycaemic responses, but this is not a consistent finding (Table 2.9). The lack of consistency may relate to the fact that methodology used to test the effect of volume varies widely. Perhaps one of the most important variables is the nature of the carbohydrate in the meal, particularly whether it is soluble, i.e. sugars dissolved in water, or readily hydrated (e.g. cooked potato starch), as opposed to relatively insoluble form, i.e. solid test meal to which water is added.

Schwartz *et al.* (1994) studied the effect of increasing the volume of a 50 g glucose solution from 150 to 450 ml in 132 pregnant women. In the 107 normal women, increasing the volume increased the rise in plasma glucose at 30 min by 12%, but had no effect at 60 min (+0.5%, ns). In the 25 women with gestational diabetes, increasing the volume significantly increased the rise in plasma glucose at 30 min by 17% and at 60 min by 11%. Vuksan's group in Toronto has done a series of studies on the effect on glucose responses of diluting solutions of sugars. In the first study (Sievenpiper *et al.*, 1998), increasing the volume of solutions containing 25 g glucose, sucrose or fructose from 200 to 600 ml significantly increased the incremental area under the finger-prick capillary blood glucose response curve by 30–60% in normal subjects. The results of the second study (Sievenpiper *et al.*, 2000) were consistent with those of the first in showing that as the volume of water in which 75 g glucose was dissolved was increased from 300 to 600 to 900 ml, the area under the finger-prick capillary blood glucose response curve in normal subjects increased by 20% for every doubling of the volume. Each of the ten subjects repeated each volume three times, and the reproducibility of the test was not affected by the volume. The results of the third study differed

**Table 2.9.** Effect of volume of test meal on glycaemic responses.

| Volume (ml) | Test meal | Osmolarity (mOsm/l) | Subjects (*n*) | % Change in AUC | Reference[a] |
|---|---|---|---|---|---|
| 150 → 450 | 50 g glucose | 1852 → 617 | N preg (107) | +9 | 1 |
| 150 → 450 | 50 g glucose | 1852 → 617 | GDM (25) | +14 | 1 |
| 200 → 600 | 25 g glucose | 694 → 232 | Normal (8) | +27 | 2 |
| 200 → 600 | 25 g sucrose | 366 → 122 | Normal (8) | +33 | 2 |
| 200 → 600 | 25 g fructose | 694 → 232 | Normal (8) | +67 | 3 |
| 300 → 600 | 75 g glucose | 1389 → 694 | Normal (10)[b] | +18 | 3 |
| 300 → 900 | 75 g glucose | 1389 → 463 | Normal (10)[b] | +44 | 3 |
| 300 → 600 | 75 g glucose | 1389 → 694 | Lean (11)[b] | −18[c] | 4 |
| 300 → 900 | 75 g glucose | 1389 → 463 | Lean (11)[b] | −37[c] | 4 |
| 300 → 600 | 75 g glucose | 1389 → 694 | Normal (12)[b] | −27[c] | 4 |
| 300 → 900 | 75 g glucose | 1389 → 463 | Normal (12)[b] | −13[c] | 4 |
| 300 → 600 | 75 g glucose | 1389 → 694 | Obese (12)[b] | −3[c] | 4 |
| 300 → 900 | 75 g glucose | 1389 → 463 | Obese (12)[b] | −3[c] | 4 |
| 0 → 300 | Potato/meat | Na | Normal (7) | +68 | 5 |
| 0 → 300 | Potato/meat | Na | T2DM (20) | +40 | 5 |
| 90 → 600 | Bread/butter | Na | T2DM (10) | −12 | 6 |
| 50 → 250 | Test wafer | Na | Normal (12)[d] | +11 | 7 |
| 50 → 500 | Test wafer | Na | Normal (12)[d] | +13 | 7 |
| 50 → 750 | Test wafer | Na | Normal (12)[d] | +12 | 7 |
| 50 → 1000 | Test wafer | Na | Normal (12)[d] | 0 | 7 |

[a]1. Schwartz *et al.* (1994); 2. Sievenpiper *et al.* (1998); 3. Sievenpiper *et al.* (2000); 4. Sievenpiper *et al.* (2001); 5. Torsdottir and Andersson (1989); 6. Gregerson *et al.* (1990); 7. Young and Wolever (1998).
[b]Each subject repeated each test three times.
[c]Difference in increment at 45 min.
[d]Each subject repeated each test two times.

from those of the first two in showing that increasing the volume of 75 g glucose solutions from 300 to 900 ml significantly *decreased* postprandial glucose responses in lean, athletic subjects ($n = 11$) and normal lean subjects ($n = 12$) and had no effect in obese normal subjects ($n = 12$) (Sievenpiper *et al.*, 2001). Although, in this last study, glucose was measured in venous plasma as opposed to finger-prick capillary blood, it is difficult to see how this could explain the completely different results.

Torsdottir and Andersson (1989) studied the effect of adding 300 ml water to a test meal of meat and potatoes in normal subjects and subjects with type 2 diabetes divided into those who were well controlled or poorly controlled. Water had the marked effect of increasing the area under the glycaemic response curve in normal subjects by 65%, and in subjects with well-controlled diabetes by 40%. There was no effect of water in subjects with poorly controlled diabetes. The results of this study do not agree with those of another in which either 90 or 600 ml water was added to a meal of rye bread, butter and tomatoes taken by ten subjects with type 2 diabetes (Gregerson *et al.*, 1990). Here, the increase in volume tended, if anything to reduce the area under the glucose response curve by 12%, but the difference was not statistically significant. These results are similar to ours (Young and Wolever, 1998) in which we studied the effect of consuming 50, 250, 500, 750 or 1000 ml water with a solid test meal bar in 12 normal subjects. We found that volume significantly affected the shape of the glucose response curve, but not the IAUC (Fig. 2.20). Increasing volume from 50 to 500 ml tended to increase the area under the glycaemic response curve by 13% (not significant), but the glycaemic response area after 1000 ml water was exactly the same as that after 50 ml. This suggests that the effect of changing volume on glycaemic responses is not linear; as volume increased from 50 to 500 ml, blood glucose at 30 min (peak) increased, and blood glucose at 120 min decreased; but these effects began to reverse as volume continued to increase from 500 to 1000 ml (Fig. 2.21).

Taken together, the above results suggest that large changes in the volume of drink taken with a

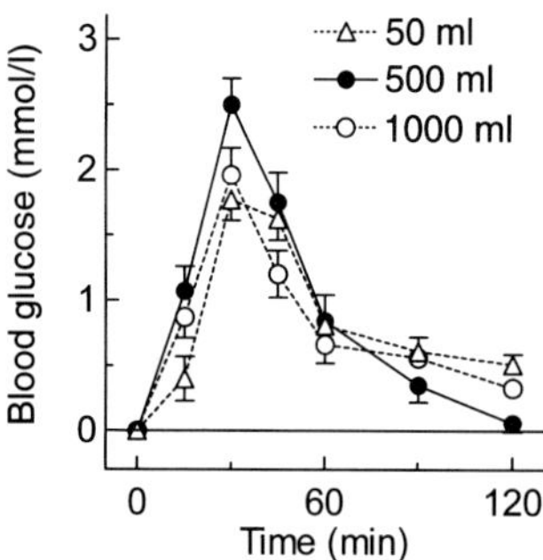


**Fig. 2.20.** Mean ± SEM blood glucose responses of normal subjects after consuming a standardized solid mixed meal in the form of a wafer with 50, 500 or 1000 ml water. Data from Young and Wolever (1998).

test meal influence glycaemic responses, probably through effects on gastric emptying. This provides a rationale for providing subjects with a drink of a standard volume. If test meals to be compared have large differences in volume, it may be worthwhile controlling for the volume difference.

### *2.2.8.2 Type of drink*

Coffee and tea are popular drinks and for many subjects, a drink of hot tea or coffee with the test meal may make the experience of participating as a subject in glycaemic response tests more pleasant than if they were allowed to drink only water. Coffee and tea contain caffeine and related compounds which have many effects on the human body (Donovan and DeVane, 2001; Armstrong, 2002; Heaney, 2002; Smith, 2002; Nawrot *et al.*, 2003). Of particular relevance to the testing of glycaemic responses is the fact that caffeine acutely decreases insulin sensitivity in humans (Graham *et al.*, 2001; Keijzers *et al.*, 2002). Graham *et al.* (2001) gave subjects 5 mg/kg caffeine (average of 385 mg, range 317–468 mg) 1 h before a 75 g oral glucose load, and found a significantly increased plasma insulin response after caffeine compared to placebo. Keijzers *et al.* (2002) administered caffeine intravenously with a 3 mg/kg loading dose followed by continuous infusion at a rate of 0.6 mg/kg/h for 2 h for a total dose of 4.2 mg/kg. Compared to placebo, caffeine impaired whole-body insulin sensitivity, measured with a euglycaemic, hyperinsulinaemic clamp, by about 15% ($P < 0.05$). Both studies demonstrated significant counterregulatory effects of caffeine with significant increases in plasma free-fatty acids (FFAs) and epinephrine.

However, the results of these studies may not necessarily be relevant to the question of whether a drink of coffee or tea should be allowed when determining the GI of foods. The amount of caffeine in tea and coffee varies depending on the nature of preparation, but instant or brewed coffee contains about 65–100 mg per 250 ml cup and brewed black tea 50 mg per 250 ml cup (US Department of Agriculture, 2004). These amounts are only about 15–35% of those used in the caffeine studies cited above. In addition, coffee and tea contain more than just caffeine, and the methods of administration used in these studies may not reflect the pharmacokinetics of caffeine obtained from a drink of coffee or tea taken with a test meal. Thus, it would seem more instructive to look at the effects of coffee or tea on postprandial responses.

Coffee and tea stimulate gastric secretions (Dubey *et al.*, 1984; Coffey *et al.*, 1986; Boekema *et al.*, 1999), reduce glucose-dependent insulinotropic polypeptide (GIP), increase glucagon-like peptide 1 (GLP-1) secretion (Johnston *et al.*, 2003) and may accelerate gastric emptying (Lien *et al.*, 1995). When we compared the effect taking 250 ml water, coffee or tea with a standardized solid test meal bar, we found that blood glucose at 45 min was significantly higher after coffee and

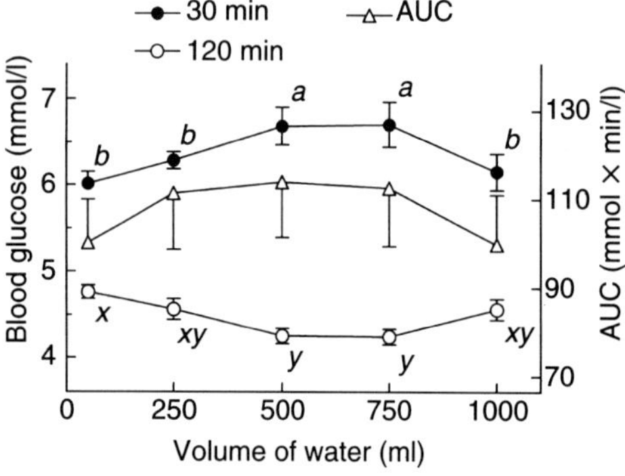


**Fig. 2.21.** Effect of consuming different volumes of water with a standardized solid test meal on blood glucose concentrations at 30 and 120 min and incremental area under the blood glucose response curve in normal subjects. Values are mean ± SEM. Means with different letters differ significantly ($P <$ 0.05). Data from Young and Wolever (1998).

tea compared to water, but there was no significant effect on the incremental area under the glycaemic response curve (Fig. 2.22; Young and Wolever, 1998).

These results are similar to those from Johnston *et al.* (2003) who found significantly higher plasma glucose 30 min after coffee containing 25 g glucose, compared to 25 g glucose dissolved in water, but no significant effect on the incremental area under the glycaemic response curve.

In terms of determining the GI of foods, the question is not so much whether coffee and tea influence glycaemic responses, but whether they influence either the mean or the variability of the GI. Unfortunately, there are no data addressing this issue. However, if coffee had the same relative effect on postprandial glycaemic responses of all test meals, it would have no effect on the calculated GI value, because the AUC of both the test food and the reference food would be increased to the same extent: i.e. $A/B = kA/kB$, where $A$ and $B$ are the AUC values for the test and reference foods, respectively, and $k$ is the effect of coffee on AUC. It is possible that the effect of coffee and tea on postprandial responses may differ for different carbohydrate sources, but this has not been investigated. Coffee and tea might conceivably influence the variation of glycaemic responses by stimulating gastric activity and making subjects feel better, but data here are also lacking.

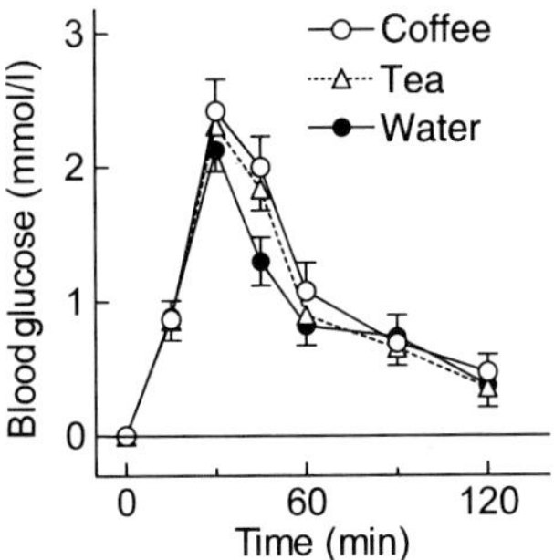


**Fig. 2.22.** Effect of consuming 250 ml coffee or tea compared to 250 ml water with a standardized solid test meal bar on blood glucose responses in normal subjects. Blood glucose at 45 min was significantly higher after coffee and tea than water, but there was no significant effect on incremental area under the curve (Young and Wolever, 1998).

### 2.2.9 Time to consume test meal

It is known that consuming glucose (Jenkins *et al.*, 1990), liquid test meals (Wolever, 1990a) or solid test meals (Jenkins *et al.*, 1982b, 1992; Bertelsen *et al.*, 1993; Segura *et al.*, 1995) in small divided doses over a period of 3–4 h has a marked effect in flattening the glycaemic response compared to consuming exactly the same test meal over 10–15 min. However, the effect of varying the time of ingestion of solid meals over periods of less than 30 min has not been investigated. Heine *et al.* (1983) showed in healthy volunteers that consuming 75 g glucose or hydrolysed starch in 300 ml water over 1 min, as compared to 10 min, reduced the netAUC by about 50%. For these reasons, it appears appropriate to recommend that the test meal is consumed in about 10–15 min, depending on the type of food.

## 2.3 Conclusions

If the GI is to become a useful marker of the biological effects of carbohydrate foods, the first thing we must be clear about is what it means. Nutrition scientists and professionals must appreciate the difference between the 'glycaemic index' and a 'glycaemic response'. The GI is determined by measuring the glycaemic responses elicited by feeding reference and test foods to human subjects on separate occasions. There are many ways to measure glycaemic responses, and methodological differences may or may not influence the results. Factors, which affect the glycaemic responses will, therefore, affect the GI values obtained. If the GI is to be practically useful, it must be a function of the carbohydrate food which can be measured reproducibly. Thus, standardized methodology is required. However, this does not necessarily mean that every experimental variable must be rigidly controlled. This could lead to methods which are so difficult and restrictive that they would render the GI practically useless because it was too expensive to measure. Some things which might seem to be very important to control (e.g. the type of subject studied) may have little impact on the results obtained or may actually tend to make the results worse (e.g. standardized meal the night before). Some things which might not even be considered (e.g. the type of blood sampling) may actually be quite important to the results obtained. Thus, we need to understand the sources of error in the methodologies used and how these errors affect the results obtained. Methods can then be developed with an appropriate balance of cost vs precision. There are many more questions about methodology for which we have no answers than there are questions about which we have some information. However, since studies on methodological factors have often produced surprising results, I would strongly recommend that changes to GI methodology should not be translated into practice until the effects of such changes on the results obtained have been investigated, particularly for changes which make it more expensive or difficult to carry out GI tests.

# 3

# The Insulin Response to Carbohydrate Foods: Critical Evaluation of the Insulinaemic Index

Shortly after the GI emerged, it was suggested that knowledge of the glycaemic effects of foods alone is insufficient and that a measure of the insulin response elicited by foods is also required (Coulston *et al.*, 1984b). It was noted that insulin responses were sometimes quite divergent in the face of similar glycaemic responses (Crapo *et al.*, 1977, 1981; Coulston *et al.*, 1980, 1981). Measurement of insulin responses was considered possibly to be of more clinical significance in the population without diabetes than measurement of glucose because of data showing that high plasma insulin contributed to hypertriglyceridaemia (Farquhar *et al.*, 1966) and was a primary risk factor for cardiovascular disease (Ducimetiere *et al.*, 1980). Subsequent work has reinforced the role of hyperinsulinaemia in the development of chronic 'Western' diseases (Reaven, 1988). More recently, it has again been alleged that the correlation between the glucose and insulin responses of foods is not good, and thus, it is not possible to use the GI to choose foods on the basis of their insulin response (Pi-Sunyer, 2002).

There are two general reasons why it might be desirable to measure insulin responses: to help understand the mechanism by which glucose responses are altered, and to provide information which is clinically useful for diet planning. From a scientific point of view, it is always useful to have as much information about a phenomenon as possible to help understand what is going on. However, I would like to focus here on the practical question of whether measuring the insulin response elicited by foods has any clinical utility by asking several questions. Do foods with high insulin responses contribute to high plasma insulin concentrations and insulin resistance? Do the insulin responses of individual foods reflect their effects when incorporated into mixed meals? Can the insulin responses of foods be measured with a reasonable degree of precision and accuracy? Are the results of insulin response test the same in all subjects regardless of their glucose tolerance status or degree of insulin sensitivity? In addition, I will examine the question of whether measuring insulin responses provides useful information which cannot be gained by measuring glucose responses. First, however, I will review briefly the meaning of the terms 'insulin sensitivity' and 'insulin resistance' and their role in human disease.

## 3.1 Insulin Sensitivity

Insulin sensitivity is the degree to which a given rise in plasma insulin stimulates an increase in the rate of uptake of glucose from the blood (Bergman *et al.*, 1985). If an individual is insulin-sensitive (i.e. low insulin resistance), the individual's tissues are sensitive to insulin and a high rate of glucose uptake is achieved at a normal concentration of plasma insulin. If an individual is insulin-resistant (i.e. low insulin sensitivity), a high concentration of insulin is required to obtain a normal rate of glucose disposal (Kahn *et al.*, 1993). Thus, in an individual with normal blood glucose, insulin resistance is usually associated with a high concentration of plasma insulin. Nevertheless, this is not always the case, and in a large European cohort of 1308 subjects, only 60% of the cohort of subjects in the lowest quartile of clamp-derived insulin sensitivity was also part of the cohort of subjects in the highest quartile of fasting plasma insulin (Ferrannini and Balkau, 2002).

### 3.1.1 Use of the term 'insulin sensitivity'

The terms 'insulin resistance' and 'insulin sensitivity' are used rather loosely in the literature. Ideally insulin sensitivity is determined by measuring directly the ability of insulin to stimulate the *rate* of uptake of glucose from the bloodstream. A number of dynamic experimental procedures have been used for this purpose all of which involve intravenous (IV) injection or infusion of insulin to change the plasma insulin concentration followed by a direct or indirect measure of the rate of glucose uptake from the blood. Although these tests do not yield exactly the same results, they do, at least, attempt to make a direct measurement of insulin sensitivity by raising plasma insulin and measuring the *rate* of glucose uptake.

However, a number of tests have been described to estimate insulin sensitivity from measures of fasting or postprandial plasma glucose and insulin concentrations. The first of these was homeostasis model assessment (HOMA) (Matthews *et al.*, 1985) in which an insulin resistance index was calculated as $G \times I/22.5$ and β-cell function as $20 \times I/(G-3.5)$ where $I$ is fasting plasma insulin in μU/ml and $G$ is fasting glucose in mmol/l. Other ways of using fasting glucose and insulin to estimate insulin sensitivity such as QUICKI (Katz *et al.*, 2000) have been proposed. Since fasting glucose is largely determined by the rate of endogenous glucose production, which, in turn, is largely determined by the rate of output of glucose from the liver, indices of insulin resistance based on fasting glucose and insulin are really a measure of hepatic insulin sensitivity (Matsuda and DeFronzo, 1999). This is not the same thing as whole body insulin sensitivity since most insulin-stimulated glucose uptake occurs in muscle. Although a rise in plasma insulin is associated with a reduction in hepatic glucose output, which contributes to a reduction in blood glucose concentration, there is evidence that insulin *per se* is not entirely responsible for this effect (Lewis *et al.*, 1996, 1997, 1998).

Insulin sensitivity has also been estimated by a variety of methods from plasma glucose and insulin concentrations after a 75 g oral glucose tolerance test (OGTT) (Phillips *et al.*, 1995; Matsuda and DeFronzo, 1999; Caumo *et al.*, 2000; Della Man *et al.*, 2002). Since insulin resistance is part of the pathogenic process causing glucose intolerance, it is not surprising that it correlates with oral glucose tolerance. However, the problem with using postprandial glucose and insulin responses to assess insulin sensitivity is that the rate of glucose uptake from the circulation cannot be determined because the rate of glucose entry into the blood after a meal is not known (although steps have been taken to improve on the validity of the estimates used) (Della Man *et al.*, 2004). The amount of glucose injected intravenously as a bolus, or the rate of glucose infusion can be known exactly. However, the rate at which glucose enters the circulation after oral glucose depends on a number of gastrointestinal factors which likely vary not only from person to person but also within an individual from day to day. Thus, measures of insulin sensitivity derived from postprandial glucose and insulin responses are not true measures of insulin sensitivity.

The term 'insulin resistance syndrome' or 'metabolic syndrome' is used to describe individuals with abnormalities in blood pressure, body fat distribution, blood lipids or blood glucose presumed to be due to reduced insulin sensitivity. However, it has been argued that just because hypertension, abdominal obesity and dyslipidaemia tend to cluster in the same individuals does not necessarily mean that they have the same aetiology (i.e. insulin resistance) (Ferrannini and Balkau, 2002). Indeed, the presence of insulin resistance or high-plasma insulin is not necessary to identify an individual as having the metabolic syndrome. In addition, there is controversy about how the metabolic syndrome is defined (Balkau *et al.*, 2002). The WHO (World Health Organization, 1999) defines it as being the presence of impaired glucose regulation or diabetes and/or insulin resistance plus two or more of hypertension, high triglycericides and/or low HDL cholesterol, abdominal obesity and increased urinary albumin excretion (Table 3.1). In the USA (Expert Panel on Detection, Evaluation, and Treatment of High Blood Cholesterol in Adults, 2001), the syndrome is defined as the presence of any

**Table 3.1.** Comparison of definitions of metabolic syndrome according to WHO and NCEP.

| Factor | World Health Organization | Adult Treatment Panel III |
|---|---|---|
| A. Hyperglycaemia (plasma glucose) | Fasting ≥6.1 mmol/l and/or 2 h after 75 g glucose ≥7.8 mmol/l | Fasting ≥110 mg/dl (6.1 mmol/l) |
| B. Insulin resistance | <25 percentile of glucose uptake under euglycaemic hyperinsulinaemic conditions | – |
| C. Hypertension | ≥140/90 mmHg | ≥130/≥85 mmHg |
| D. High triglycerides | ≥1.7 mmol/l | ≥150 mg/dl (1.69 mmol/l) |
| E. Low HDL cholesterol | ♂: <0.9 mmol/l<br>♀: <1.0 mmol/l | ♂: <40 mg/dl (1.03 mmol/l)<br>♀: <50 mg/dl (1.30 mmol/l) |
| F. Abdominal obesity | ♂: waist to hip ratio >0.90<br>♀: waist to hip ratio >0.85 and/or BMI >30 kg/m$^2$ | ♂: waist circumference >102 cm<br>♀: waist circumference >88 cm |
| G. Microalbuminuria | Albumin excretion ≥20 μg/min or albumin:creatinine ratio ≥30 mg/g | – |
| Definition: | A and/or B<br>Plus any 2 of the 4 factors: C, D and/or E, F, G | Any 3 of the 5 factors: A, C, D, E and/or F |

three of the following: abdominal obesity, high triglycerides, low HDL cholesterol, hypertension or high fasting glucose (Table 3.1).

While it is undoubtedly true that individuals with the metabolic syndrome are at high risk for cardiovascular disease (Isomaa *et al.*, 2001), and perhaps other conditions, the metabolic syndrome is not the same thing as insulin resistance. For example, in a recent study, 65 normal subjects had insulin sensitivity measured using a recognized dynamic test and 16 were deemed to be insulin-resistant (Ascaso *et al.*, 2003); about one-third of the insulin-resistant individuals did not have the metabolic syndrome, and of the individuals with metabolic syndrome about one third did not have insulin resistance.

A final problem with insulin sensitivity as a concept is that it has been defined as the extent to which insulin increases glucose disposal. However, insulin does more than just stimulate glucose uptake, it also influences fat and protein metabolism. It is not fully known whether individuals who are insulin-resistant with respect to glucose metabolism are similarly resistant to the effects of insulin on protein and lipid metabolism (Maheux *et al.*, 1997).

### 3.1.2 Measurement of insulin sensitivity

Several methods have been used to measure insulin sensitivity, and these will be reviewed briefly. For a more complete review of the historical aspects, physiological principles and methods used to measure insulin sensitivity, see Bergman *et al.* (1985).

#### *3.1.2.1 Short insulin tolerance test*

The first method was to inject intravenously a small amount of insulin as a bolus and to measure the rate at which blood glucose fell over the next 15–20 min (Himsworth, 1932, 1935, 1936). This method is still used today and is known as the short insulin tolerance test (SITT) (Bonora *et al.*, 1989; Akinmokun *et al.*, 1992). If the concentration of insulin in the plasma is not measured (and often it is not), then the measure of insulin sensitivity derived is only relative. An absolute measure of insulin sensitivity would indicate the change in rate of glucose uptake per unit change in insulin concentration. In addition, the fall in plasma glucose after insulin injection is not only due to an increased rate of uptake in tissues but also to a reduced rate of output of glucose from the liver.

Thus, SITT, strictly, does not really measure insulin sensitivity. Nevertheless, it is very simple to do, and correlates with other measures in insulin resistance in many (Bonora *et al.*, 1989; Akinmokun *et al.*, 1992), but not all (Särnblad *et al.*, 2002) populations.

### *3.1.2.2 Insulin suppression test*

Another relatively simple method developed by Reaven and colleagues (Shen *et al.*, 1970; Reaven *et al.*, 1976) was the insulin suppression test in which subjects received pharmacologic inhibition of endogenous insulin secretion together with exogenous glucose and insulin infusion. Insulin secretion was inhibited either with adrenaline (epinepherine) and propranolol or with somatostatin (Nagulesparan *et al.*, 1979). In order to compare insulin sensitivity in different groups of subjects, it was necessary to choose an insulin infusion rate to achieve a plasma insulin concentration, which was approximately equal in all subjects. The insulin infusion rate was chosen to raise plasma insulin by about 100 μU/ml. Plasma glucose tended to rise after the start of the combined infusion reaching a plateau after about 90–120 min. The measure of insulin sensitivity was the steady-state plasma glucose (SSPG), defined as the average plasma glucose concentration achieved during a steady-state observation period. SSPG has been shown to be inversely proportional to the glucose disposal rate measured during a euglycaemic, hyperinsulinaemic clamp (Section 3.1.2.3) (Mimura *et al.*, 1994). Thus, the higher the SSPG value, the lower the insulin sensitivity (or the higher the insulin resistance). The protocol we used (Chiasson *et al.*, 1996) was to infuse 260 mg/min/m$^2$ glucose, 25 μU/min/m$^2$ insulin and 5 μg/min somatostatin and measure SSPG as the average plasma glucose at 120, 150 and 180 min after the start of the infusion (Fig. 3.1).

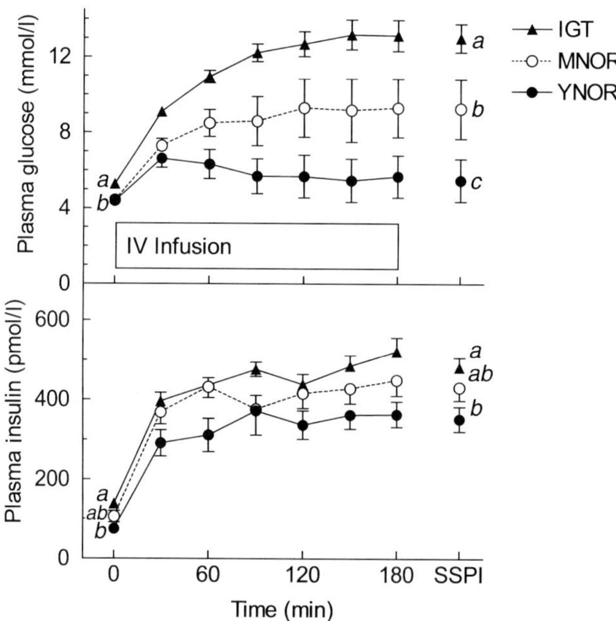


**Fig. 3.1.** Measurement of insulin sensitivity using the insulin suppression test in young lean subjects (YNOR; $n = 10$; age, 30 ± 2 years; BMI, 24 ± 1 kg/m$^2$), middle-aged obese subjects (MNOR; $n = 8$; age, 45 ± 3 years; BMI, 30 ± 2 kg/m$^2$) and subjects with impaired glucose tolerance (IGT; $n = 21$; age, 56 ± 3 years; BMI, 31 ± 1 kg/m$^2$). IV infusion contained 260 mg/min/m$^2$ (body surface area) glucose, 25 μU/min/m$^2$ insulin and 5 μg/min somatostatin. SSPG, steady-state plasma glucose; SSPI, steady-state plasma insulin. Values are means ± SEM. Means with different letter superscripts differ significantly, $P < 0.05$ (Chiasson *et al.*, 1996).

The problem with this method, it was subsequently discovered, was that not all glucose uptake depends on insulin; indeed, it has been estimated that about 40% of glucose uptake in normal individuals occurs in the absence of insulin, the so-called non-insulin-mediated glucose uptake (Bergman, 1989). Since the rate of non-insulin-mediated glucose uptake is directly related to the plasma glucose concentration, the contribution of non-insulin-mediated glucose uptake varies at different levels of SSPG. Thus, the insulin suppression test measures a combination of insulin sensitivity and glucose effectiveness (i.e. the ability of glucose to stimulate its own disposal); for this reason, this test has not been used much since the mid-1990s.

#### *3.1.2.3 Euglycaemic hyperinsulinaemic clamp*

The 'gold-standard' method is the glucose clamp in which both glucose and insulin are infused intravenously for 2–3 h. This technique was developed by Andres and colleagues about 30 years ago (DeFronzo *et al.*, 1979). The rate of insulin infusion is fixed to maintain a constant plasma insulin concentration. The plasma glucose concentration is measured regularly and the rate of glucose infusion adjusted to maintain constant plasma glucose. When steady state is reached (after hepatic glucose output has been reduced to a minimum), the rate of glucose infusion is equal to the rate of whole body glucose uptake. In this method, both glucose and insulin can be clamped at any level desired. However, usually insulin is infused to achieve a very high insulin concentration and glucose is clamped at a normal fasting concentration, hence 'hyperinsulinaemic euglycaemic' clamp. The reason for the often non-physiologically high insulin concentration is to measure the maximum insulin action, and the reason for clamping glucose at a normal fasting level is to minimize the effect of non-insulin-mediated glucose uptake. However, the latter still occurs, and so even the euglycaemic hyperinsulinaemic clamp does not distinguish between insulin-mediated and non-insulin-mediated glucose uptake (Bergman *et al.*, 1985).

#### *3.1.2.4 Minimal model*

In an attempt to distinguish between insulin-mediated and non-insulin-mediated glucose uptake, Bergman and colleagues developed the so-called 'minimal model'. This is an equation (i.e. mathematical model) to describe changes in blood glucose with time, which includes both insulin sensitivity and glucose effectiveness as factors influencing glucose uptake. It is described as 'minimal' because each of these two effects is described by a single parameter. Originally, the method involved IV injection of a bolus of glucose with frequent measurement of plasma glucose and insulin over the next 3 h. This so-called frequently sampled intravenous glucose tolerance test (FSIGTT) was validated in dogs (Finegood *et al.*, 1984), but in humans, FSIGTT-derived measures of insulin sensitivity did not correlate well with those derived from the glucose clamp due to low plasma insulin responses (Foley *et al.*, 1985). However, it was found that the addition of an injection of tolbutamide, 20 min after the glucose injection, increased the plasma insulin response and resulted in estimates of insulin sensitivity which correlated with the glucose clamp in humans better than in dogs (Bergman *et al.*, 1987). To enable the modified FSIGTT to be used in subjects with type 1 diabetes, in whom tolbutamide would not increase plasma insulin, it was found that an injection of insulin could be used instead of tolbutamide (Finegood *et al.*, 1990). Injection of insulin instead of tolbutamide was also shown to be valid in subjects without diabetes (Welch *et al.*, 1990).

In addition to measures of insulin sensitivity and glucose effectiveness, a measure of insulin secretion can be derived by calculating the area under the plasma insulin response curve after the glucose injection (Fig. 3.2). The FSIGTT is attractive because, from a single procedure, measures of insulin sensitivity, β-cell function and glucose effectiveness are derived. Although the index of glucose effectiveness has been shown to relate to diabetes risk (Martin *et al.*, 1992; Osei *et al.*, 2004), recent questions have arisen about its validity (Quon *et al.*, 1994; Finegood and Tzur, 1996). Nevertheless, the indices of insulin sensitivity and β-cell function derived from the FSIGTT procedure are considered to be valid and used extensively by many investigators.

### 3.1.3 Clinical utility of insulin sensitivity

Despite some problems, the concept of insulin resistance is very popular because it is such an

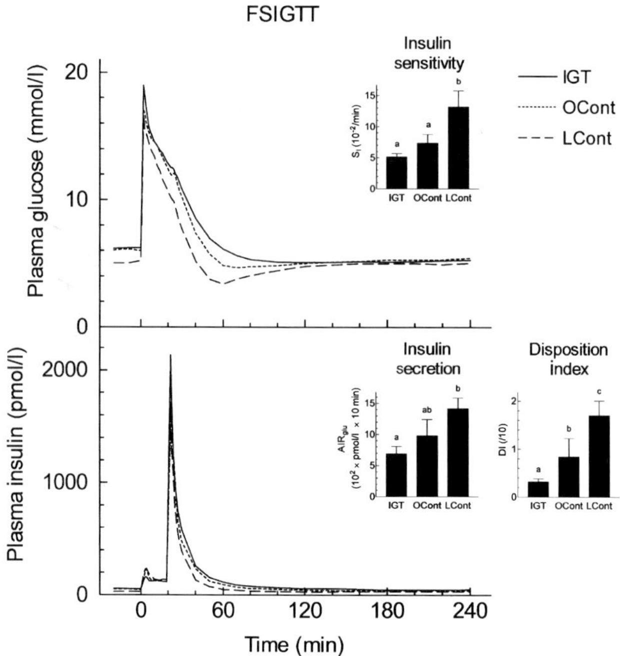


**Fig. 3.2.** Measurement of insulin sensitivity ($S_I$), insulin secretion ($AIR_{glu}$) and disposition index ($DI = S_I \times AIR_{glu}$) in lean controls (LCont; $n = 8$; age, 33 ± 4 years; BMI, 22.9 ± 0.9 kg/m$^2$), obese controls (OCont; $n = 7$; age, 59 ± 6 years; BMI, 29.3 ± 0.8 kg/m$^2$) and subjects with impaired glucose tolerance (IGT; $n = 35$; age, 57 ± 2 years; BMI, 29.9 ± 1.0 kg/m$^2$). A bolus of glucose (50% glucose solution, 25.1 ml/m$^2$ body surface area) was given intravenously at 0 min and a bolus of insulin (1.6 U/m$^2$) was given intravenously at 20 min. Values are means ± SEM. Means with different letter superscripts differ significantly ($P < 0.05$).

elegant explanation for the different plasma glucose and insulin responses of individuals at various stages in the development of type 2 diabetes. For example, Fig. 3.3 shows glucose and insulin responses after 75 g oral glucose in subjects with various degrees of glucose intolerance (Wolever

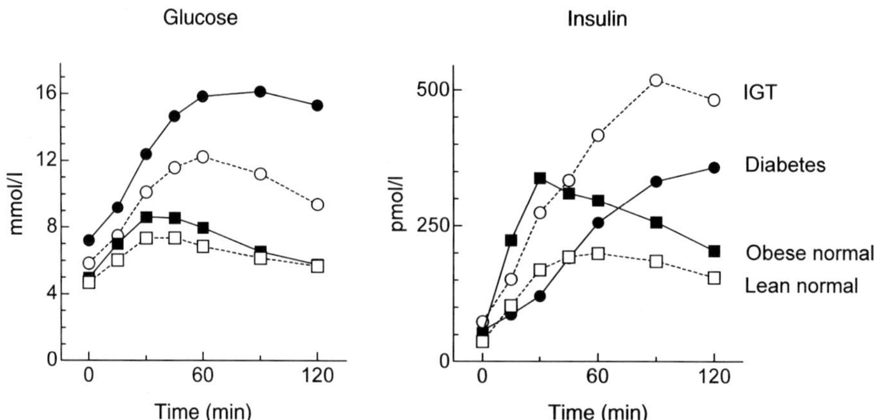


**Fig. 3.3.** Mean plasma glucose (left) and insulin (right) responses after 75 g oral glucose of ten lean normal (□) and nine obese normal subjects (■), nine subjects with impaired glucose tolerance (○) and eight subjects with mild type 2 diabetes (●).

*et al.*, 1998a). Lean normal subjects are insulin sensitive and have low (i.e. normal) plasma glucose and insulin responses. Middle-aged obese subjects are somewhat insulin-resistant, but maintain normal plasma glucose responses because of an increased rate of rise and an increased absolute rise in plasma insulin. Subjects with IGT are even more insulin-resistant and have fasting and postprandial hyperinsulinaemia. However, indicative of reduced first-phase insulin secretion, the rate at which plasma insulin increases in subjects with IGT is reduced compared to obese normal subjects, and so postprandial plasma glucose is increased. IGT progresses to diabetes because of a further decline in β-cell function. This results in a rate of rise of plasma insulin in subjects with diabetes which is less than that of lean normal subjects despite two- to threefold higher concentrations of plasma glucose and a fourfold higher rise in plasma glucose (Fig. 3.3).

Individuals become insulin-resistant because of genetic (Martin *et al.*, 1992; Zimmet, 1995; Hong *et al.*, 1998) and environmental factors. Lack of exercise (Goodyear and Kahn, 1998) and central obesity (Després, 1998) are the environmental factors for which there is most evidence. Insulin resistance is thought to be involved in the pathogenesis of type 2 diabetes (Ferrannini, 1998; Gerich, 1998), CHD (Reaven and Laws, 1994), colon cancer (McKeown-Essen, 1994) and hypertension (DeFronzo and Ferrannini, 1991). The reason for this is, however, not clear.

## 3.2 Are High Postprandial Insulin Responses Harmful?

It is difficult to answer this question. It has been argued that hyperinsulinaemia *per se* is the cause of, or at least contributes to, the deleterious health outcomes associated with insulin resistance (Reaven, 1988, 1994). Since administering insulin to normal subjects has been shown to increase insulin resistance (Del Prato *et al.*, 1994), presumably by downregulating insulin receptors, a vicious cycle could be set up with insulin resistance, leading to hyperinsulinaemia which, in turn, leads to more insulin resistance, etc. However, an alternate interpretation is that hyperinsulinaemia is a normal physiologic response to insulin resistance and is desirable, and, indeed necessary, to maintain homeostasis. The question of whether hyperinsulinaemia is harmful or beneficial has been a matter of debate for a number of years (Fontbonne, 1994; Jarrett, 1994; Reaven and Laws, 1994; Stern, 1994) and the issue has not been fully resolved.

The evidence that a dietary-induced increase in postprandial insulin is harmful and is even more ambiguous. For example, it has been suggested that a high-carbohydrate diet is deleterious for people with insulin resistance because it raises plasma insulin concentrations to a greater extent than in subjects who are insulin-sensitive (Jeppesen *et al.*, 1997). However, this could merely reflect a fixed percentage increase of postprandial plasma insulin induced by an increased carbohydrate intake; a given percentage increase in insulin response would result in a greater absolute increase in postprandial insulin concentration subjects with higher baseline insulin concentrations.

### 3.2.1 Hyperinsulinaemia and cardiovascular disease

In arguing that high postprandial insulin is deleterious, the Reaven group put much weight on the concept that the increase in insulin contributes to the hypertriglyceridaemia which is consistently associated with a high-carbohydrate diet, at least in their hands (Farquhar *et al.*, 1966; Coulston *et al.*, 1983; Liu *et al.*, 1983; Jeppesen *et al.*, 1997). The role of high insulin in causing hypertriglyceridaemia is based on correlations between insulin sensitivity, very low-density lipoprotein (VLDL) secretion rates and plasma triglyceride concentrations (Reaven *et al.*, 1967), and the fact that a high-carbohydrate diet increased hepatic VLDL secretion (Chen *et al.*, 1995). High-serum triglycerides, in turn, are related to increased risk for cardiovascular disease (Austin, 2000). However, hyperinsulinaemia actually reduces hepatic VLDL triglyceride and VLDL apolipoprotein B (apoB) production in normal subjects (Lewis *et al.*, 1993, 1995); this suggests that high postprandial insulin, *per se*, is not the cause of hypertriglyceridaemia. It is of interest that there was resistance to the VLDL apoB reducing effect of insulin in obese subjects (Lewis *et al.*, 1993). In addition, FFAs are a potent stimulus to hepatic VLDL production, even in the presence of insulin

(Lewis *et al.*, 1992). Thus, a more likely explanation of the mechanism by which a carbohydrate diets raise serum triglycerides is an increased incorporation of FFA into VLDL due to a combination of increased fatty acid synthesis from carbohydrate (Hudgins *et al.*, 2000) and reduced oxidation of FFA in liver (Mittendorfer and Sidossis, 2001). However, the effect of this on cardiovascular risk remains unresolved (Hellerstein, 2002).

High-plasma insulin has been suggested to be atherogenic via mechanisms other than raising triglycerides, namely by direct effects on vascular endothelium (Stout, 1990) and by promoting hypertension by stimulating sodium reabsorption in the kidney (DeFronzo and Ferrannini, 1991). However, if high-plasma insulin *per se* caused atherosclerosis, then treatments which raise plasma insulin would be expected to increase the risk of myocardial infarction. The UK Prospective Diabetes study showed that treatments which increase plasma insulin such as sulphonylureas or insulin itself had no deleterious effects. They improved glycaemic control and reduced overall diabetes complications (Anonymous, 1998b). There was a significant reduction in microvascular complications and a trend toward a reduction in myocardial infarction. This is not consistent with a deleterious effect of hyperinsulinaemia on cardiovascular disease risk. However, it could be argued that the reduction in cardiovascular disease was due to improved glycaemic control. Indeed, when considering the treatment of overweight patients metformin, sulphonlyureas and insulin improved glyaemic control to a similar extent; metformin significantly reduced myocardial infarction, whereas the effect of sulphonylureas and insulin was intermediate between that of the control- and metformin-treated groups (Anonymous, 1998b). Nevertheless, the differences were not statistically significant, so it is not possible to draw any conclusion except that sulphonylureas and insulin did not have any deleterious effect.

The Lyon diet–heart study (de Lorgeril *et al.*, 1999) and the more recent Indo-Mediterranean diet–heart study (Singh *et al.*, 2002) showed that a 'Mediterranean' diet reduced the incidence of CHD by over 50%. The beneficial effects of these diets are generally ascribed to the increased intake of ω–3 fatty acids, but it is noteworthy that both treatment diets were higher in carbohydrate than the control diets, with dietary carbohydrate intake increasing from 56% to 60% of energy in the Indo-Mediterranean diet–heart study.

### 3.2.2 Hyperinsulinaemia and type 2 diabetes

Type 2 diabetes involves abnormalities of insulin resistance and insulin secretion (DeFronzo, 1988), and a major question has been which is the primary defect. The so-called two-step model (Saad *et al.*, 1991) suggested that insulin resistance is the primary problem. According to this model, the first step is transition from normal to impaired glucose tolerance, for which insulin resistance due to obesity is the main determinant, and the second and later step is worsening from IGT to diabetes, in which β-cell dysfunction plays a critical role. If this model is correct, then high post-prandial insulin concentrations may contribute to the development of diabetes by exacerbating insulin resistance (Del Prato *et al.*, 1994), and it may be important, therefore, to categorize the insulinaemic index (II) of foods.

However, the primacy of insulin resistance in the aetiology of type 2 diabetes has been questioned recently (Ferrannini, 1998). Experimentally induced abnormalities in the pattern of insulin secretion can produce hyperglycaemia in lean normal subjects (Basu *et al.*, 1996). New evidence suggests that β-cell dysfunction and insulin resistance coexist in the prediabetic state, and exacerbate each other through multiple feedback mechanisms (Cavaghan *et al.*, 2000). Indeed, we found that reduced insulin secretion was a much more prominent defect than insulin resistance in about one third of a group of 34 subjects with IGT (Fig. 3.4). A recent longitudinal study in Pima Indians compared the results of 31 subjects with normal glucose tolerance at baseline and who remained normal throughout, with 17 individuals who had normal glucose tolerance initially, but developed IGT and type 2 diabetes during the course of follow-up (Weyer *et al.*, 1999). The people who eventually developed diabetes had impaired β-cell function at baseline (when they had normal glucose tolerance) compared to the 31 normal subjects who did not progress to diabetes. As the 17 subjects progressed from normal to impaired glucose tolerance, and then to diabetes,

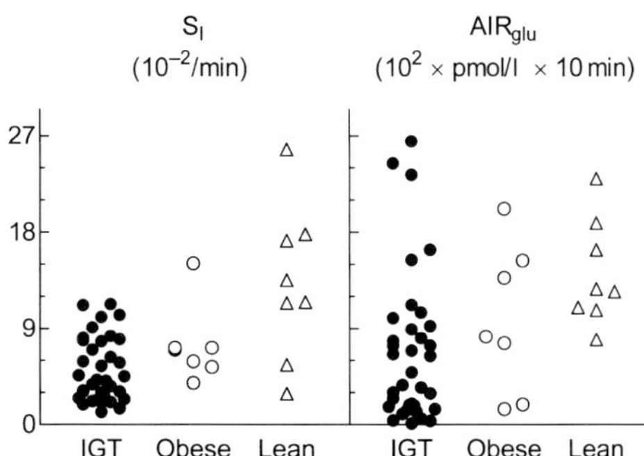


**Fig. 3.4.** Individual values of insulin sensitivity ($S_I$) and insulin secretion ($AIR_{glu}$) in eight lean controls (age, 33 ± 4 years; BMI, 22.9 ± 0.9 kg/m$^2$), seven obese controls (age, 59 ± 6 years; BMI, 29.3 ± 0.8 kg/m$^2$) and 35 subjects with impaired glucose tolerance (IGT; age, 57 ± 2 years; BMI, 29.9 ± 1.0 kg/m$^2$). Data from Fig. 3.2.

insulin sensitivity became somewhat worse, but reduced insulin secretion appeared to be a much more prominent feature both in the conversion from normal to impaired glucose tolerance and in the conversion from IGT to diabetes. The progression of diabetes itself also appears to be due to a continuous decline in insulin secretion rather than further deterioration of insulin sensitivity (Anonymous, 1995). These data would suggest, therefore, that far from being deleterious, in the presence of insulin resistance or diabetes, hyperinsulinaemia is desirable and necessary to maintain normal glucose tolerance.

### 3.2.3 Hyperinsulinaemia and obesity

One popular theory about the development of obesity is that a high level of plasma insulin causes obesity because insulin is the body's anabolic hormone which promotes fat storage. Therefore, if this were so, one would expect that insulin-resistant subjects with high-plasma insulin would gain more weight than insulin-sensitive subjects with low plasma insulin. In fact, however, most studies show that insulin-resistant adults gain less weight than insulin-sensitive adults (Swinburn *et al.*, 1991a; Valdez *et al.*, 1994; Hoag *et al.*, 1995; Schwartz *et al.*, 1995). In addition, treatment of diabetes with the insulin sensitizer, pioglitazone for 2 years was associated with reduced insulin resistance, reduced plasma insulin concentrations and improved glycaemic control compared to treatment with the insulin secretogog gliclazide; nevertheless, subjects on pioglitazone gained more weight than those on gliclazide (Tan *et al.*, 2005). These results would suggest that, far from promoting obesity, insulin resistance and hyperinsulinaemia may protect against excess weight gain. The role of hyperinsulinaemia in the development of obesity is discussed in more detail in Chapter 7.

## 3.3 Determinants of Postprandial Insulin Responses

Each of the three main macronutrients, protein, fat and carbohydrate, affect postprandial insulin. The effects of fat and protein are reviewed in more detail in Chapter 5.

### 3.3.1 Dietary protein and acute insulin responses

Protein is well known to stimulate insulin secretion when added to oral carbohydrate loads, but different proteins have different effects, at least in part due to differences in their absorption (Gannon *et al.*, 1988). This is likely due to a potentiating effect of amino acids on the β-cell. However, if β-cell function is reduced, the effects of protein on insulin secretion may become attenuated (Chapter 5, this volume). Thus, it may become difficult to make general conclusions about the effect of dietary protein on insulin responses. In addition, while studies on the effects of protein on postprandial insulin responses are of physiologic interest, I do not believe the study designs used have very much relevance to normal diets. Most studies compare the effects of a meal with 0 g protein to the one with 30–50 g of protein. However, diets do not contain no protein, and the question of whether it is beneficial to increase protein intake from 80 to 200 g per day is not addressed by a study which compares the effect of 0 g protein to 50 g protein. Indeed, there is some evidence to suggest that increasing the protein content of a test meal from 0 to 15 g doubles insulin secretion, but a further increase in protein intake from 15 to 50 g has no further effect (Spiller *et al.*, 1987).

### 3.3.2 Dietary fat and acute insulin responses

Fat acutely delays gastric emptying and thus reduces the rate of glucose absorption and the rise in postprandial insulin (Welch *et al.*, 1987). However, the amount of fat which must be added to 50 g carbohydrate to see these effects, 30–50 g, contributes 50–65% of total energy, which is much larger than is typically recommended. It is not clear what effect smaller amounts of fat have and there is fairly good evidence that fat has no effect on postprandial glucose or insulin responses in subjects with diabetes (Gannon *et al.*, 1993). In addition, the effect of fat on gastrointestinal motility in normal subjects may depend on external factors such as habitual fat intake (Morgan *et al.*, 1988a,b). Thus, it may be difficult to generalize about the effects of dietary fat on postprandial insulin responses.

### 3.3.3 Dietary carbohydrate and insulin responses

#### *3.3.3.1 Amount of carbohydrate*

As the amount of dietary carbohydrate consumed increases postprandial glucose and insulin responses increase (Wolever and Bolognesi, 1996a; Lee and Wolever, 1998) (Fig. 3.5). However, the dose–response relationship differs for plasma glucose and insulin. The IAUC for plasma glucose increases nearly linearly with the dose of carbohydrate up to about 50 g, but then flattens off. By contrast, the IAUC for plasma insulin continues to increase nearly linearly from 0 to 100 g carbohydrate. Similar dose–response relationships hold for sugars and starches (Lee and Wolever, 1998).

#### *3.3.3.2 Source of carbohydrate*

Plasma glucose and insulin responses are also affected by the source of dietary carbohydrate (Wolever and Bolognesi, 1996a; Lee and Wolever, 1998). Figure 3.6 shows the plasma glucose and insulin responses of 50 g carbohydrate portions of seven different starchy foods and sugars. Both the glucose and insulin responses vary over a fourfold range, and the correlation between the relative glucose and insulin responses was very close ($r$ = 0.94). Data from other laboratories suggest that glucose and insulin responses are linearly related to each other regardless of whether the portion sizes of the different foods tested contained equal amounts of carbohydrate (Brand Miller *et al.*, 1995) (Fig. 3.7) or equal amounts of energy (Holt *et al.*, 1996) (Fig. 3.8). The latter study involved portion sizes of foods tested containing 1000 kJ with the amount of carbohydrate contained in the test meals varying from 0 to about 50 g. This raises the question of the effect of varying both source and amount of carbohydrate on insulin and glucose responses.

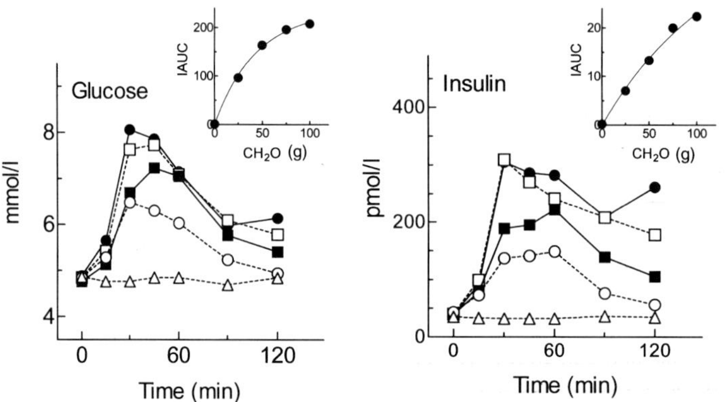


**Fig. 3.5.** Mean plasma glucose (left) and insulin (right) responses of eight normal subjects after consumption of 0 g (△), 25 g (○), 50 g (■), 75 g (□) or 100 g (●) available carbohydrate portions of white bread. Insets: relationship between available carbohydrate intake and incremental area under the plasma glucose and insulin response curves.

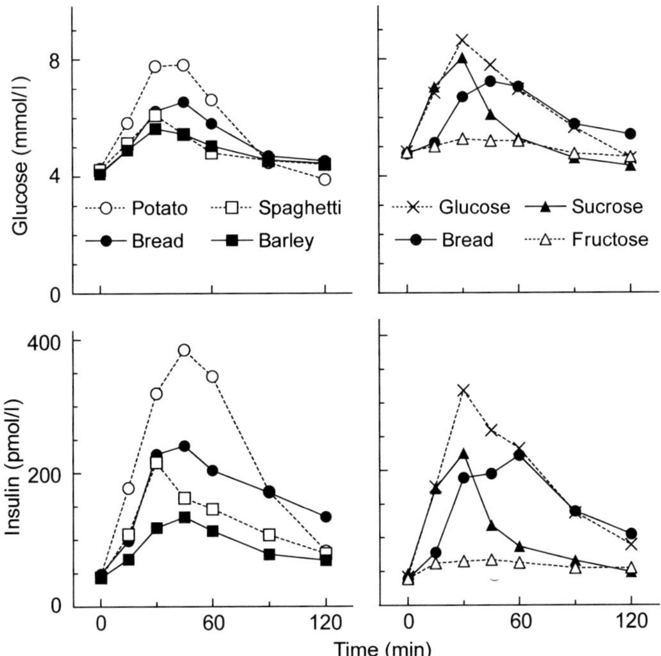


**Fig. 3.6.** Mean plasma glucose (top) and insulin (bottom) after consumption of 50 g available carbohydrate portions of starchy foods (instant mashed potato (○), white bread (●), spaghetti (□) and pearled barley (■)) (left) and pure sugars (glucose (×), sucrose (▲) and fructose (△)) compared to bread (●) (right).

### 3.3.3.3 *Varying both amount and source of carbohydrate*

Plasma glucose and insulin responses are influenced by both the source and the amount of carbohydrate, but the dose–response relationships are not the same for glucose and insulin. Over the range of carbohydrate intake from 0 to 50 g both glucose and insulin responses increase approximately linearly, but as carbohydrate intake

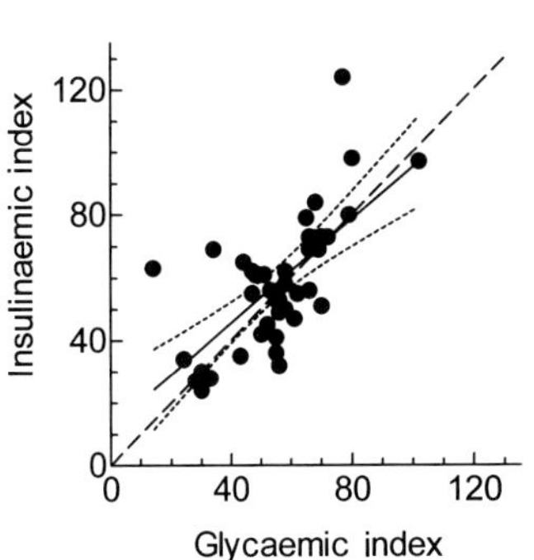


**Fig. 3.7.** Relationship between glycaemic index and insulinaemic index values of 50 g available carbohydrate portions of 41 different foods. Drawn from data given by Brand Miller *et al.* (1995). The dashed line is the line of identity and the solid line is the regression line with 95% confidence intervals shown as dotted lines ($r = 0.676$, $P < 0.001$).

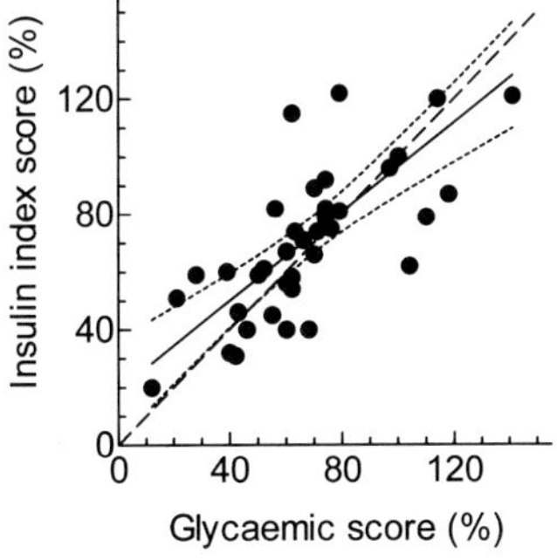


**Fig. 3.8.** Relationship between the mean blood glucose and insulin responses of 1000 kJ portions of 38 different foods. Drawn from data given by Holt *et al.* (1996). Glucose and insulin responses are expressed as a percentage of the response to bread. The dashed line is the line of identity and the solid line is the regression line with 95% confidence intervals shown as dotted lines ($r = 0.741$, $P < 0.001$).

increases from 50 to 100 g there is only a small increase in glucose response, but the insulin response nearly doubles (Fig. 3.5). Thus, with wide variation in both source and amount of carbohydrate, the relationship between glucose and insulin responses would not be expected to be linear. This is illustrated by data from my laboratory (Wolever and Bolognesi, 1996a; Lee and Wolever, 1998) showing the relationship between the relative glucose and insulin responses elicited by test meals containing carbohydrate foods varying in GI from 20 to 100 and varying in dose of available carbohydrate from 0 to 100 g (Fig. 3.9). The shape of the dose–response curve is exponential. This will be explored in more detail below. What I would like to point out here is that the responses for fructose, sucrose, glucose and starchy foods all fall along the same line.

### 3.3.4 Dietary sucrose and fructose and insulin responses

It has been suggested that fructose is insulinogenic (Reiser *et al.*, 1987); I disagree with this for several reasons. To determine the insulin responses that would be expected from starchy carbohydrate foods, plasma glucose and insulin responses elicited by various doses of different starchy carbohydrate foods were fit using non-linear regression analysis to derive equations expressing relative

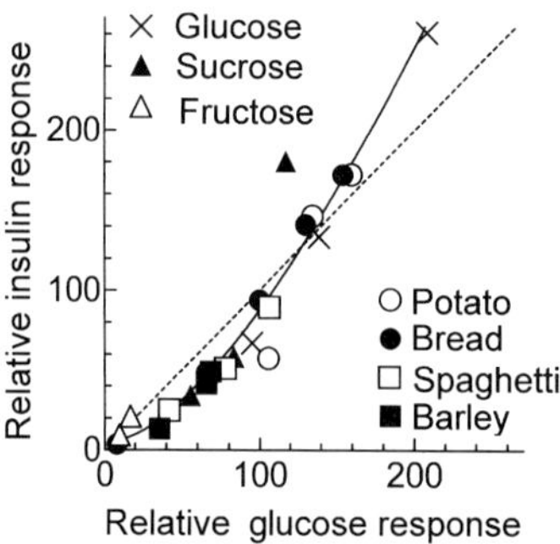


**Fig. 3.9.** Relationship between mean plasma glucose and insulin response areas under the curve elicited by 50 g available carbohydrate portions of various starchy foods (potato (○), bread (●), spaghetti (□), barley (■)) and pure sugars (glucose (×), sucrose (▲), fructose (△)). Data from Wolever and Bolognesi (1996a) and Lee and Wolever (1998).

glucose and insulin responses as a function of the amount of carbohydrate consumed and its GI (Wolever and Bolognesi, 1996a). By applying the same methods to the data from a study where different doses of glucose, sucrose and fructose and white bread were fed (Lee and Wolever, 1998), equations were derived which described the glucose and insulin responses elicited by the glucose-containing carbohydrates (glucose and bread) equally well as the fructose-containing carbohydrates (sucrose and fructose) (Fig. 3.10). This suggests that the plasma insulin response elicited by sugars is appropriate for their glycaemic responses.

Reiser *et al.* (1987) concluded that fructose was 'insulinogenic' based on the results of a study in which subjects consumed 1 g/kg glucose or 1 g/kg glucose followed 20 min later by 1.75 g/kg fructose. Fructose was considered insulinogenic because glucose- plus fructose-raised plasma insulin compared to glucose alone, but had no effect on plasma glucose (Fig. 3.11). However, the consumption of the second meal of fructose was not controlled for by the consumption of the same amount of another type of carbohydrate such as glucose. Thus, responses of unequal amounts of carbohydrate (1 vs 2.75 g/kg) were compared. The data shown in Fig. 3.10 suggest that the 'insulinogenic' effect of fructose occurred because of the difference in the shape of the dose–response curves for plasma glucose and insulin. Assuming the subjects weighed an average of 68 kg, they consumed either 68 g glucose (GI = 100) or 187 g carbohydrate consisting of 36% glucose (68 g) and 64% fructose (119 g). The GI of this test meal is $100 \times 0.36 + 24 \times 0.64 = 51$. Figure 3.12 shows how the plasma glucose and insulin responses of a meal with a GI of 100 and a meal with a GI of 51 would be expected to vary at different levels of carbohydrate intake based on the regression equations derived in Fig. 3.10. A meal with a GI of 51 and containing 187 g carbohydrate would be expected to produce a lower glucose and higher insulin response than a meal of 68 g carbohydrate with a GI of 100. The percentage differences in glucose and insulin predicted by this model are virtually identical to those actually observed.

Similarly, Crapo *et al.* (1976) concluded that sucrose elicited a similar glucose response but a 20% greater plasma insulin response than glucose. This is surprising because most other studies have

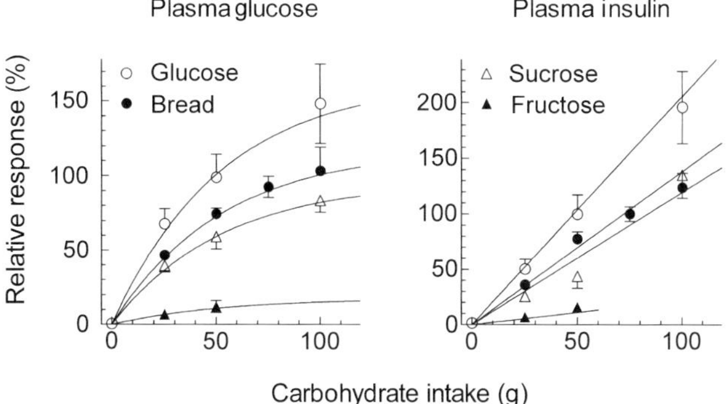


**Fig. 3.10.** Plasma glucose and insulin response areas under the curve, expressed as a percentage of that after a 50 g carbohydrate portion of glucose, of normal subjects after consumption of different amounts of glucose (○), white bread (●), sucrose (▲) and fructose (△) (Lee and Wolever, 1998). Values are means ± SEM. Lines represent non-linear regression equations derived for pooled data. The equation for glycaemic responses is: GR = 1.64 × GI × $(1–e^{-0.0191g})$ where GR = the incremental area under the glycaemic response curve expressed as a percentage of that for 50 g carbohydrate from glucose, GI = glycaemic index and g = grams of carbohydrate consumed. Similarly, the equation for insulinaemic responses is: IR = 51.3 × GI × $(1–e^{-0.000366g})$ where IR is the incremental area under the insulinaemic response curve expressed as a percentage of that after 50 g carbohydrate from glucose, GI = glycaemic index and g = grams of carbohydrate consumed.

shown that sucrose elicits lower glucose and insulin responses than does glucose (Foster-Powell *et al.*, 2002). However, the results of Crapo *et al.* (1976) are explained by the fact that the effects of 50 g glucose were compared with those of 100 g sucrose. Assuming that sucrose has a GI of 65, the model in Fig. 3.10 predicts that 100 g sucrose would elicit glucose and insulin responses 91% and 120% of those elicited by 50 g glucose; values almost identical to those actually obtained by Crapo *et al.* (1976).

Thus, fructose and sucrose, like all carbohydrate foods, stimulate a rise in blood insulin, but the rise is no more than that would be expected for the same amount of carbohydrate from another source with the same GI.

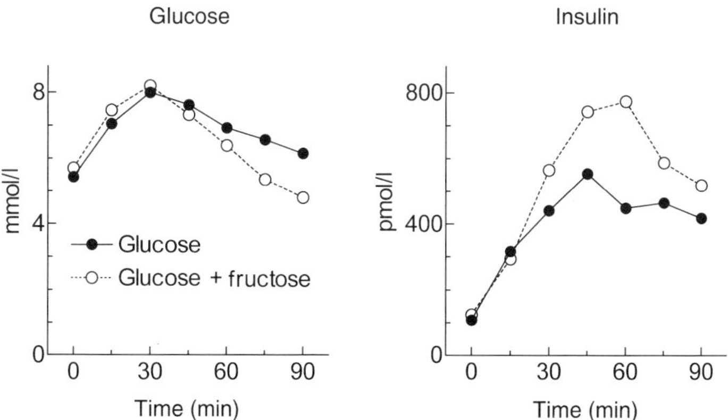


**Fig. 3.11.** Plasma glucose (left) and insulin (right) responses after normal subjects consumed either 1 g/kg glucose (●) or 1 g/kg glucose followed by 1.75 g/kg fructose 20 min later (○). Redrawn from Reiser *et al.* (1987).

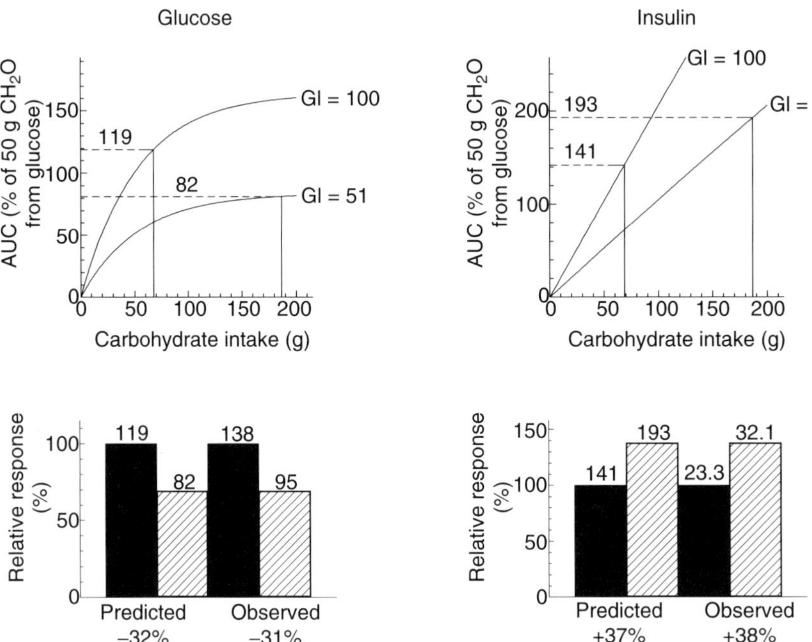


**Fig. 3.12.** Explanation of results shown in Fig. 3.11. Top: curves showing expected relative glycaemic (left) and insulinaemic (right) responses of test meals with a GI of 100 and 51 containing 0–200 g carbohydrate. The glucose test meal (GI = 100) containing 68 g carbohydrate has expected relative glucose and insulin responses of 119 and 141, respectively. The glucose plus fructose test meal (GI = 51) containing 187 g carbohydrate results in expected relative glucose and insulin responses of 82 and 193, respectively. Bottom: the glucose plus fructose meal is predicted to have a 32% lower glycaemic response and a 37% higher insulinaemic response than the glucose meal, values are very similar to the percentage differences between the observed incremental areas under the curves.

### 3.3.5 Relationship between glucose and insulin responses of foods

One of the major recent criticisms of the GI is that it does not allow prediction of the insulin responses of foods (Pi-Sunyer, 2002). This, certainly, has not been our experience, and data from our laboratory has generally indicated that the glucose and insulin responses elicited by relatively small number of starchy foods or sugars are very closely related to each other. For example, we fed test meals of bread, rice, spaghetti or barley to which cheese and tomato were added to a group of normal subjects (Wolever *et al.*, 1988b). The mean insulin response AUC values were almost perfectly proportional to the mean glucose AUC (Fig. 3.13), and both, in turn were closely related to the rates of digestion of the foods *in vitro*.

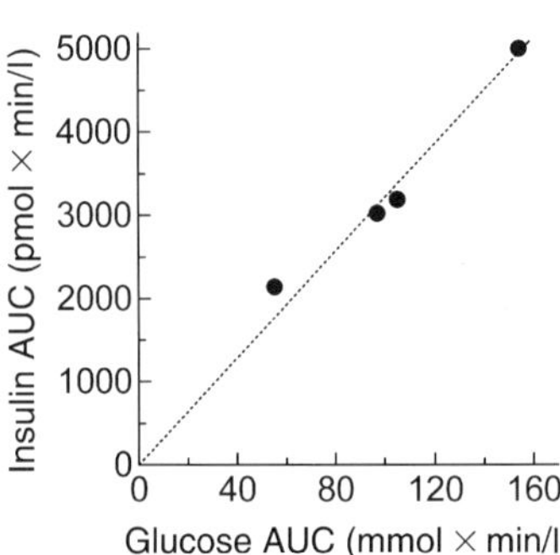


**Fig. 3.13.** Relationship between incremental areas under the plasma glucose and plasma insulin response curves (AUC) of normal subjects after consuming four starchy foods to which cheese and tomato had been added (Wolever *et al.*, 1988b). The dotted line is the line of identity.

Pi-Sunyer (2002) cites one of our studies (Lee and Wolever, 1998) as evidence that insulin responses increase more rapidly than glucose responses. In this study, we fed 25, 50 and 100 g of glucose, sucrose, fructose or bread on separate occasions to normal volunteers. The graph of insulin AUC on glucose AUC did have an exponential shape (Fig. 3.7), but this was due to the different doses of carbohydrate. Figure 3.14 shows the data from this study with each dose of carbohydrate represented by a different symbol. Within each dose of carbohydrate, the relationship between glucose AUC and insulin AUC for the different sources of carbohydrate is absolutely linear. But the slope of the line increases with the dose of carbohydrate from 0.057 for 25 g carbohydrate ($r$ = 0.97, $P$ = 0.02) to 0.078 for 50 g carbohydrate ($r$ = 0.98, $P$ = 0.02) to 0.094 for 100 g carbohydrate ($r$ = 0.91, $P$ = 0.09). The same is so for the comparison of four starchy foods, barley, spaghetti, bread and instant potato fed at portion sizes containing 25, 50 or 100 g carbohydrate (Fig. 3.15) (Wolever and Bolognesi, 1996a). Here the slope of the regression line of insulin AUC on glucose AUC at 25 g carbohydrate is 0.072 ($r$ = 0.93, $P$ = 0.07), at 50 g carbohydrate the slope is 0.14 ($r$ = 0.95, $P$ = 0.05), and at 100 g carbohydrate the slope is 0.19 ($r$ = 0.98, $P$ = 0.01). These analyses suggest that at a given dose of carbohydrate, the GI of a single starchy food or sugar predicts 83–97% of the insulin response. However, GI does not predict insulin responses as accurately when the amount of carbohydrate consumed varies.

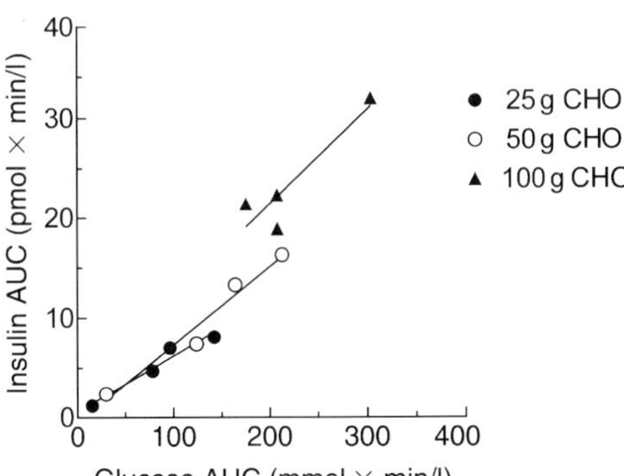


**Fig. 3.14.** Relationship between incremental areas under the plasma glucose insulin response curves (AUC) for portions of white bread, glucose, sucrose or fructose containing 25, 50 or 100 g available carbohydrate (CHO). Slopes of lines: 25 g CHO, 0.057 ($r$ = 0.97, $P$ = 0.02); 50 g CHO, 0.078 ($r$ = 0.98, $P$ = 0.02); 100 g CHO, 0.094 ($r$ = 0.91, $P$ = 0.09). Data from Lee and Wolever (1998).

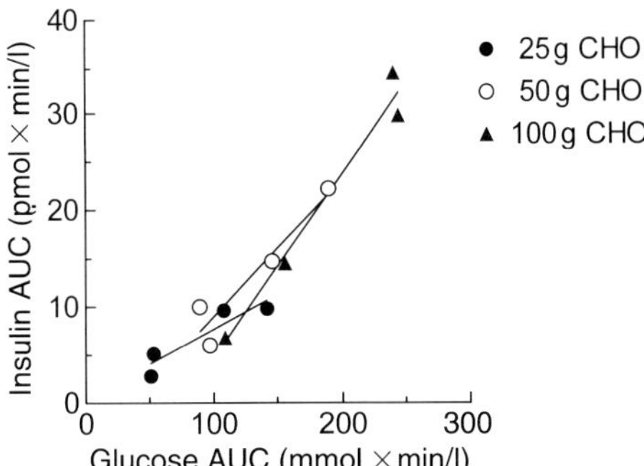


**Fig. 3.15.** Relationship between incremental areas under the plasma glucose insulin response curves (AUC) for portions of four starchy foods containing 25, 50 or 100 g available carbohydrate (CHO). Slopes of lines: 25 g CHO, 0.072 ($r$ = 0.93, $P$ = 0.07); 50 g CHO, 0.14 ($r$ = 0.95, $P$ = 0.05); 100 g CHO, 0.19 ($r$ = 0.98, $P$ = 0.01). Data from Wolever and Bolognesi (1996a).

Pi-Sunyer (2002) cited Holt *et al.* (1997) as evidence that the glucose responses of foods only predicted 23% of the variation of the insulin responses of the same foods. However, the value of 23% is cited incorrectly. In fact, Holt *et al.* (1997) report several different correlation coefficients between various different measures of glucose and insulin responses; none of them yield coefficients of determination ($r^2$) as low as 0.23 (or 23%). They report correlations of $r$ = 0.67 ($r^2$ = 0.45) for insulin AUC on glucose AUC, $r$ = 0.57 ($r^2$ = 0.32) for insulin peak concentration vs glucose peak; and $r$ = 0.70 ($r^2$ = 0.49) for insulin score (IS) on glucose score (GS). In an accompanying figure, they report the correlation between IS and GS to be 0.74 ($r^2$ = 0.55), which agrees with what I calculate from the data given in the paper (Fig. 3.8). I do not know how Dr Pi-Sunyer came up with a value of 23% from this paper. Since the 38 foods examined in this study were tested in groups of different subjects with somewhat different glucose and insulin responses after the reference food, white bread, the comparison of IS with GS is considered the best because IS and GS are measures of the insulin and glucose responses elicited by 1000 kJ of the test foods expressed as a percentage of that elicited by white bread in each subject group. Thus, I conclude that Holt *et al.* (1997) show that 55% of the variation in insulin responses elicited by 1000-kJ portions of foods is predicted by their glucose responses.

The 38 foods tested by Holt *et al.* (1997) varied in their contents of fat (0–20 g), protein (1–56 g) and carbohydrate (sum of starch and sugars, 0–59 g). In a multiple regression model, the amounts of fat, protein and carbohydrate only explained 15% of the variation in insulin response. GS alone explained 54.9% of the IS, and adding fat, protein and carbohydrate to the model with GS only explained 55.3% of the variation in IS. This suggests that, at least for these 38 foods, GS is a much better predictor of IS than the amounts of fat, protein or carbohydrate they contain. However, 45% of the variation in IS remains unexplained. If GS perfectly predicted IS, it would be expected that the ratio of IS:GS would be 1, and a ratio different from 1 indicates that the glucose response does not predict the insulin response. In this study, the IS:GS ratio tends to be high with low-carbohydrate, high-protein foods, but there is no relationship with fat intake (Fig. 3.16). This is consistent with an insulin-stimulating effect of protein.

Brand Miller's laboratory have also determined the glucose and insulin responses of 50 g available carbohydrate portions of 42 foods (Brand Miller *et al.*, 1995) and calculated GI and II values. They did not report the correlation between the mean GI and II values, but it can be calculated from the results given in the paper,

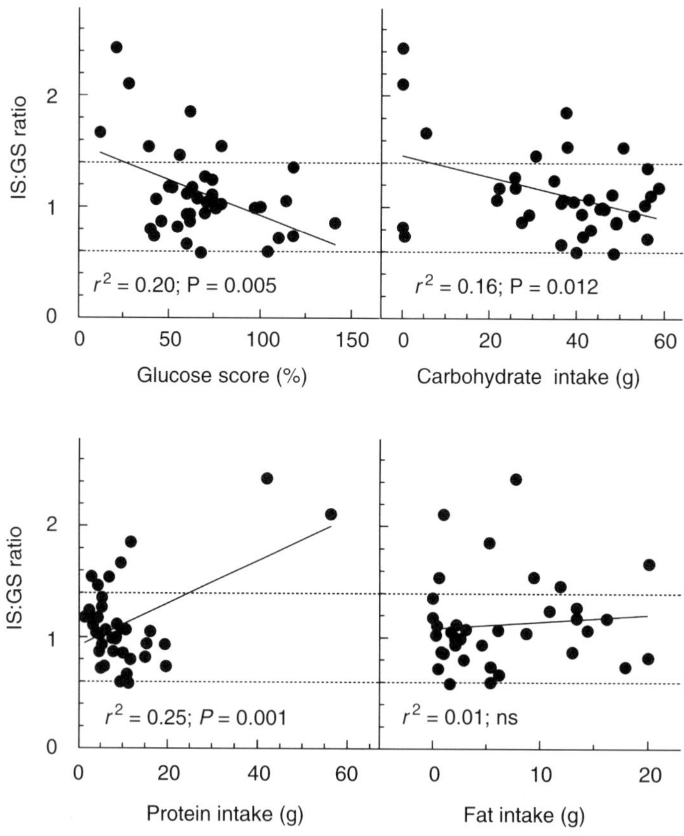


**Fig. 3.16.** Relationship between ratio of insulin score (IS) and glucose score (GS) and GS and carbohydrate, protein and fat intakes for portions of 38 foods containing 1000 kJ. IS and GS are the glucose and insulin response areas elicited by the food expressed as a percentage of that elicited by white bread. Data from Holt *et al.* (1997).

and I found it to be $r = 0.676$ ($r^2 = 0.46$, $P < 0.001$; Fig. 3.8). It has been suggested that milk is a particularly insulinogenic food, with II values for milk products being much greater than their corresponding GI values (Östman *et al.*, 2001; Hoyt *et al.*, 2005). In Fig. 3.17, the results for milk are shown as open circles and triangles superimposed on the results of Brand Miller *et al.* (1995, closed circles). Björck's group (Östman *et al.*, 2001) tested lactose, and found it to have a GI of about 70 and II of about 50, whereas milk and fermented milk products are the three open circles with GI values <30 and II values >80. Hoyt *et al.* (2005) found that the II of whole and skimmed milks were about 3.5 times those of their GI values. It is of interest that two of the apparent three outlying points from the Brand Miller *et al.* (1995) data (point a = aspartame-sweetened low-fat yogurt and point b = sugar-sweetened chocolate milk) are milk products having considerably higher II values than GI values. However, two other milk products (point c = aspartame-sweetened chocolate milk and point d = sugar-sweetened low-fat yogurt) have similar II and GI values. If the GI and II values for the four milk products are excluded from the regression analysis, the resulting coefficient of determination is 0.600. In other words, GI predicts 60% of the variation II responses of foods other than milk products.

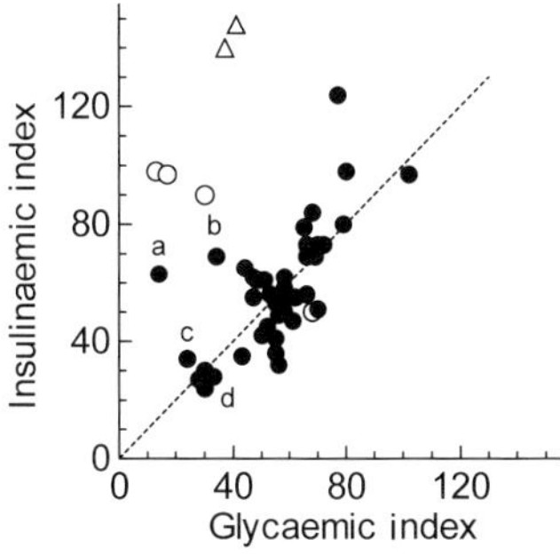


**Fig. 3.17.** Relationship between glycaemic index and insulinaemic index values of 50 g available carbohydrate portions of 41 different foods (Brand Miller *et al.*, 1995; closed circles), lactose and three milk products (Östman *et al.*, 2001; open circles), and whole and skimmed milk (Hoyt *et al.*, 2005; open triangles). a = aspartame-sweetened low-fat yogurt; b = sugar-sweetened chocolate milk; c = aspartame-sweetened chocolate milk; d = sugar-sweetened low-fat yogurt.

Presumably, the reason why milk elicits a high-insulin response is due to its content of protein. However, whether there is anything special about the insulinogenic effect milk protein compared to other sources is difficult to tell. Björck's group went on, in a further study, to determine the effect of adding milk to bread and spaghetti (Liljeberg-Elmstal and Björk 2001). When added to bread, 200 and 400 ml milk increased the insulin AUC from 13.5 to 16.7 and 22.3 (increased by 24% and 65%, respectively). When added to spaghetti, milk increased the insulin response from 3.5 to 11.6 and 10.9 (increased by 231% and 211%, respectively). The increase in insulin when milk was added to bread is similar to that found for other protein sources in other studies, but the effect with spaghetti is larger (Fig. 5.9, study 'f').

A final study relevant to this discussion was conducted by Hertzler and Kim (2003) who measured the glucose and insulin responses of 20 normal subjects after 60 g portions of three different energy bars or chicken. The best correlation between glucose and insulin response of the 20 subjects was for the high-carbohydrate bar (39 g carbohydrate, 9 g protein and 2 g fat; $r = 0.722$). However, there was no significant correlation for the medium carbohydrate bar (26 g carbohydrate, 17 g protein and 7 g fat; $r = 0.044$). Although there were significant correlations between glucose and insulin responses after the low-carbohydrate bar (3 g carbohydrate, 20 g protein, 10 g fat; $r = 0.596$) and chicken (0 g carbohydrate, 18 g protein, 5 g fat; $r = 0.659$), each of these two correlations was driven by single outlying point, the removal of which would reduce the correlation coefficients to near 0.

The discussion in this section therefore suggests that when carbohydrate is the predominant energy source in a test meal, there is a good correlation between glucose and insulin responses. However, if high amounts of protein and fat are present in test meals the relationship between glucose and insulin responses is less predictable.

## 3.4 Plasma Insulin Responses of Mixed Meals and Whole Diets

As we have seen above, the glucose responses of single sugars or starchy carbohydrate foods are good predictors of their insulin responses.

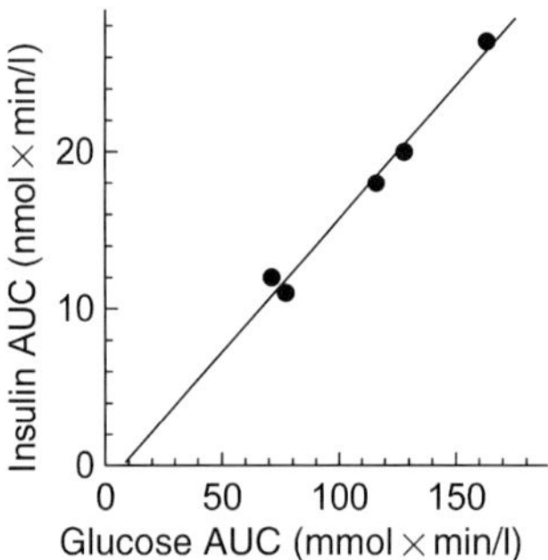


**Fig. 3.18.** Relationship between mean incremental areas under the plasma glucose and insulin response curves (AUC) elicited by five different meals varying in energy, protein, fat, carbohydrate and glycaemic index (Wolever and Bolognesi, 1996b; $r = 0.992$, $P = 0.0009$). The solid line is the regression line ($y$-intercept not significantly different from 0).

However, the predictability is reduced when one includes carbohydrate foods containing higher amounts of fat and protein such as dairy products, baked goods and energy bars. Thus, the ability of GI to predict insulin responses may not apply in mixed meals containing variable amounts of fat and protein. To test this, we designed five test meals which varied to a considerable extent in energy (1650–2550 kJ), fat (8–24 g), protein (12–25 g), carbohydrate (38–104 g) and GI (43–99) but still represented 'normal' meals made up of normal foods (Wolever and Bolognesi, 1996b). In this study, the mean AUC under the glucose curve accounted for 98% of the variation in the mean AUC under the insulin curve (Fig. 3.18). Longer-term studies have shown that a low-GI diet reduces urinary c-peptide excretion, a marker of insulin secretion, in both normal (Jenkins *et al.*, 1987a) and diabetic subjects (Wolever *et al.*, 1992b), and reduces mean day-long plasma insulin in diabetic subjects (Järvi *et al.*, 1999). In each case, the percentage reduction in insulin was almost exactly the same as the percentage reduction in diet GI (Table 3.2).

This does not mean to say that the insulin responses of meals with more extreme variations in protein and fat are able to be predicted from their glucose responses. Indeed, in Chapter 5, we will see that the effect of adding protein or fat to carbohydrate on glucose and insulin responses is highly variable from study to study, and may depend not only on the nature of the fat and protein added, but also the carbohydrate food to which it is added, the method of incorporating the protein and fat and the type of subject studied.

## 3.5 Relevance of GI to Insulin Sensitivity and Related Outcomes

There is evidence that reducing diet GI reduces the area under the plasma insulin response curve after 75 g oral glucose in subjects with CHD (Frost *et al.*, 1996), and improves insulin sensitivity in subjects with diabetes (Järvi *et al.*, 1999) or CHD (Frost *et al.*, 1998). Prospective epidemiologic studies show that a low-diet GI is associated with a reduced risk of developing diabetes in men (Salmerón *et al.*, 1997a) and women (Salmerón *et al.*, 1997b). Most recently, it was demonstrated that there was an inverse relationship between diet GI and serum high-density lipoprotein (HDL) cholesterol (Frost *et al.*, 1999). The associations between diet GI and both diabetes risk and serum HDL could be explained by improved insulin sensitivity. Thus, there is increasing

**Table 3.2.** Relationship between change in diet glycaemic index and change in insulin secretion.

| | Diet glycaemic index | | | Insulin secretion | | |
|---|---|---|---|---|---|---|
| | High GI | Low GI | Change | Measure[a] | Change | Reference |
| Normal ($n = 6$) | 104 | 63 | −39% | Day-time UC-P/Cr | −39%[b] | Jenkins *et al.* (1987a) |
| Diabetic ($n = 15$) | 87 | 60 | −31% | Day-time UC-P/Cr | −30%[c] | Wolever *et al.* (1992b) |
| Diabetic ($n = 20$) | 83 | 57 | −31% | Plasma insulin AUC | −27%[b] | Järvi *et al.* (1999) |

[a]Day-time UC-P/Cr = urinary c-peptide:creatinine ratio from 7 am to 11 pm. Plasma insulin AUC = incremental area under the plasma insulin curve from 7 am to 7 pm.
Significance of differences: [b]$P < 0.01$; [c]$P < 0.02$.

evidence that the GI of dietary carbohydrate affects insulin sensitivity and features of the insulin resistance syndrome. It is not known whether the mechanism for these effects is related to reductions in acute glucose and insulin responses, alterations in gut hormones (Collier *et al.*, 1984; Elliott *et al.*, 1993), increased colonic fermentation (Royall *et al.*, 1990) or some other effect. However, because of the relationship between the glycaemic and insulinaemic responses to foods, it seems unlikely that knowledge of the II will provide significantly better information than the GI about the effect of different carbohydrate foods on insulin sensitivity.

## 3.6 Variation of Plasma Glucose and Insulin

Plasma glucose and insulin concentrations vary from day to day within the same subject. For normal subjects and those with IGT and diabetes, the within-subject variation of concentrations of fasting and postprandial insulin is two to three times greater than the variation of plasma glucose measured in the same sample (Wolever *et al.*, 1998a). One reason why plasma insulin varies to a greater extent than plasma glucose is that insulin is secreted in a pulsatile fashion, resulting in minute-to-minute variation in plasma glucose and insulin concentrations (Lang *et al.*, 1981; Matthews *et al.*, 1983). The magnitude of the insulin fluctuations is two to three times greater than that for glucose (Abdallah *et al.*, 1997). In addition, analytic variation for plasma insulin is two to three times greater than that for plasma glucose (Wolever *et al.*, 1998a).

The magnitude of variation and the number of subjects studied determine the difference in response between foods which can be detected in a study (i.e. statistical power); for a given number of subjects, the larger the variation, the larger the minimum statistically significant difference which can be detected. Some studies comparing the plasma glucose and insulin responses of different foods or meals have detected larger and more statistically significant differences in insulin than glucose (Bolton *et al.*, 1981; Coulston *et al.*, 1981). Results like these suggest the need to measure both glucose and insulin responses. However, in most studies, differences in insulin are accompanied by differences in glucose. Because of greater variation of plasma insulin than glucose, we uniformly find that differences in glycaemic response are more statistically significant than differences in plasma insulin when comparing test meals consisting of sugars (Lee and Wolever, 1998), starchy foods (Wolever and Bolognesi, 1996a) and mixed test meals (Wolever *et al.*, 1988b; Wolever and Bolognesi, 1996b), regardless of whether the tests are done in lean or obese normal subjects, or in those with IGT or diabetes (Wolever *et al.*, 1998b). Figure 3.19 shows the sources of variation of blood and plasma glucose and plasma insulin response areas under the curve after different subjects took different doses of different foods. The proportion of variation of plasma insulin response arising from differences between foods is about half that for capillary glucose, with the proportion from random error being about the same. Thus, for comparisons between foods with relatively small differences, the difference in glucose response is more likely to be statistically significant than the difference in insulin response.

## 3.7 Cost of Measuring Glucose and Insulin

It is more difficult and costly to measure insulin than glucose responses. Glucose can be measured in whole blood very accurately from a two-drop capillary blood sample, which can be obtained

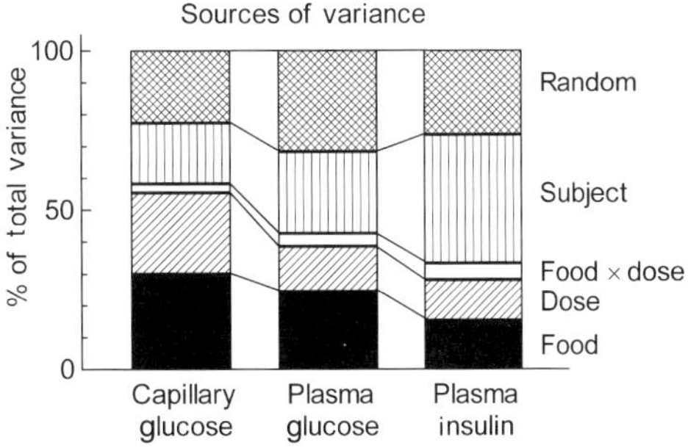


**Fig. 3.19.** Partitioning of variance from repeated measures analysis of variance of incremental areas under the capillary blood glucose, plasma glucose and plasma insulin response curves of normal subjects consuming 25, 50 or 100 g carbohydrate from barley, spaghetti, bread or instant potato (Wolever and Bolognesi, 1996a).

from a finger-prick by an unassisted, trained subject. We find measurement of glucose in whole capillary blood to be more reproducible than measurement of glucose in simultaneously obtained venous plasma (Fig. 3.19). Routine insulin measurement of insulin at the Core Diabetes Laboratory at my institution requires 1 ml of serum or plasma, which has to be separated from the blood by centrifugation. Blood for this purpose is normally obtained by venepuncture which requires a specially trained technician or nurse. Capillary blood can be used but the volume of blood able to be obtained is limited. Insulin can be measured in as little as 50–100 μl of serum but the small volume requires special handling and reduces the accuracy because of the smaller volumes of sample and reagent used. To obtain 100 μl of serum requires about 250 μl of blood which is about five whole drops, or two times more than required for glucose, which may require multiple finger-sticks to obtain. The cost of the reagents for measuring insulin is also more than those for glucose.

## 3.8 Clinical Utility of II

For valid clinical utility, the GI and II of foods should be the same in different individuals regardless of their glucose tolerance status. This has proven to be true for the GI, which is similar in normal and diabetic individuals (Foster-Powell and Brand Miller, 1995) and in subjects with type 1 and type 2 diabetes (Wolever *et al.*, 1987). There are no studies where the formally derived II values of the same foods have been compared in different subjects. However, we determined the glucose and insulin responses of a standardized starchy test meal containing 50 g glycaemic carbohydrate, relative to those of 75 g oral glucose in lean and obese normal subjects and subjects with IGT and diabetes. The RGR did not differ in the different groups (41–54%) but there were significant differences in relative insulinaemic responses, with type 2 diabetics having a higher value, 84 ± 7%, than both IGT subjects, 69 ± 5%, and obese normal subjects, 50 ± 5% ($P = 0.0003$) (Wolever *et al.*, 1998b).

More recently, we compared the glucose and insulin responses of low- and high-fibre breakfast cereals in 35 men with fasting plasma glucose <7.0 mmol/l and normal fasting plasma insulin (≤40 pmol/l; controls) and 42 men with fasting glucose <7.0 mmol/l and high fasting insulin (>40 pmol/l; hyper[I]) (Wolever *et al.*, 2004). The overall mean glycaemic response elicited by the high-fibre cereal was 12% ($P = 0.036$) less than that elicited by the low-fibre cereal, with the magnitude of the reductions being equivalent in control (13 ± 8%) and hyper[I] (11 ± 9%) subjects. Thus there was no correlation between fasting insulin and RGR (Fig. 3.20). However, the

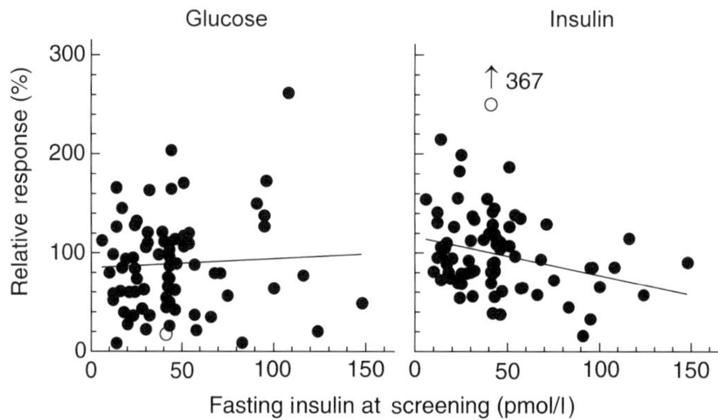


**Fig. 3.20.** Areas under the glucose (left) and insulin (right) response curves after consuming a high-fibre cereal expressed as a percentage of those after a low-fibre cereal in 77 non-diabetic men, plotted against fasting plasma insulin at screening. Lines are regression lines. The open circle represents an outlying value (5.4 × SD from the mean). Relative glucose response vs fasting insulin, $r = 0.056$ (ns). Relative insulin response vs fasting insulin; excluding outlier, $r = -0.297$ ($P = 0.009$); including outlier, $r = -0.240$ ($P = 0.036$). Redrawn from Wolever *et al.* (2004).

postprandial insulin response after the high-fibre cereal, expressed as a percentage of that after the low-fibre cereal, was significantly lower in hyper[I] than control subjects ($90 \pm 6\%$ vs $109 \pm 7\%$, $P = 0.026$) and there was a significant correlation between fasting insulin and relative insulin response (Fig. 3.20). These data support the concept and clinical utility of the GI, but suggest that the II is less clinically useful because it varies in different groups of subjects.

## 3.9 Conclusions

The blood glucose responses elicited by different carbohydrate foods are classified using the GI. It has been suggested that the GI on its own is insufficient and that a measure of the II is also needed. In this chapter, arguments are presented against this view. A focus on reducing plasma insulin would be important if one believes that hyperinsulinaemia *per se* is involved in the pathogenesis of dyslipidaemia, atherosclerosis, hypertension, obesity and cancer. However, an alternate interpretation is that hyperinsulinaemia is a normal physiologic response to insulin resistance and is desirable to prevent the development of diabetes. The insulinaemic responses elicited by different foods were closely related to their glycaemic responses. This was equally so for sugars and starches, and surprisingly, was true whether the portion sizes of different foods tested contained equal amounts of carbohydrate or equal amounts of energy. Relative insulinaemic responses were accurately predicted from the amount of carbohydrate and its GI, even for mixed meals and whole diets. Compared to measuring blood glucose, measurement of plasma insulin is more difficult, more expensive and less reliable because of greater within-subject variation. Finally, the GI values of foods were the same regardless of the glucose tolerance status of the subject tested, but there is evidence that the II values obtained differ in different subjects making the II less universally valid than the GI. Measurement of plasma insulin is important for research purposes. However, for routine evaluation of high-carbohydrate foods, measurement of insulin may not be necessary or even valid.

## Notes

### Definition of metabolic syndrome

A new consensus definition of the metabolic syndrome was published recently (International Diabetes Federation, 2005) which requires the presence of central obesity (defined as waist circumference $\geq 94$ cm for Europid men and $\geq 80$ cm for Europid women with ethnicity-specific values for other groups) plus any two of the following: raised triglycerides ($>1.7$ mmol/l or specific treatment for this lipid abnormality), low HDL cholesterol ($<0.9$ mmol/l in men or $<1.1$ mmol/l in women, or specific trement for this lipid abnormality), raised blood pressure ($\geq 130/85$ mm Hg or treatment for hypertension) or raised fasting glucose ($\geq 5.6$ mmol/l or previously diagnosed diabetes mellitus).

### Indo-Mediterranean diet–heart study

Section 3.2.1 discusses the impact of a high carbohydrate diet on risk for cardiovascular disease based on the results of the Indo-mediterranean diet–heart study. Serious concerns about the reliability of the data from this study been raised (Horton, 2005) which cast doubt about its reliability. Nevertheless, what is said about the effect of a high carbohydrate diet on cardiovascular risk is illustrated equally well by the results of the Lyon diet–heart study (also referred to in section 3.2.1.) about which no doubts exist.

# 4

# Mechanisms by which Different Carbohydrates Elicit Different Glycaemic Responses

Carbohydrates include a wide range of different compounds which elicit different glycaemic responses. There are four basic mechanisms by which different dietary carbohydrates may influence blood glucose: the nature of the monosaccharides absorbed, the amount of carbohydrate which is absorbed, the amount of carbohydrate which is metabolized and the rate of absorption.

## 4.1 The Monosaccharides Absorbed

Carbohydrates in the diet exist as monosaccharides, disaccharides, oligosaccharides and polysaccharides. However, in the normal human intestine, only monosaccharides can be absorbed (Wright *et al.*, 2003). Thus, before di-, oligo- or polysaccharides can raise blood glucose they must be broken down to their component monosaccharides via the process of digestion, which has been reviewed elsewhere (Asp, 1995; Cummings and Englyst, 1995). The majority of digestible carbohydrates commonly consumed in the diet consist of the disaccharides sucrose (glucose plus fructose) and lactose (glucose plus galactose) and the polysaccharide starch (a polymer of glucose). In Western diets, starch makes up about 40–60% of the available carbohydrate consumed, with most of the remainder consisting of mono- or disaccharides of which glucose (either as a monosaccharide or part of a disaccharide) comprises 40–60%. Thus, a large majority (70–85%) of dietary available carbohydrate is absorbed as glucose and the rest is primarily a mixture of fructose and galactose. The sugar alcohols, or polyols, are present in small amounts in some fruits (e.g. apples and pears) (Dikeman *et al.*, 2004), but are becoming more common in the food supply to replace sucrose in 'sugar-free' confectionary and other products.

### 4.1.1 Glucose, fructose and galactose

Glucose has a high GI (GI = 100), fructose a low GI (GI = 23) and sucrose, comprised of glucose and fructose, has a GI almost exactly the average of those for glucose and fructose (GI = 65) (Foster-Powell *et al.*, 2002). Lactose, a disaccharide of glucose and galactose, has a GI of 46. This value could be less than that of sucrose either because lactose is less well absorbed than sucrose or because galactose elicits a lower glycaemic response than fructose. The latter is more likely. In newborn infants, IV infusion of galactose raised blood glucose about 20% as much as an equal amount of glucose (Pribylová and Kozlová, 1979), and more than an equal amount of intravenous fructose (Pribylová *et al.*, 1979). However, in adult men, intravenous galactose raised blood glucose only about 5% as much as intravenous glucose (Ganda *et al.*, 1979). In normal subjects, consumption of 50 g galactose elicited virtually no rise in plasma glucose (Gannon *et al.*, 2001b).

Major dietary sources of naturally occurring sugars are fruits and dairy products, all of which have relatively low GI values. Dairy products (whose carbohydrate is lactose), such as milk and yogurt, have GI values similar to lactose itself (Foster-Powell and Brand Miller, 1995; Foster-Powell *et al.*, 2002). Fruits contain mixtures of fructose, sucrose and glucose in varying proportions. The GI of fruits and fruit juices are generally with the range of

30–60 and tend to be lower than the GI values of most starchy foods. The sugars content of fruits predicts, to some extent, their GI values (Wolever *et al.*, 1993). Ironically, sucrose-sweetened breakfast cereals have lower GI values than unsweetened ones because sucrose has a lower GI than that of the highly processed starch it replaces (Brand Miller and Lobbesoo, 1994).

Fructose does not raise blood glucose appreciably because it is converted to glucose in the liver, and only a small proportion of this glucose is released into the circulation (Delarue *et al.*, 1993; Nuttall *et al.*, 2000). Sucrose has a low GI because only half of the molecule is glucose and the other half is fructose. So sugars with a low GI are considered to have a low GI primarily because they contain less glucose than starch rather than because they are slowly absorbed. Indeed, blood glucose responses elicited by pure sugars and fruits suggest rapid absorption because the blood glucose concentration rises more quickly and falls more rapidly than after bread (Wolever *et al.*, 1993; Lee and Wolever, 1998).

Further evidence that sugars are rapidly absorbed is provided by recent studies indicating that the switch from oxidation of fat to carbohydrate after an overnight fast occurs more rapidly after a high-sucrose meal than a high-starch meal, with the increase in carbohydrate oxidation being sustained for longer after the starch than the sucrose meal (Daly *et al.*, 2000). This study showed that over 6 h, total carbohydrate oxidation was higher after the sugar than the starch meal. In addition, the oxidation of fructose in the sucrose meal was much faster than the oxidation of the glucose moiety and it appeared that the fructose in sugar delayed the oxidation of glucose. Thus, it would be difficult from this study to conclude that the carbohydrate energy in a meal of sucrose runs out more quickly than that after starch – but the starch sources in this study were bread and maize starch (in custard), both of which have a high GI.

### 4.1.2 Polyols

Polyols, or sugar alcohols, are saccharide derivatives in which a ketone or aldehyde group is replaced by a hydroxyl group (Zumbé *et al.*, 2001). They are classified according to the number of saccharide units in the molecule. Common monosaccharide sugar alcohols are sorbitol, mannitol and xylitol, derived from glucose, mannose and xylose, respectively. They are naturally present in some fruits and vegetables, but are produced commercially by hydrogenation of the sugars from which they are derived. Common disaccharide polyols include maltitol (derived from maltose), lactitol (derived from lactose) and isomalt (also known as palatinit), a 1:1 mixture of α-D-glucopyranosyl-[1–6]-D-sorbitol and α-D-glucopyranosyl-[1–6]-D-mannitol. Oligo- and polysaccharide sugar alcohols are derived from hydrogenation of starch hydrolysates. Sugar alcohols are only partly digested and/or absorbed from the human small intestine. The percentage absorption derived from some studies is about 0% for lactitol, 50–60% for isomalt, 50–75% for maltitol, 50% for mannitol, 50–80% for sorbitol and 50% for xylitol (Patil *et al.*, 1987; Würsch *et al.*, 1989; Beaugerie *et al.*, 1990; Langkilde *et al.*, 1994). Polyols are also only partly metabolized and the percentage of the ingested dose which is excreted in the urine ranging from nearly 0% for lactitol (which is not absorbed) to 90% for erythritol (Livesey, 1992, 2003). In deriving energy values for sugar alcohols, Livesey (1992, 2003) has estimated the fractional small intestinal absorption of energy from sugar alcohols and fractional availability of the proportion absorbed (Table 4.1). These values have been used to calculate the proportion of 'available carbohydrate' from sugar alcohols which I suggest should be used for the purpose of determining GI values of the sugar alcohols or foods containing them.

Sorbitol, lactitol and xylitol elicited little or no rise in plasma glucose after either oral or IV administration in either normal (Macdonald *et al.*, 1978; Akgün and Ertel, 1980; de Kalbermatten *et al.*, 1980; Natah *et al.*, 1997) or diabetic subjects (Akgün and Ertel, 1980; Hassinger *et al.*, 1981). However, maltitol elicits a moderate glycaemic response, about 33% of that seen after administration of an equal amount of glucose (Secchi *et al.*, 1986) and 64% of that after an equal amount of sucrose (Felber *et al.*, 1987). Livesey (2003) provides a comprehensive review of over 50 articles of which the glycaemic responses of various polyols were determined. In these studies, the glycaemic responses of sugar alcohols were compared with an equal amount of glucose or sucrose. Livesey (2003) provides a table of the 'GI' values of polyols, but the values are not adjusted for the fact that polyols are not completely available. To be

**Table 4.1.** Relative glycaemic response (RGR) and estimated 'available carbohydrate' content of various sugar alcohols.

| Sugar alcohol | RGR[a] | Absorbed (g/100 g) | Excreted in urine (g/100 g) | Estimated available carbohydrate (g/100 g) |
|---|---|---|---|---|
| Erythritol | 0 | 90 | 10 | 0 |
| Xylitol | 13 | 50 | <2 | 50 |
| Mannitol | 0 | 25 | 25 | 0 |
| Sorbitol | 9 | 25 | <2 | 25 |
| Lactitol | 6 | 2 | <2 | 0 |
| Isomalt | 9 | 10 | <2 | 10 |
| Maltitol | 35 | 40 | <2 | 40 |
| Maltitol syrup[b] | 51 | 50 | <2 | 50 |
| Maltitol syrup[c] | 36 | 40 | – | 40 |
| Polyglycitol | 39 | 40 | <2 | 40 |

Data from Livesey (1992, 2003).
[a]Mean AUC after sugar alcohol expressed as % of mean AUC after same amount of glucose.
[b]Regular, intermediate and high-maltitol syrups.
[c]High polymer maltitol syrup.

consistent with GI methodology, these values should be adjusting for the amount of available carbohydrate they contain. This is complex since glycaemic responses do not increase linearly with the amount of carbohydrate (Fig. 4.1). This will be discussed in Section 4.2.2.4.

## 4.2 The Amount of Carbohydrate Metabolized

The amount of carbohydrate metabolized can be influenced by one or more of the following: the amount consumed, the proportion of the amount consumed which is absorbed or the proportion of the amount absorbed which is metabolized.

### 4.2.1 The amount of carbohydrate consumed

There have been a number of attempts to study the dose–response effect of carbohydrate, i.e. the effect of consuming different amounts of carbohydrate on glycaemic responses (Staub, 1921; Castro *et al.*, 1970; Sisk *et al.*, 1970; Christensen *et al.*, 1972; Toeller and Knußmann, 1973; de Nobel and van't Laar, 1978; Jenkins *et al.*, 1981a; Gannon

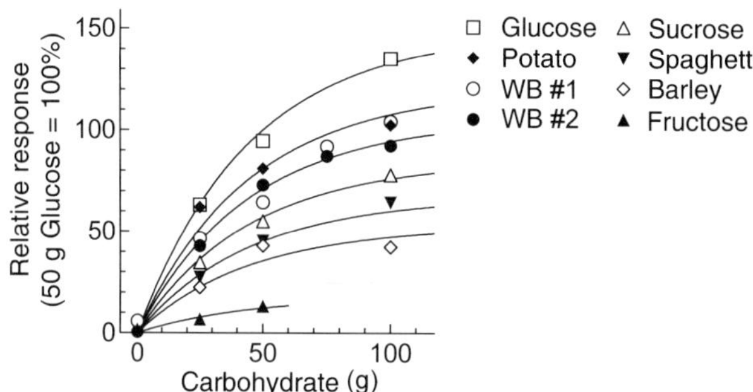


**Fig. 4.1.** Incremental area under the blood glucose curves in normal subjects after consuming various amounts of seven different carbohydrate foods, expressed as a percentage of the response elicited by 50 g glucose. Values are means. Lines represent the equation RR = 1.49 × GI × $(1 - e^{-0.0222g})$, where RR = relative response, GI = glycaemic index (glucose = 100) and g = grams of available carbohydrate consumed. The model explains 96% of the variation in observed mean glycaemic responses. Data from Wolever and Bolognesi (1996a) and Lee and Wolever (1998).

*et al.*, 1989; van Amelsvoort *et al.*, 1989; Rasmussen, 1993a,b). All of these studies clearly show that the glycaemic responses increase as the amount of carbohydrate consumed increases. However, the question arises as to the shape of the dose–response curve. This is an important question, especially with the introduction of the concepts such as the glycaemic load (GL) (Salmerón *et al.*, 1997a,b) and glycaemic glucose equivalents (GGE) (Monro, 2002) which attempt to model the actual glycaemic potency of foods taking into account both their GI and the amount of carbohydrate they contain. These calculations assume that glycaemic responses are directly proportional to the amount of carbohydrate consumed. However, this has not been proven and most existing studies on the effect of consuming different doses of carbohydrate suffer from one or more drawbacks, such as a small number of different doses or a narrow range of carbohydrate intakes, which limits their ability to be used to determine the shape of the dose–response curve. In addition, the studies are difficult to compare, at least directly, because of differences in the methods used to analyse the data, such as methods of calculating AUC, time over which glucose is measured, etc. As discussed in Chapter 2, these factors can have a major effect on the interpretation of the results obtained. It is quite possible that applying different methods of data analysis to the same set of data might yield quite different conclusions as to the shape of the dose–response curve. We did two studies which attempted to determine how GI and the grams of carbohydrate consumed influenced blood glucose and insulin responses; one study looked at the effect of different doses of four different starchy foods (instant potato, bread, spaghetti and barley) (Wolever and Bolognesi, 1996a) and the other studied different doses of bread and three different sugars (glucose, sucrose and fructose) (Lee and Wolever, 1998). These studies showed that, in normal subjects, the incremental area under the blood glucose response curve (AUC) over 2 h increased non-linearly across the range of intakes from 0 to 100 g carbohydrate. The results were very similar for starchy foods and sugars (Fig. 4.1).

These dose–response studies can be used to estimate the theoretic effect on glycaemic responses of replacing part of the available carbohydrate in a food with an unavailable carbohydrate which has no effect on the digestion and absorption of the available carbohydrate (see below). As the dose–response of AUC on dose of carbohydrate is not linear (Fig. 4.1), the effect of reducing the amount of carbohydrate on the RGR depends on the level of available carbohydrate being consumed. The dose–response equation (Fig. 4.1) is:

$$\mathrm{RGR} = \mathrm{GI} \times 1.49 \times (1 - e^{-0.0222g})$$

where RGR is the AUC relative to that elicited by 50 g glucose, GI is glucose-based GI (GI of glucose = 100) and g is grams of available carbohydrate. This equation predicts that the effect of a 25% reduction in available carbohydrate from 15 g (the amount in one slice of bread) to 11.25 g results in a 22% reduction in glycaemic response, a 25% reduction in available carbohydrate from 50 to 37.5 g results in a 16% reduction in glycaemic response and a reduction from 90 to 67.5 g has only a 10% effect.

It is of interest that the dose–response equation developed for Fig. 4.1 accounts for 96–97% of the variability of mean blood glucose responses of subjects with diabetes who consumed 0, 25, 50, 75 or 100 g carbohydrate from white bread (Wolever *et al.*, 1994a), normal subjects who consumed 25, 50, 100 or 200 g glucose (Christensen *et al.*, 1972), and normal subjects who consumed various doses of glucose, bread and lentils from the original GI paper (Jenkins *et al.*, 1981a) (Fig. 4.2). It is also of interest that the AUC for plasma insulin in normal subjects increased linearly with increased doses of carbohydrate either from starch or sugars (Fig. 4.3). However, since the relationship between glucose and insulin responses is not linear, and also varies in different subjects, it is not possible to produce a model to predict insulin responses simply from GI and grams carbohydrate which is valid in all situations.

Our studies on the dose–response of carbohydrates (Wolever and Bolognesi, 1996a; Lee and Wolever, 1998) have a number of drawbacks, including the use of a small number of doses (4–5; 0, 25, 50 and 100 g carbohydrate for all carbohydrates, with an additional dose of 75 g carbohydrate from bread) and the fact that blood glucose and insulin responses were only measured for 2 h after eating, by which time blood glucose and insulin had not returned to baseline after the highest doses of carbohydrate. However, this does not account entirely for the non-linear nature of the dose–response curve for glucose. Christensen *et al.* (1972) measured the glucose and insulin

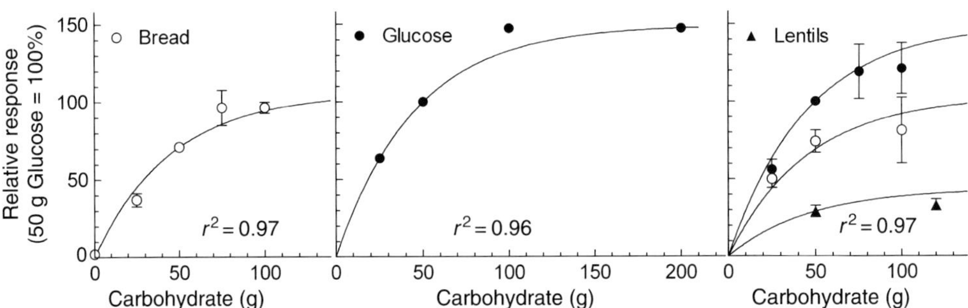


**Fig. 4.2.** Goodness-of-fit of equation developed in Fig. 4.1 (RGR = GI × 1.49 × (1–e$^{-0.0222g}$)) in explaining the dose–response relationship from previously published dose–response studies: left, different doses of white bread taken by subjects with type 2 diabetes (Wolever *et al.*, 1994a); centre, different doses of glucose taken by normal subjects (Christensen *et al.*, 1972); right, different doses of oral glucose, bread or lentils (Jenkins *et al.*, 1981a). The solid lines represent GI × 1.49 × (1–e$^{-0.0222g}$) where the GI values used for glucose, bread and lentils were 100, 71 and 29, respectively.

responses of normal subjects for 6 h after they consumed 25, 50, 100 or 200 g glucose (Fig. 4.4). Figure 4.5 shows the IAUC values for glucose and insulin calculated from the mean glucose and insulin concentrations given in the paper using the data from 0 to 2 h, 0 to 3 h, 0 to 4 h and 0 to 6 h. As the amount of time included in the AUC calculation increases, the degree of curvature of the dose–response curve becomes less, but there is still a noticeable curve even when the AUC measure is extended to 6 h, by which time plasma glucose had returned to baseline for all treatments (Fig. 4.4). For doses of glucose between 0 and 50 g, the shape of the dose–response curve is not affected by measuring glucose and insulin for longer than 2 h. Extending the period of measurement beyond 2 h only begins to influence the AUC values by more than ~10% at doses of carbohydrate >100 g. The remarkable similarity between the rate constant for the 0–2 h AUC values derived from Christensen *et al.* (1972) (Fig. 4.5), 0.0223, and that derived from our studies with sugars and starchy foods

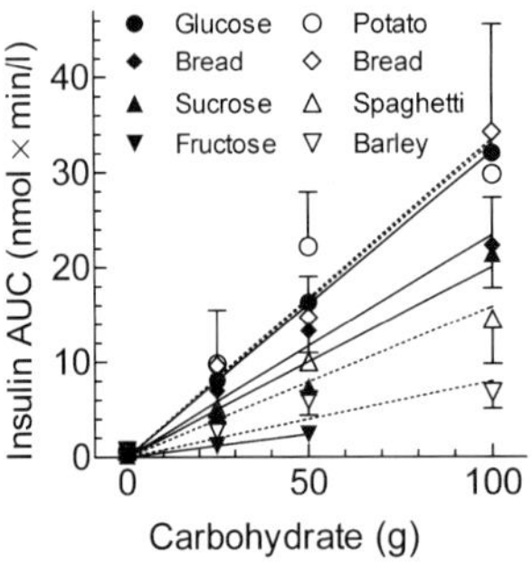

**Fig. 4.3.** Incremental area under the plasma insulin response curves elicited by various amounts of different carbohydrates consumed by normal subjects; open symbols, four starchy foods (Wolever and Bolognesi, 1996a); closed symbols, bread plus three sugars (Lee and Wolever, 1998).

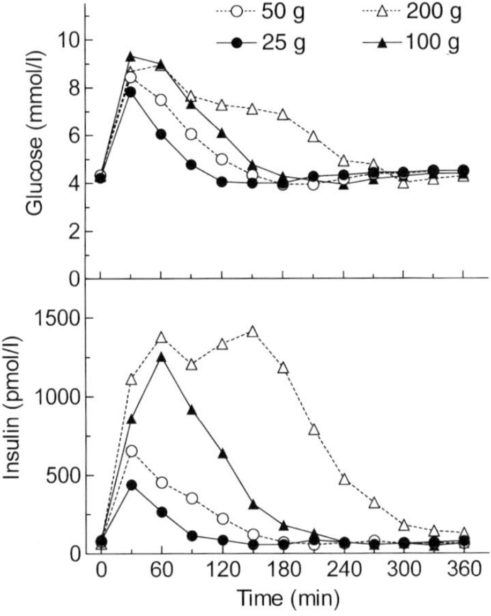


**Fig. 4.4.** Mean plasma glucose and insulin responses of eight normal subjects after consuming 25, 50, 100 or 200 g glucose. Redrawn from Christensen *et al.* (1972).

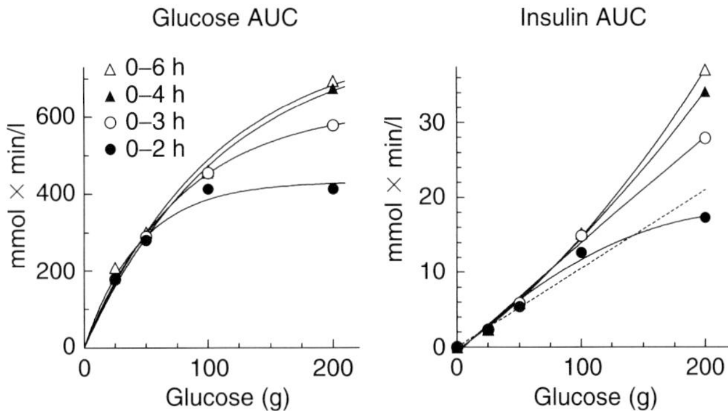


**Fig. 4.5.** Incremental areas under the curve (AUC) of mean glucose and insulin responses measured for 6 h in normal subjects after consuming various doses of glucose (data shown in Fig. 4.4; Christensen *et al.*, 1972). AUC values are shown using the data from 0 to 2 h, 0 to 3 h, 0 to 4 h and 0 to 6 h. Solid lines represent the results of non-linear regression analysis with the model for glucose being one-phase exponential association [0–2 h AUC = $432 \times (1-e^{-0.0223g})$; 0–3 h AUC = $627 \times (1-e^{-0.0128g})$; 0–4 h AUC = $807 \times (1-e^{-0.00881g})$; 0–6 h AUC = $811 \times (1-e^{-0.00925g})$] and the model for insulin being a second-order polynomial (0–2 h AUC = $0.158g - 3.35 \times 10^{-4} g^2$; 0–3 h AUC = $0.151\ g - 3.19 \times 10^{-5} g^2$; 0–4 h AUC = $0.128\ g + 2.30 \times 10^{-4} g^2$; 0–6 h AUC = $0.115\ g + 3.62 \times 10^{-4} g^2$), where g = grams of glucose. The dotted line on the insulin graph is a linear regression: 0–2 h AUC = 0.105 g. Note that the rate constant for the 0–2 h AUC glucose curve, 0.0223, is within 1% of that derived in Fig. 4.1.

(Fig. 4.1), 0.0222, suggest that these conclusions regarding the effect of time over which glucose responses are measured can be applied to other types of carbohydrates.

### 4.2.2 The proportion of carbohydrate absorbed

Certain carbohydrates are not digested or absorbed in the human small intestine and are termed 'unavailable carbohydrates'. By definition, unavailable carbohydrates do not provide glucose to the body, and thus, do not raise blood glucose. Carbohydrates can be unavailable because humans lack the enzymes necessary to hydrolyse them into their component monosaccharides; examples of these include fructo-oligosaccharides, RS and NSP. Alternatively, monosaccharides may be unavailable because they are incompletely transported into the intestinal cells and blood stream; examples of these include sorbitol, xylose (Caspary, 1972) and mannose. The sugar alcohols have been discussed above. The discussion below will include sections on the availability of lactose and fructose, which are partially digested/absorbed in certain individuals or in certain circumstances, fructo-oligosaccharides and starch.

#### *4.2.2.1 Lactose and fructose*

Some individuals, particularly Africans and Asians, have low intestinal lactase activity, and hence, are either partly or totally unable to digest lactose. Thus, milk elicits a much lower glycaemic response relative to glucose in African subjects (Walker and Walker, 1984) than in Europeans (Jenkins *et al.*, 1981a). This is an example of one situation in which the GI of foods differs in different individuals, i.e. when the digestion and/or absorption of the test food in the different groups of subjects differs from that of the reference food.

Fructose absorption is poorly understood, but it appears to be passively absorbed across the apical surface of the enterocyte through GLUT5 transporters, and across the basolateral membrane through GLUT2 transporters (Corpe *et al.*, 1999). Thus, the amount of fructose which is absorbed depends on how much is consumed and whether it is consumed alone or with other nutrients. When fructose is consumed alone in aqueous solution, it is partly malabsorbed, as judged by the production of breath hydrogen. The proportion of adult subjects with malabsorption increased from 0% to 80% as the amount of a 10% fructose solution consumed increased from 200 to 500 ml, but the proportion of subjects varied in different populations (Fig. 4.6) (Ravich *et al.*, 1983; Rumessen and

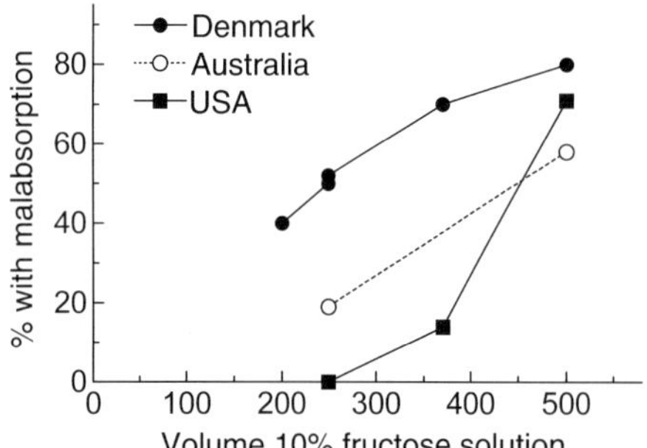


**Fig. 4.6.** Percentage of subjects from different populations with malabsorption after consuming various volumes of 10% (1 g/10 ml) fructose solution. Malabsorption was judged by a significant increase in breath hydrogen. Data from Denmark, Rumessen and Gudmand-Høyer (1986); Australia, Truswell *et al.* (1988); USA, Ravich *et al.* (1983).

Gudmand-Høyer, 1986, 1988; Truswell *et al.*, 1988). Interestingly, diluting the strength of the fructose solution appeared to reduce the percentage of subjects with malabsorption from 71% for 50 g fructose in 250 ml to 37% for 50 g fructose in 500 ml. Adding glucose (Fig. 4.7) or starch (Riby *et al.*, 1993) to fructose increased its absorption, and indeed, there was no malabsorption in most studies after adding an equal amount of glucose to fructose, or after consuming sucrose (Ravich *et al.*, 1983; Rumessen and Gudmand-Høyer, 1986, 1988; Truswell *et al.*, 1988). Thus Riby *et al.* (1993) suggested that fructose and glucose were co-trans ported. However, subsequently it was observed

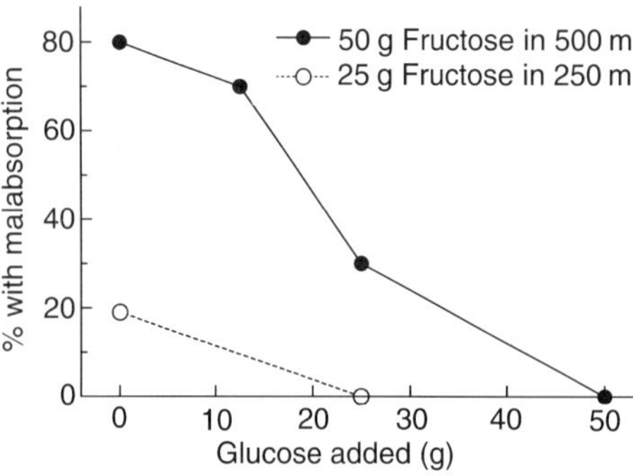


**Fig. 4.7.** Effect of adding various amounts of glucose to fructose on the proportion of subjects with malabsorption (Rumessen and Gudmand-Høyer, 1986; Truswell *et al.*, 1988).

that amino acids also enhance fructose and sorbitol absorption (Hoekstra and van den Aker, 1996), s uggesting that the facilitating effect of glucose on fructose absorption is partly a consequence of glucose-induced streaming of water through the mucosal layer, the so-called phenomenon of solvent drag. In addition, osmotic absorption of water related to the absorption of other nutrients may increase in intraluminal fructose concentration, thus enhancing its absorption (Corpe *et al.*, 1999).

#### *4.2.2.2 Resistant oligosaccharides*

Common unavailable oligosaccharides include inulin and oligofructose which are present naturally in many plant foods. Most of the inulin and oligofructose commercially available as food ingredients are produced either by extraction from chicory roots or synthesis from sucrose (Niness, 1999). Inulin is a mixture of linear fructose polymers and oligomers linked by β(2-1) bonds which are unable to be hydrolysed by human small intestinal enzymes. Therefore, inulin is not digested and absorbed in the small intestine. A glucose unit usually resides at the end of each fructose chain and is linked by an α(1-2) bond, as in sucrose. The chain lengths of these fructans vary from 2 to 60 units (Niness, 1999). Although not an oligosaccharide, lactulose, a disaccharide of galactose and fructose, behaves similarly, and is often used experimentally as a model of an unabsorbed carbohydrate. Studies in ileostomy subjects show that inulin and oligofructose pass through the small intestine without being degraded and without influencing the absorption of starch and other nutrients (Andersson *et al.*, 1999). In humans with an intact colon, fructo-oligosaccharides appear to be completely fermented in large intestine (Alles *et al.*, 1996).

Although dispersible in water, fructans have little or no effect on viscosity and would be predicted to have little or no effect on the rates of digestion and absorption of dietary carbohydrates (Schneeman, 1999). Indeed, when added to carbohydrate foods, neither lactulose nor inulin had any acute effect on glycaemic or insulinaemic responses (Jenkins *et al.*, 1991; Ritz *et al.*, 1993; Brighenti *et al.*, 1999).

#### *4.2.2.3 Starch*

At the time of the publication of the first paper on GI (Jenkins *et al.*,1981a), it was generally thought that most dietary starches were virtually completely digested in the human small intestine. However, shortly thereafter, it began to be appreciated that a portion of dietary starch in common foods escaped digestion in the small intestine (Anderson *et al.*, 1981; Stephen *et al.*, 1983), leading to the classification of starch as readily digestible starch (RDS), partially resistant starch (PRS) and resistant starch (RS) (Table 4.2) and the development of methods to measure these fractions (Englyst *et al.*, 1982, 1992; Englyst and Cummings, 1984, 1985, 1987). RS is naturally present in variable amounts in foods, and the amounts may be increased or decreased by various normal food processing methods such as storing (e.g. ripening of banana), hydration, drying, cooking or cooling. Recently, resistant starches have been developed as functional food ingredients to replace conventional starch in baked goods and other manufactured products, however, their digestibility appears to vary.

Completely indigestible resistant starches would not be expected to influence either the viscosity of the small intestinal contents or the digestion and absorption of other nutrients. For example, lintner starch was similar to cellulose in eliciting neither a glycaemic response when fed alone, nor influencing the glycaemic response when added to glucose (Ranganathan *et al.*, 1994). Raw banana starch did not appear to influence the small intestinal absorption of nutrients (Langkilde *et al.*, 2002). However, some resistant starches are only partly resistant (Schweizer *et al.*, 1990; Raben *et al.*, 1994; Champ *et al.*, 1998), and may, therefore, raise blood glucose to some extent. Replacement of conventional starch by RS in bread or muffins reduces the glycaemic response (Jenkins *et al.*, 1998; Hoebler *et al.*, 1999), but does it reduce the GI? This can only be sorted out properly if, in addition to determining the glycaemic response elicited by the control product and an amount of test product containing the same amount of total carbohydrate, an additional trial is done with an amount of test product containing the same amount of available carbohydrate as the control product. Jenkins *et al.* (1998) did this and found that when the RS they used was added to the control muffin (instead of being substituted for conventional flour), there was no effect on the glycaemic response. Thus, the reduced glycaemic effect was due to a reduction in the amount of starch absorbed without any effect on the GI.

However, when Hoebler *et al.* (1999) tested high-amylose bread, the portion of high-amylose bread contained the same amount of total carbohydrate as the reference food, and thus, less available carbohydrate. Therefore, their conclusion that the high-amylose bread had a low 'GI' was an incorrect use of the term, since the amounts of available carbohydrate were not equal. These authors fed three test meals, control bread containing 92 g available starch and 1.3 g RS, a test bread containing 74 g available starch and 16.5 g RS, and spaghetti containing 95 g available starch

**Table 4.2.** Nutritional classification of starch.[a]

| Type of starch | Physical form | Present in | Fate in small intestine |
|---|---|---|---|
| *Readily digestible starch (RDS)* | | | |
| RDS1 | Dispersed starch | Freshly cooked foods | Rapidly digested |
| RDS2 | Crystalline starch with X-ray diffraction pattern A | Most uncooked cereals and gelatinized starch dried at high temperatures | Slowly but virtually completely digested |
| *Partially resistant starch (PRS)* | | | |
| PRS 1 | Physically inaccessible starch | Whole or partly milled grains and legumes | Partly digested |
| PRS 2 | Starch granules with X-ray diffraction pattern B or C | Raw potato and banana | Partly digested |
| PRS 3 | Mainly retrograded amylopectin | Cooled cooked potato | Partly digested |
| *Resistant starch (RS)* | | | |
| RS | Mainly retrograded amylose | Cooled cooked potato, breads and maize flakes | Resists digestion totally |

[a]Englyst and Cummings (1987).

and 2.5 g RS. The mean areas under the glycaemic response curve were reduced by 40% and 17% after the test bread and spaghetti, respectively, compared to control. Since the spaghetti meal contained the same amount of available carbohydrate as the bread meal, its low glycaemic response can be said to be due to a lower GI. However, there was 20% less available carbohydrate in the RS bread, so its lower glycaemic response cannot be said to be only due to a low GI. Using the equation shown in Section 4.2.1, reducing available carbohydrate intake from 92 to 74 g would be expected to reduce the glycaemic response by 10% which only explains a small amount of the 40% reduction in glycaemic response observed. Thus, the test bread probably has a lower GI than the control bread, but this would need to be determined in a properly controlled experiment.

#### *4.2.2.4 Polyols*

Polyols are only partly absorbed (Table 4.1). Several authors have given 'GI' values for polyols (Foster-Powell *et al.* 2002; Livesey, 2003) by expressing the blood glucose AUC elicited by various polyols as a percentage of that elicited by the same amount of sucrose or glucose. Since only a portion of the carbohydrate in polyols is available, these values should not be termed 'GI' because the GI is based on equal amounts of available carbohydrate in the test and reference foods. We can refer to these 'GI' values of polyols more correctly as RGR (Table 4.1). The true GI values for polyols could be estimated by adjusting the RGR values for the unavailable carbohydrate. But, since the dose–response curve of glucose AUC on dose of carbohydrate is not linear, the factor used to adjust the RGR values for incomplete absorption varies depending on the amount of carbohydrate fed (Table 4.3). Therefore, the estimated GI value of polyols varies depending on the amount of carbohydrate fed (Table 4.4).

It can be seen from Table 4.4 that GI values should not be ascribed to erythritol, mannitol and lactitol because these polyols contain no available carbohydrate being either virtually entirely malabsorbed or non-metabolized. For the other

**Table 4.3.** Effect of partially available carbohydrate on glycaemic response AUC relative to fully absorbed carbohydrate and adjustment factor for estimating GI.

| Fed (g) | % Available | Absorbed (g) | RGRab | RGRfed | Adjustment factor |
|---|---|---|---|---|---|
| 50 | 10 | 5 | 15.7 | 99.9 | 6.38 |
| 50 | 25 | 12.5 | 36.1 | 99.9 | 2.77 |
| 50 | 40 | 20 | 53.4 | 99.9 | 1.87 |
| 50 | 50 | 25 | 63.5 | 99.9 | 1.57 |
| 50 | 100 | 50 | 99.9 | 99.9 | 1.00 |
| 30 | 10 | 3 | 9.6 | 72.4 | 7.55 |
| 30 | 25 | 7.5 | 22.9 | 72.4 | 3.17 |
| 30 | 40 | 12 | 34.8 | 72.4 | 2.08 |
| 30 | 50 | 15 | 42.2 | 72.4 | 1.72 |
| 30 | 100 | 30 | 72.4 | 72.4 | 1.00 |
| 20 | 10 | 2 | 6.5 | 53.4 | 8.26 |
| 20 | 25 | 4 | 12.7 | 53.4 | 4.22 |
| 20 | 40 | 8 | 24.2 | 53.4 | 2.20 |
| 20 | 50 | 10 | 29.7 | 53.4 | 1.80 |
| 20 | 100 | 20 | 53.4 | 53.4 | 1.00 |
| 10 | 10 | 1 | 3.3 | 29.7 | 9.07 |
| 10 | 25 | 2.5 | 8.0 | 29.7 | 3.69 |
| 10 | 40 | 4 | 12.7 | 29.7 | 2.34 |
| 10 | 50 | 5 | 15.7 | 29.7 | 1.89 |
| 10 | 100 | 10 | 29.7 | 29.7 | 1.00 |

RGRab = $149 \times (1-e^{-0.0222g})$ where g = amount absorbed; RGRfed = $149 \times (1-e^{-0.0222g})$ where g = amount fed (Fig. 4.1). Adjustment factor = RGRfed/RGRab; the value by which to multiply *X* to estimate GI, where *X* is the AUC after the partly available carbohydrate expressed as percentage of that after the same amount of glucose (see text, Section 4.2.2.4). Note that for the same % availability, the adjustment factor varies for different amounts of carbohydrate fed.

**Table 4.4.** Glycaemic index of various sugar alcohols estimated from the literature.

| | | | Intake (g)[c] | | | |
|---|---|---|---|---|---|---|
| Sugar alcohol | RR[a] | % Av. CHO[b] | Mean | Minimum | Maximum | GI[d] |
| Erythritol | 0 | 0 | 41 | 17 | 64 | na |
| Xylitol | 13 | 50 | 34 | 20 | 50 | 21 |
| Sorbitol | 9 | 25 | 36 | 20 | 50 | 28 |
| Mannitol | 0 | 0 | 25 | – | – | na |
| Isomalt | 9 | 10 | 44 | 20 | 70 | 60 |
| Lactitol | 6 | 0 | 33 | 25 | 50 | na |
| Maltitol | 35 | 40 | 44 | 20 | 50 | 69 |
| HM syrup[e] | 48 | 50 | 32 | 10 | 50 | 82 |
| IM syrup[f] | 53 | 50 | 44 | 25 | 50 | 87 |
| RM syrup[g] | 52 | 50 | 42 | 20 | 66 | 85 |
| HP syrup[h] | 36 | 40 | 50 | 50 | 50 | 67 |
| Polyglycitol | 39 | 40 | 30 | 25 | 35 | 80 |

[a]RR = relative response; mean AUC after sugar alcohol expressed as % of mean AUC after glucose (GI according to Livesey, 2003).
[b]From Table 4.1.
[c]Intake = mean and range of intakes of polyol and reference carbohydrate for the different studies reported by Livesey (2003).
[d]GI mean for all studies on each sugar alcohol of RR × RGRfed/RGRab, where RGRfed = 149 × $(1-e^{-0.0222g})$ where g = amount fed and RGRab = 149 × $(1-e^{-0.0222g})$ where g = amount absorbed. 'na' = GI is not applicable for non-glycaemic carbohydrates.
[e]HM = high-maltitol syrup.
[f]IM = intermediate malitol syrup.
[g]RM = regular maltitol syrup.
[h]HP = high polymer maltitol syrup.

polyols, it could be asked whether the adjustment for available carbohydrate is necessary, for sorbitol, for example, what is the difference between saying that 50 g sorbitol has an RGR of 9, or saying that 50 g sorbitol contains 12.5 g available carbohydrate which has a GI of 36? These statements seem to be equivalent, and having to adjust for the amount of available carbohydrate seems very complicated. However, the distinction becomes important when considering mixed meals.

## 4.3 Rate of Carbohydrate Absorption

Several lines of evidence suggest that slowing the rate of absorption of carbohydrate reduces glycaemic responses. These include addition of viscous fibre, correlation between the rates of digestion of starches *in vitro* and their glycaemic responses *in vivo*, the use of inhibitors of digestive enzyme activity, reducing the rate of consumption of carbohydrate, the use of stable isotopes, and, most recently, the euglycaemic hyperinsulinaemic clamp plus oral carbohydrate loading. However, before reviewing this evidence, it should be acknowledged that while these lines of evidence show that slowing absorption reduces glycaemic responses and that low-GI foods are actually slowly absorbed *in vivo* in the human, they do not prove that *complete* carbohydrate absorption occurs. In addition, the statement that delayed absorption reduces blood glucose responses depends on what is meant by 'reduced glycaemic response'. Slowing absorption reduces the peak rise of blood glucose, but delays the return of blood glucose to baseline, possibly for several hours. Thus, slowing the absorption of carbohydrate, for example, by increasing meal frequency, may not actually reduce the average blood glucose concentrations throughout the day in normal (Jenkins *et al.*, 1989) or diabetic subjects (Jenkins *et al.*, 1992). Nevertheless, reducing glucose fluctuations throughout the day may be beneficial, even if there is no reduction in mean blood glucose (Muggeo *et al.*, 1997, 2000; Ceriello, 1998; Risso *et al.*,2001). In addition, when judged according to GI methodology (i.e. IAUC measured over 2 h in normal subjects or 3 h in subjects with diabetes), there is a reduction in glycaemic response.

### 4.3.1 Addition of viscous fibre

The classic studies of Jenkins *et al.* (1978b) suggested that the ability of dietary fibres to reduce glycaemic responses was related to their viscosity. This has been verified in numerous studies (reviewed by Wolever and Jenkins, 1993). The exact mechanism by which viscous fibres reduce the glycaemic response is a matter of debate and the hypothesized mechanisms include: an increase in the thickness of the unstirred layer in the small intestine (Elsenhaus *et al.*, 1980), inhibition of the effects of intestinal motility on fluid convection in the lumen of the intestine (Blackburn *et al.*, 1984), increased contractile activity in the small intestine (Cherbut *et al.*, 1994) or a reduced rate of gastric emptying (Holt *et al.*, 1979; Di Lorenzo *et al.*, 1988). Although all these mechanisms ultimately result in a reduction in the rate of carbohydrate absorption, direct proof of this is lacking.

### 4.3.2 Rate of starch digestion *in vitro*

Traditionally, there have been two conflicting views of starch digestion. One school of thought held that pancreatic α-amylase is present in high activity in the small intestine (Dahlqvist and Borgstrom, 1961; Fogel and Gray, 1973) and that this enzyme was not rate limiting in determining the overall rate of starch digestion and absorption (Lütjens *et al.*, 1975). In contrast, the other school of thought held that the size of the carbohydrate molecule did influence the postprandial glucose and insulin response such that the more complex carbohydrates (starches) elicited lower responses (Crapo *et al.*, 1976). The latter hypothesis was disproved when it was shown that the glycaemic responses elicited by glucose, maltose or soluble glucose polymers were virtually identical (Wahlqvist *et al.*, 1978; Jenkins *et al.*, 1987b). Nevertheless, recent work suggests that enzymatic hydrolysis of starch is a limiting factor in carbohydrate digestion because of factors related to the physicochemical properties of starch which influence the adsorption of amylase to starch, and hence the reaction velocity (Slaughter *et al.*, 2001).

Numerous studies have shown that the rates of digestion of different starchy foods differ, and that these differences are related to the glycaemic responses of the carbohydrate foods *in vivo* (Jenkins *et al.*, 1980a, 1982a; O'Dea *et al.*, 1981; Heaton *et al.*, 1988; Bornet *et al.*, 1989; Granfeldt *et al.*, 1992; Noah *et al.*, 1998). This has lead to the development of techniques for measuring rapidly available glucose (RAG) and slowly available glucose (SAG) *in vitro* (Englyst *et al.*, 1996b, 1999, 2003). The existence of correlations between *in vitro* measurements of starch digestibility and *in vivo* glycaemic responses provides evidence, but not proof, that slow digestion and absorption occurs *in vivo*. Nevertheless, the fact that the correlations from such completely different types of measurements are often quite good (Fig. 4.8) is impressive and convincing.

The reasons for the differences in starch digestion have been reviewed elsewhere (Würsch, 1989; Biliaderis, 1991; Björck *et al.*, 1994, 2000) and will not be reviewed in detail here. Nevertheless, some factors influencing the rate of starch digestion and/or glycaemic response include particle size (Jenkins *et al.*, 1988; Liljeberg *et al.*, 1992), the degree of gelatinization (Ross *et al.*, 1987; Holm *et al.*, 1988; Panlasigui *et al.*, 1991), the ratio of amylose to amylopectin (Behall *et al.*, 1988), starch–protein (Jenkins *et al.*, 1987c) and starch–lipid interactions (Merier *et al.*, 1980; Eliasson *et al.*, 1981), and various processing methods which either influence starch structure (Englyst and Cummings, 1986; Holm *et al.*, 1989) or preserve or add compounds which may inhibit gastric emptying or starch digestion such as phytate (Yoon *et al.*, 1983; Thompson *et al.*, 1987), tannins (Thompson *et al.*, 1984), saponins (Onning and Asp, 1995), lectins (Rea *et al.*, 1985) or organic acids (Brighenti *et al.*, 1995; Liljeberg and Björck, 1996, 1998).

There has been some suggestion that the glycaemic responses of starchy foods are related to their rates of gastric emptying (Torsdottir *et al.*, 1984). Although this mechanism may contribute to reduced glycaemic responses, or even be the predominant reason in some cases (e.g. Liljeberg and Björck, 1996, 1998), it is probably not a major factor for most low-GI foods. When gastric emptying and *in vitro* digestion rates of three different starches were measured in the same study, the rate of starch digestion was the major determinant of their glycaemic responses (Bornet *et al.*, 1990).

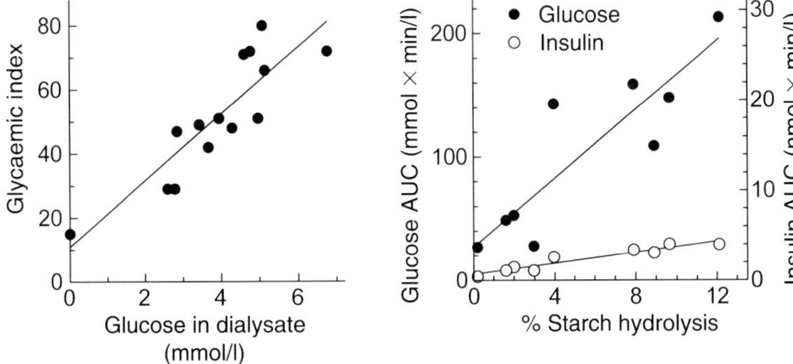


**Fig. 4.8.** Examples of correlations between rates of digestion of carbohydrate foods or starches *in vitro* and blood glucose and insulin responses *in vivo*. Left, Jenkins *et al.* (1982a) ($r = 0.87$); right, Bornet *et al.* (1989) ($r = 0.88$ for glucose, $r = 0.95$ for insulin).

### 4.3.3 Enzyme inhibitors

Various α-glucosidase inhibitors such as acarbose (Clissold and Edwards, 1988; Chiasson *et al.*, 1994), miglitol (Chiasson *et al.*, 2001) and voglibose (Vichayanrat *et al.*, 2002) have been developed for the treatment and/or prevention of diabetes (Mooradian and Thurman, 1999; Scheen, 2003). These, and other glucosidase inhibitors, have proven useful models for the effects of slowing carbohydrate absorption on postprandial glycaemic responses. In rats, there was a nearly linear relationship between dose of an intestinal sucrase inhibitor and the net incremental area under the glucose response curve (Fig. 4.9; Robinson *et al.*, 1990). In humans, it was shown that a large dose of acarbose (200 mg) reduced the area under the blood glucose response curve by 89% after 50 g sucrose, and breath hydrogen measurements suggested that this was accompanied by almost complete malabsorption of the oral sucrose load. However, with 50 mg acarbose, there was smaller reduction in the glycaemic response, but no significant increase in breath hydrogen, suggesting no significant amount of carbohydrate malabsorption (Jenkins *et al.*, 1981b). This suggests that, at large doses, α-glucosidase inhibitors reduce glycaemic responses by inducing carbohydrate malabsorption, but at lower doses do so by slowing the rate of carbohydrate absorption without significant malabsorption.

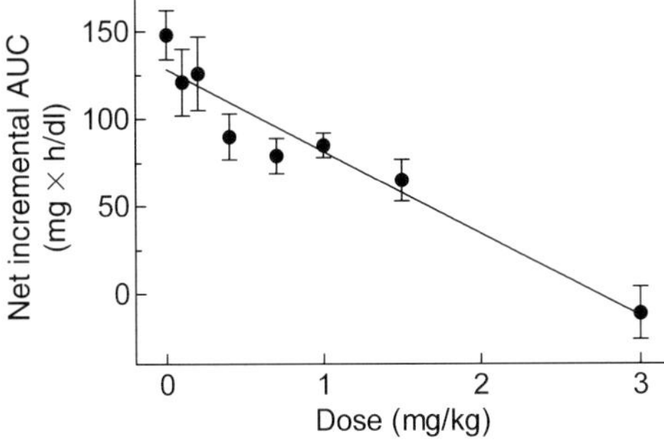


**Fig. 4.9.** Relationship between dose of the intestinal sucrase inhibitor castanospermine and glycaemic response to sucrose in rats (Robinson *et al.*, 1990).

### 4.3.4 Reducing the rate of carbohydrate consumption

Reducing the rate of carbohydrate consumption by eating multiple small meals instead of a few large ones, i.e. nibbling vs gorging, was shown in both normal (Jenkins *et al.*, 1989, 1990; Wolever, 1990a) and diabetic subjects (Jenkins *et al.*, 1992; Bertelsen *et al.*, 1993) to reduce incremental blood glucose and insulin responses. Indeed, in subjects with type 2 diabetes, the incremental blood glucose response decreased in a linear fashion as the number of meals increased from 3, to 6, 9 and 12 per day (Segura *et al.*, 1995). This model was hypothesized as being able to prove that slowing the rate of carbohydrate absorption without altering the amount absorbed reduced glycaemic responses. However, in many of these studies, nibbling continued throughout the entire period of time when blood glucose was measured. Under these circumstances, it is likely that some of the nibbled carbohydrate will have remained in the stomach, and therefore, not have been absorbed by the time of the last blood sample. Thus, it is possible to argue that this experimental model does not actually prove that slow but complete absorption of carbohydrate reduces glycaemic responses.

In this context, the results of studies in which identical amounts of glucose were infused intravenously at different rates into normal subjects are of interest (Chen and Porte, 1975; Fig. 4.10). When 20 g glucose was infused over 12 min, the rate of rise of plasma glucose was much slower than when 20 g was infused in 0.3 min, although peak plasma glucose did not differ significantly. Over the period during which the infusions occurred, 0–13 min, the incremental area under the plasma glucose curve was reduced by about 45%. However, over the entire 2 h experimental period, both the TAUC and IAUC of plasma glucose were virtually identical. On the other hand, plasma insulin concentrations were reduced by reducing the rate of glucose infusion, both over the acute period of the infusion, and on average over the entire 2-h period (Fig. 4.10). These results are consistent with the results of studies of nibbling vs gorging (Table 4.5). Peak rises of plasma glucose were reduced by nibbling, but average blood glucose over the entire day was no different during nibbling than gorging, nevertheless, mean plasma insulin over the entire 12 h day was reduced.

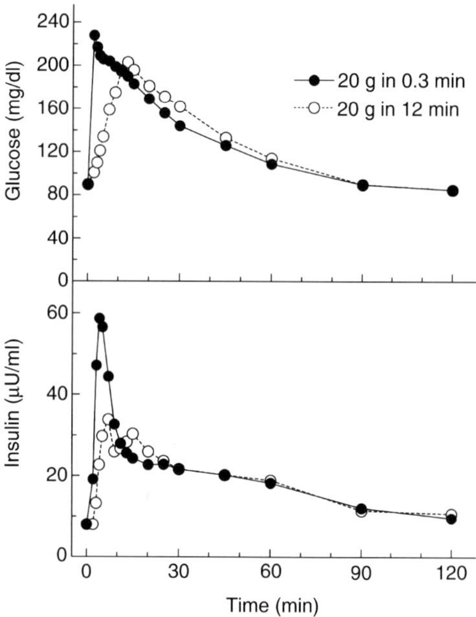


**Fig. 4.10.** Plasma glucose (top) and insulin (bottom) of human subjects after IV infusion of 20 g glucose at different rates (Chen and Porte, 1975).

### 4.3.5 Studies using stable isotopes

Enrichment of carbohydrates with stable isotopes allows one to study the fate of the labelled substrates in the body. Maize starch is naturally enriched with $^{13}C$, a stable isotope of carbon, and Normand *et al.* (1992) compared the appearance of $^{13}C$ in plasma glucose and breath $CO_2$ during feeding with crackers, polenta or pasta made from maize starch. They found no significant differences in the rates of $^{13}C$ appearance in plasma glucose or breath $CO_2$, or carbohydrate oxidation between the different foods. However, they also found no significant difference between the areas under the glucose response curve elicited by the different foods. Thus, the results were unable to contribute to our understanding of the mechanism by which different starchy foods elicit different glycaemic responses.

### 4.3.6 The euglycaemic hyperinsulinaemic clamp

The euglycaemic hyperinsulinaemic clamp is a technique originally developed for measuring whole-body insulin sensitivity (Bergman *et al.*, 1985). In this technique, insulin is infused intravenously into human (or animal) subjects at a rate necessary to raise plasma insulin to a high physiological concentration (about 800 pmol/l), and maintained for several hours. Glucose is simultaneously infused at a variable rate as necessary to maintain plasma glucose at a normal fasting level, normally about 5 mmol/l. The high-plasma insulin concentration acts to stimulate glucose uptake by peripheral tissues and inhibit hepatic glucose output. After a period of about 2 h, 'steady state' is achieved – at which time, it is assumed that hepatic glucose output is completely suppressed, and the only input of glucose into the circulation (at least in normal subjects) is from the intravenous

**Table 4.5.** Effect of nibbling (>6 meals/12 h) vs gorging on mean plasma glucose and insulin concentrations.

| | | | Mean glucose (mmol/l) | | Mean insulin (pmol/l) | | |
|---|---|---|---|---|---|---|---|
| No. of meals | Subjects | Duration (h) | Gorg. | Nib. | Gorg. | Nib. | Reference |
| 1 vs cont. | 9 N | 4 | 5.2 | 5.3 | 140 | 83* | Jenkins *et al.* (1990) |
| 3 vs 17 | 7 N | 12 | 5.5 | 5.3* | 153 | 104* | Jenkins *et al.* (1989) |
| 3 vs cont. | 7 N | 12 | 5.3 | 5.0 | 360 | 240* | Wolever (1990a) |
| 2 vs 6 | 12 2DM | 8 | 9.9 | 9.5 | 273 | 237* | Bertelsen *et al.* (1993) |
| 3 vs 13a | 11 2DM | 10 | 11.1 | 9.6* | 336 | 276* | Jenkins *et al.* (1992) |
| 3 vs 6 | 9 2DM | 12 | 14.1 | 13.8 | 154 | 133* | Segura *et al.* (1995) |
| 3 vs 9 | 9 2DM | 12 | 14.1 | 13.1 | 154 | 145 | Segura *et al.* (1995) |
| 3 vs 12 | 9 2DM | 12 | 14.1 | 13.2 | 154 | 139* | Segura *et al.* (1995) |

Cont. = continuous sipping; N = normal subjects; 2DM = subjects with type 2 diabetes mellitus.
*$P < 0.05$.
[a]In this study, during 'nibbling', subjects ate only 11 of the 13 snacks during the period when blood glucose and insulin were measured.

glucose infusion. Since, during steady state, the concentration of glucose in the plasma is not changing, the rate of glucose removal from the blood must be equal to the rate at which it is being infused. Thus, the rate of glucose infusion is a measure of insulin-stimulated glucose uptake by the tissues of the body, i.e. a measure of insulin sensitivity. This method has been used to measure the rate of glucose uptake from the intestine. The principle is that, if after steady state has been achieved, glucose begins to enter the blood stream from the intestine, the rate of intravenous glucose infusion has to be reduced to maintain the steady-state plasma glucose concentration, with the reduction in glucose infusion being equal to the amount of glucose appearing in the blood from the intestine (Ludvik *et al.*, 1995, 1997).

In several elegant studies, the oral–carbohydrate–hyperinsulinaemic euglycaemic clamp technique was used to compare the posthepatic glucose appearance after consumption of maize starch vs mung bean starch, the latter of which has a lower GI than the former. After validation in pigs (Lang *et al.*, 1999b), Lang *et al.* (1999c) showed in humans that the cumulative appearance of glucose in the peripheral circulation 4.5 h after maize starch, 73% of the amount consumed was similar to that after oral glucose, 79%. After these meals, glucose absorption was estimated to be completed after about 3 h, with the remaining 21–27% of the oral load being taken up by liver and intestine. Only 36% of the carbohydrate in mung bean starch had appeared in the peripheral circulation by 4.5 h – thus directly showing, for the first time, a reduced rate of starch absorption *in vivo* in human subjects. However, carbohydrate from mung bean starch was still appearing in the circulation at a slow rate at the end of the experiment, and authors were unable to account for 64% which had not appeared in the peripheral circulation. The unaccounted-for carbohydrate could still have been in the intestine (i.e. not absorbed) or could have been taken up by the liver (i.e. absorbed but retained in the splanchnic bed). In a validation study in pigs (Lang *et al.*, 1999b), the authors showed that hepatic uptake of carbohydrate after slowly absorbed mung bean starch was the same as that after rapidly absorbed maize starch. However, Livesey *et al.* (1998) suggested that, in humans, there is a large difference in the amount of glucose retained in the splanchnic bed depending on the site of absorption, with 98% of glucose infused into the duodenum appearing in peripheral blood, compared to only 35% of glucose infused into the mid-jejunum. If this was so, it would account almost exactly for the unaccounted for carbohydrate in the study by Lang *et al.* (1999c). Nevertheless, the fact remains that this study was unable to account for the fate of the slowly absorbed carbohydrate.

What, then, is the predominant mechanism for low-GI foods: slow absorption or malabsorption?

## 4.4 Is Carbohydrate Malabsorption the Mechanism for Low-GI Foods?

Since it has not been possible to prove that slow carbohydrate absorption occurs in the absence of malabsorption, it could be argued that that low-GI foods elicit low glycaemic responses because a proportion of their carbohydrate is not absorbed. It has recently been suggested that naturally occurring foods contain as much as 40% of their total starch as RS (Englyst *et al.*, 1992), and this has not usually been taken into account when calculating the portion size to use in determining the GI. Thus, it is possible that the presence of RS reduces glycaemic responses merely by displacing available carbohydrate, and hence, reducing the amount of available carbohydrate absorbed. However, three types of evidence exist, all of which suggest that carbohydrate malabsorption is not the predominant mechanism which accounts for the low glycaemic responses of low-GI starchy foods: lack of correlation between RS in foods measured *in vitro* and GI, *in vivo* assessment of the amount of malabsorbed starch in humans and indirect assessment based on the 'second-meal' effect.

### 4.4.1 Relation between RS measured *in vitro* and GI

*In vitro* studies suggest that measures of the rate of starch digestion are more closely correlated with GI than measures of RS, or that differences in RS are not nearly large enough to account for differences in GI.

The largest study in which both RS measurements *in vitro* and GI measurements *in vivo* were performed on all products tested included a total of 23 manufactured cereal products (Englyst *et al.*, 2003) and does not support the concept that GI values are low in foods with more RS. Indeed, this study revealed a significant *positive* correlation between RS content and GI (Fig. 4.11). This seems counterintuitive, since it suggests that the lower the available carbohydrate, the higher the glycaemic response. However, the RS content of the foods was low (<5% of starch), and 5% differences in starch intake would have no detectable effect on glycaemic responses. Rather, the positive correlation between RS and GI may reflect a greater degree of processing in the higher RS foods which creates both more RS and makes the foods more susceptible to digestion. This study showed that *in vitro* measures of the rate of carbohydrate digestion, i.e. the amounts of RAG and SAG present in foods, were most closely related to the GI. RAG and SAG were closely related to each other ($r = 0.87$) and the correlations between RAG and GI ($r = 0.74$) and SAG and GI ($r = -0.80$) were highly significant.

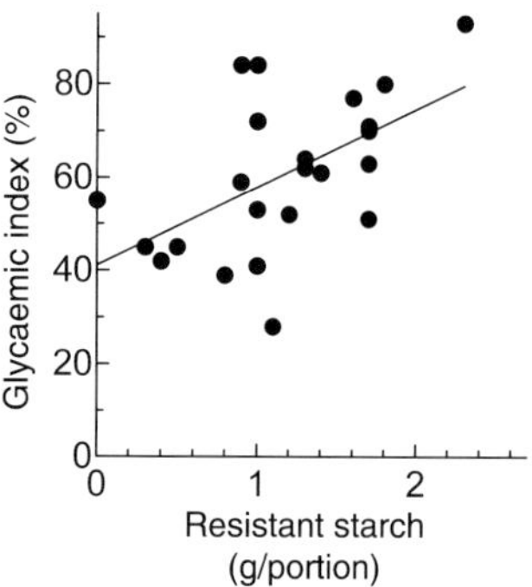


**Fig. 4.11.** Relationship between GI values of 23 manufactured foods and their content of resistant starch (Englyst *et al.*, 2003) ($r = 0.550$, $P = 0.0066$).

A number of studies have examined the effect of processing or storage on the content of RS in natural foods. For example, it has been estimated that freshly cooked potatoes contain virtually no RS, about 1.3% upon cooling, 3.3% upon a second cycle of reheating and cooling, and increasing to >5% upon four cycles of reheating and cooling (Englyst and Cummings, 1987). We recently determined the effect of cooling on the GI of boiled red potatoes (Fernandes *et al.*, 2005); when boiled red potatoes were stored in a refrigerator for 12–36 h after cooking, the mean glycaemic response was reduced by 35% compared to the same weight of boiled red potatoes consumed hot, immediately after cooking. Thus, the 1–2% increase in RS does not nearly account for the magnitude of reduction in glycaemic response.

Raben *et al.* (1994) found that 50 g raw potato starch elicited no rise in blood glucose, despite containing only 54% RS. Thus, again, the reduction in blood glucose was considerably greater than could be accounted for by the amount of RS.

The amount of RS measured *in vitro* has been shown in some studies to accurately reflect the amount of starch escaping digestion in the small intestine *in vivo* in subjects with an ileostomy (Silvester *et al.*, 1995; Englyst *et al.*, 1996a) but this is not always the case (Englyst and Cummings, 1987; Champ *et al.*, 1998).

### 4.4.2 Quantification of carbohydrate malabsorption in humans *in vivo*

Classically, the degree of malabsorption of nutrients is assessed using a balance study with the amount malabsorbed being equal to the amount consumed in the diet minus the amount excreted in the faeces. However, since many carbohydrates are partly or completely fermented in the large intestine, measurement of excretion in the faeces is not a good measure of the amount absorbed in the small intestine. Three general approaches have been taken to measure the amount of carbohydrate escaping digestion in the small intestine: the breath hydrogen method, intubation studies and studies in humans with an ileostomy.

#### *4.4.2.1 The breath hydrogen method*

It has been known for some time that breath hydrogen is a non-invasive way of detecting carbohydrate malabsorption in humans (Calloway *et al.*, 1969; Levitt and Donaldson, 1970; Bond and Levitt, 1972). Early on, the test was developed as a way to measure small intestinal transit time (Bond *et al.*, 1975) and to diagnose lactose intolerance (Calloway *et al.*, 1969; Metz *et al.*, 1976). There was interest in minimizing the production of hydrogen and methane which were potential fire hazards during colonoscopy (Bond and Levitt, 1975; Bond *et al.*, 1976) or in the enclosed environment of a capsule used in space travel (Calloway and Murphy, 1969; Calloway, 1972). Although breath hydrogen was measured after consumption of normal foods (Calloway and Burroughs, 1969; Calloway *et al.*, 1971; Hickey *et al.*, 1972a,b; Murphy and Calloway, 1972), the amounts were not quantified in the early studies. Bond and Levitt (1972) validated a method for quantifying carbohydrate malabsorption, which has been used extensively ever since (Anderson *et al.*, 1981; Jenkins *et al.*, 1981b, 1982b; Ravich *et al.*, 1983; Rumessen and Gudmand-Høyer, 1986, 1988; Levitt *et al.*, 1987; Flourié *et al.*, 1988b; Truswell *et al.*, 1988; Hamberg *et al.*, 1989; Rumessen *et al.*, 1990; Robb *et al.*, 1991; Alles *et al.*, 1996).

Breath hydrogen is measured at intervals of 8–12 h after consumption of a carbohydrate test meal in human subjects on several different days. On the first day, subjects are given a known dose of a completely malabsorbed indicator carbohydrate (typically lactulose). On each of the other days, a known amount of each test carbohydrate is given. An integrated measure of breath hydrogen 'production' (e.g. AUC or sum of concentrations) is calculated. The indicator carbohydrate is used to determine the amount of hydrogen 'produced' per gram of carbohydrate malabsorbed for each subject, and this value is divided into the amount 'produced' from the test carbohydrate to give the grams of carbohydrate malabsorbed. This method relies on a number of assumptions: the only source of hydrogen gas in the human body is the colonic fermentation of carbohydrates, hydrogen measured in breath is either quantitatively related to the amount produced in the colon and/or to the amount of carbohydrate malabsorbed, and that the stoichiometry of hydrogen production from the test source of carbohydrate is the same as that from the indicator carbohydrate.

Measurement of breath hydrogen is generally considered as a valid method (Rumessen, 1992) of assessing carbohydrate malabsorption, although various problems have been identified including large day-to-day variation (Flourié *et al.*, 1988a), the confounding effects of colonic adaptation to chronic lactulose ingestion (Florent *et al.*, 1985; Vogelsang *et al.*, 1988), previous antibiotic use (Gilat *et al.*, 1978) and the fact that certain unabsorbed carbohydrates do not elicit an increase in breath hydrogen (Wolever and Robb, 1992; Wolever *et al.*, 1992c; Livesey *et al.*, 1993; Olesen *et al.*, 1994).

We attempted to validate the breath hydrogen method by comparing results from it to those obtained by measurement of undigested available carbohydrate leaving the terminal ileum in subjects with an ileostomy (Wolever *et al.*, 1986b). The results were very comparable. The estimated mean% available carbohydrate malabsorbed from white bread, whole wheat bread and red lentils, using the breath hydrogen method were 10%, 8% and 22%, respectively, compared to 11%, 8% and 18%, respectively, in subjects with an ileostomy. However, another study suggested that breath hydrogen measures did not correlate with the amount of starch malabsorbed: mean daily breath hydrogen concentrations in normal subjects did not change significantly when switching from a low- (100 g/day) to a high-starch (300 g/day) diet, despite a significant increase in the amount of starch leaving the small intestine directly measured via intubation (Flourié *et al.*, 1988b).

#### 4.4.2.2 Intubation studies

In this type of study, human subjects swallow a radio-opaque tube which is allowed to pass down the gut until the end is in the terminal ileum, thus allowing direct sampling of luminal contents at the end of the small intestine. This is a difficult technique and so has only been used in a small number of studies (Stephen *et al.*, 1983; Flourié *et al.*, 1988b). In addition, it has been suggested that the presence of the tube reduces transit time (Read *et al.*, 1984) and, thus, may impair digestion and absorption. Nevertheless, this is the only method allowing direct measurement of the amount of carbohydrate remaining in the digesta at the end of the small intestine.

#### 4.4.2.3 Studies in human subjects with an ileostomy

The normal intestinal tract is a hollow tube with its start at the mouth and its end at the anus. The treatment of choice for some diseases of the colon, such as familial polyposis coli or ulcerative colitis, is to remove the colon, in which case the end of the small intestine is brought out onto the abdominal wall, where it empties into a bag. This is called an ileostomy. The creation of ileostomies is becoming more uncommon, as surgeons are now often able to preserve the anal musculature and, after removing the colon, fashion an artificial rectum and anus from the remaining terminal ileum.

To study the small intestinal digestion and absorption of carbohydrates and other nutrients and compounds, such as bile acids, using the ileostomy model, the experimental design usually includes a period when subjects with an ileostomy consume a control diet, perhaps free of, or low in the nutrient of interest (e.g. starch) and then another period when the nutrient of interest is added to the diet. Analysis of the diet consumed and the ileal effluent can be used to provide a direct measure of disappearance and presumed absorption of the nutrient. Apart from the difficulty in finding willing subjects, and the inconvenience of consuming restricted diets and collecting effluent, this method has the drawback that some bacterial colonization of the terminal ileum occurs, and so degradation of nutrients may occur before they are excreted, or after they are excreted while in the ileostomy bag. Nevertheless, with frequent emptying of the bag and immediate freezing of the contents, this appears to be a relatively minor problem. The main advantage of the method is that the intestinal transit time is so short that the effluent corresponding to one day's intake is completely excreted before the next morning. For this, and other reasons which are reviewed elsewhere (Andersson, 1992; Andersson *et al.*, 1999), the ileostomy model is considered to be a reliable model to study small bowel absorption.

We used the ileostomy method to compare carbohydrate malabsorption with glycaemic responses in two studies. First (Wolever *et al.*, 1986b) we studied three foods: white bread, wholemeal bread and red lentils. The mean% carbohydrate malabsorbed for these foods, 11%, 8% and 18%, respectively, was not related to the mean areas under the glycaemic response curves they elicited, 83, 82 and 20 mmol × min/l, respectively. In the second study, the digestibility and GI of a range of 20 foods was studied (Jenkins *et al.*, 1987d) in one or more ileostomate subjects. It should be noted that the 50 g available carbohydrate portion used to determine the GI of these foods included RS because values for RS were not widely available (and, so technically, perhaps, the results should not be called 'GI' according to the strict definition above). The GI values from the subject with an ileostomy were closely related to published values ($r = 0.81$). Therefore, published GI values are plotted against % carbohydrate malabsorbed for the 20 foods in Fig. 4.12. There is a significant negative linear relationship between GI and % carbohydrate malabsorbed (dashed line, $r^2 = 0.451$, $P = 0.001$), however, this does not appear to fit the data optimally. The best-fit model was a two-phase exponential decay (solid line, $r^2 = 0.513$). Also plotted on in this figure (dotted line) is the theoretical effect on glycaemic responses of reducing carbohydrate intake by an amount equal to the proportion of carbohydrate malabsorbed. It is clear that the effect of carbohydrate malabsorption *per se* (dotted line) explains only a small proportion of the reduction in

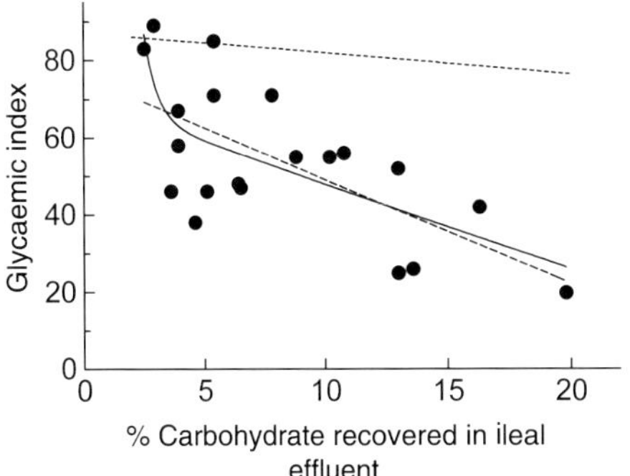


**Fig. 4.12.** Relationship between % carbohydrate malabsorbed and GI for 20 starchy foods (Jenkins *et al.*, 1987d). Dotted line, theoretical effect of reducing carbohydrate intake by an amount equal to the proportion of carbohydrate malabsorbed; dashed line, linear regression ($r^2 = 0.451$); solid line, non-linear regression model of two-phase exponential decay ($r^2 = 0.513$).

glycaemic response, at 20% malabsorption, it only explains about 15% of the reduction in GI. Therefore, these data support the suggestion that differences in GI for most starchy foods are primarily due to a mechanism distinct from differences in the amount of carbohydrate absorbed. This supports the traditional view that the 50 g carbohydrate load used to measure GI should continue to exclude unavailable carbohydrates.

It is widely appreciated that the cooling of cooked starches results in starch retrogradation and the creation of RS. It has been noted that above 1–2% of the starch in cooked potatoes is converted to RS (chemically defined) when they are cooled (Englyst and Cummings, 1987). However, when measured using the ileostomy model, the RS content of potatoes increased to 3% for freshly cooked potatoes and 12% for cooked and cooled potatoes (Englyst and Cummings, 1987). Therefore, a 50 g 'available carbohydrate' portion of hot cooked potato actually contains about 48.5 g of available carbohydrate while the portion of cooled potato contained about 44 g of available carbohydrate, a difference which would be expected to result in a 5% reduction in glycaemic response (Fig. 4.1). Thus, carbohydrate malabsorption *per se* accounts for only about 15% of the 35% reduction in glycaemic response elicited by cooled boiled red potatoes compared to freshly cooked boiled red potatoes (Fernandes *et al.*, 2005).

Englyst and Cummings (1985) determined the starch content and degree of digestibility of bananas. The starch content of banana varied with its stage of ripeness, being 46% of carbohydrate in slightly under-ripe banana (mainly yellow skin with some green at the tips), 29% for ripe banana (yellow skin) and 10% for slightly over-ripe banana (mainly yellow with a few black spots). Also, the starch in banana is very indigestible, with an average of 69% being recovered in ileal effluent (Englyst and Cummings, 1985). From this information, it can be calculated that 50 g available carbohydrate (defined as total carbohydrate minus dietary fibre) portions of under-ripe, ripe and over-ripe bananas actually contain 34, 40 and 47 g of absorbable carbohydrate. Based on the dose–response curve for carbohydrate (Fig. 4.1), 34 and 40 g of available carbohydrate would be expected to elicit glycaemic responses 82% and 91% of that elicited by 47 g. Three groups have determined the glycaemic responses of under-ripe, ripe and over-ripe bananas. Wolever *et al.* (1988c) and Hermansen *et al.* (1992) found that the mean glycaemic response elicited by under-ripe bananas was 35% and 42%, respectively, less than that elicited by over-ripe bananas (both $P < 0.05$). By contrast, Ercan *et al.* (1993) found no significant difference. The GI values of bananas from Wolever *et al.* (1988c) are plotted against the % of carbohydrate malabsorbed in Fig. 4.13. Again, it can be seen

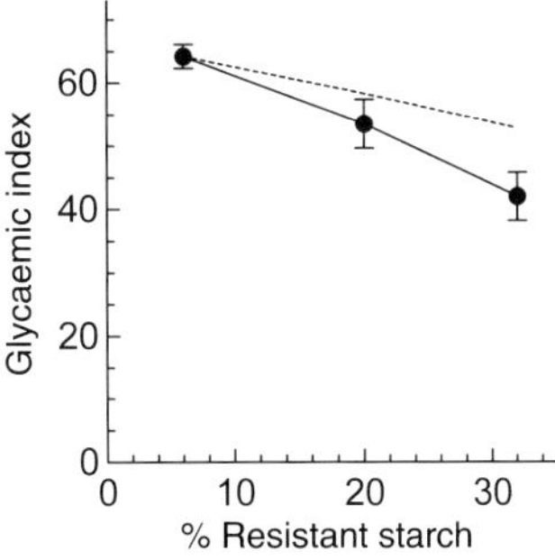


**Fig. 4.13.** GI of bananas (means ± SEM) of different degrees of ripeness plotted against % of carbohydrate malabsorbed (Englyst and Cummings, 1985; Wolever *et al.*, 1988c). Dotted line, theoretical effect of reducing carbohydrate intake by an amount equal to the proportion of carbohydrate malabsorbed.

that carbohydrate malabsorption accounted for less than half of the reduction in glycaemic response.

Schweizer *et al.* (1990) compared the digestion of starch from potatoes and beans using the ileostomy method and also measured glycaemic responses from the same foods. About 10% of dietary bean starch escaped digestion in the small intestine compared to about 2% in beans, a difference which does not explain the more than 50% reduction in peak glucose response.

## 4.5 Conclusions

Dietary carbohydrates influence glycaemic responses by at least four mechanisms: the nature of the monosaccharides absorbed, the amount of carbohydrate consumed, the proportion of the consumed carbohydrate absorbed and metabolized and the rate of carbohydrate absorption. Foods containing sugars other than glucose or maltose, which have a low GI, elicit low glycaemic responses because part or all of the monosaccharides absorbed is not glucose. Starchy foods with a low GI elicit low glycaemic responses primarily because the starch is slowly digested and absorbed. Some of the starch in foods escapes digestion in the small intestine, and the amount of undigested starch tends to be inversely related to the GI. However, a reduction in the amount of carbohydrate absorbed after low-GI foods is relatively small and only accounts for about 15–20% of the reduction in glycaemic response.

# 5

# Glycaemic Index: Application to Mixed Meals

Perhaps the major reason why the GI has not been (Hollenbeck *et al.*, 1988; American Diabetes Association, 1994) and continues (American Diabetes Association, 2002; Pi-Sunyer, 2002; Flint *et al.*, 2004) not to be accepted by everyone is the criticism, made very early on (Coulston *et al.*, 1984a,b), that the GI of individual foods does not apply in the setting of mixed meals which contain a combination of carbohydrate foods along with fat and protein. To a certain extent, one could consider the question of whether the GI can predict glycaemic responses of mixed meals to be irrelevant to the question of whether the GI is useful for the promotion of health or the prevention or treatment of diabetes or other conditions because it has been asserted by those on both sides of the GI debate that the results of acute test meal studies should not be used as evidence upon which to base nutrition recommendations for long-term health (Coulston *et al.*, 1984b; Hollenbeck *et al.*, 1986; Wolever, 1989). Nutrition recommendations should be based on the results of long-term studies in human subjects on health outcomes, pathophysiological mechanisms for disease or well-established risk factors or surrogate endpoints. Indeed, there is no paucity of such evidence for the GI, and it will be reviewed in later chapters.

However, the ability to predict postprandial glycaemic responses, *per se*, is of interest not only because it has clinical utility in some situations (e.g. selection of preprandial insulin dosage in type 1 diabetes), but also because it is an interesting area of investigation. I have been drawn into the debate not so much because I believe the outcome is critical to the GI concept, but because I feel the criticisms about the lack of utility of the GI in mixed meals are unfounded, being based on faulty methods and/or a naive treatment of what is actually an extremely complex area. Thus, although the authors of a relatively large number of papers conclude that their data show that the GI does not apply in mixed meals, I am not convinced by most of them, and in some cases I would assert that the data support the opposite conclusion! There are some good data which do not support the utility of the GI in mixed meals, and I will point them out below, but they are greatly outweighed by the supportive data.

The role of the GI in predicting the glycaemic responses of mixed meal is a very complex area. This chapter goes through, step by step, some of the major factors involved, beginning with an examination of the effects on glycaemic responses of mixing carbohydrate foods, followed by a review of the effects of adding fat and protein, and then on to consideration of mixed meals themselves. These effects may be modified in different types of subjects (e.g. those who have normal glucose tolerance, or have type 2 diabetes or type 1 diabetes) because the day-to-day variation of glycaemic responses varies in the different subject groups, or because mechanisms active in one group are not active in another (e.g. stimulation of insulin secretion).

## 5.1 Effect of Mixing Carbohydrate Foods on Glycaemic Responses

Logically, one would consider that when more than one carbohydrate foods are mixed together, the resulting glycaemic response should represent the combined effects of the amount of carbohydrate contributed by each food and the GI of each food, rather like mixing paint. This was suggested by the fact that in the original GI paper (Jenkins *et al.*, 1981a) the GI of sucrose, a disaccharide of glucose and fructose, was 59, a value which is almost exactly the average of the GI values of glucose, 100 and fructose, 20 (Fig. 5.1). When the glycaemic response elicited by 50 g sucrose was compared with that elicited by 25 g glucose plus 25 g fructose in five subjects, the curves were almost identical (Fig. 5.2). Later, we showed that the plasma glucose and insulin responses elicited by 100 g sucrose were similar to those elicited by 50 g glucose plus 50 g fructose in eight normal subjects (Fig. 5.2) (Lee and Wolever, 1998).

This led us to determine the effect on glycaemic response of mixtures of various different carbohydrate foods in normal subjects and subjects with diabetes. In one series of studies, we determined the effect of 50 g available carbohydrate from white bread, 50 g available carbohydrate from navy beans, or a meal consisting of 25 g available carbohydrate from white bread plus 25 g available carbohydrate from navy beans, in normal subjects (Wolever *et al.*, 1985), and in subjects with both type 1 and type 2 diabetes (Jenkins *et al.*, 1984). It was hypothesized that the incremental area under the glucose response curve elicited by the bread and beans mixed meals would be the average of those elicited by bread alone and beans alone. In normal subjects, navy beans elicited a glycaemic response area 56% that of bread, resulting in an expected response for the mixed meal of (100 + 56)/2 = 78%. The observed response was 77% (Fig. 5.3). Likewise, in subjects with type 2 diabetes, navy beans had a glycaemic response 41% that of bread resulting in an expected response for the mixed meal of 70.5%; the observed response, 60 ± 8%, was not significantly different from that expected (Fig. 5.3).

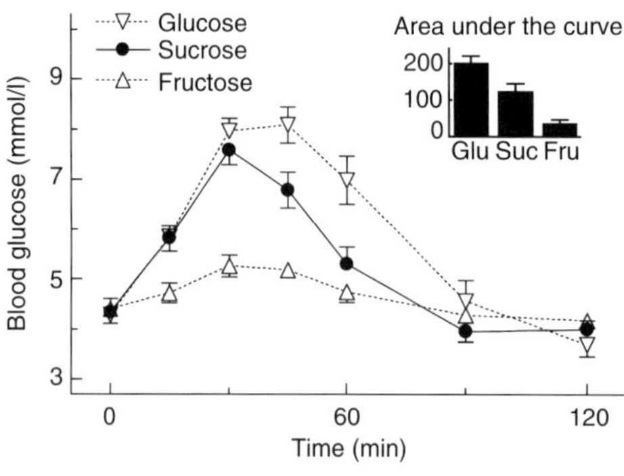


**Fig. 5.1.** Glycaemic responses and incremental areas under the curve elicited by 50 g glucose, sucrose or fructose in normal subjects. Data from Jenkins *et al.* (1981a).

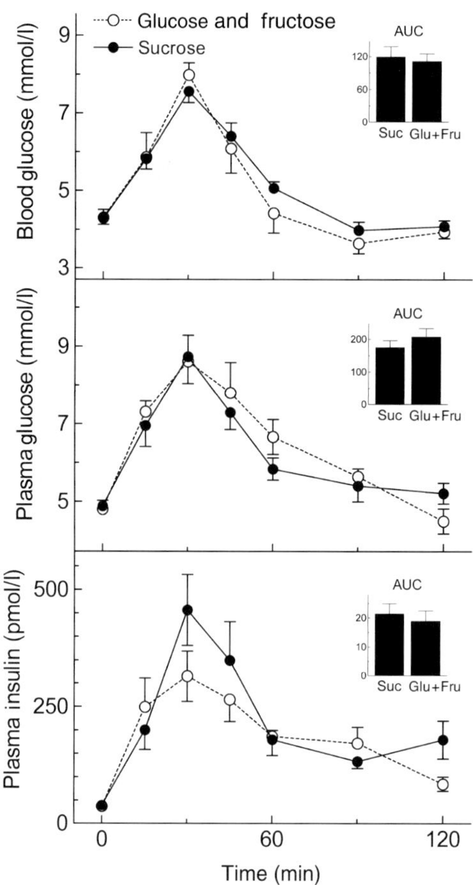


**Fig. 5.2.** Glucose and insulin responses and incremental areas under the curve (AUC) elicited by sucrose or glucose plus fructose in normal subjects. Top: 50 g sucrose vs 25 g glucose plus 25 g fructose (data for glucose/fructose obtained from the same subjects who tested sucrose (Jenkins *et al.*, 1981a) but results were not included in the original publication). Middle (plasma glucose) and bottom (plasma insulin): 100 g sucrose vs 50 g glucose plus 50 g fructose (Lee and Wolever, 1998).

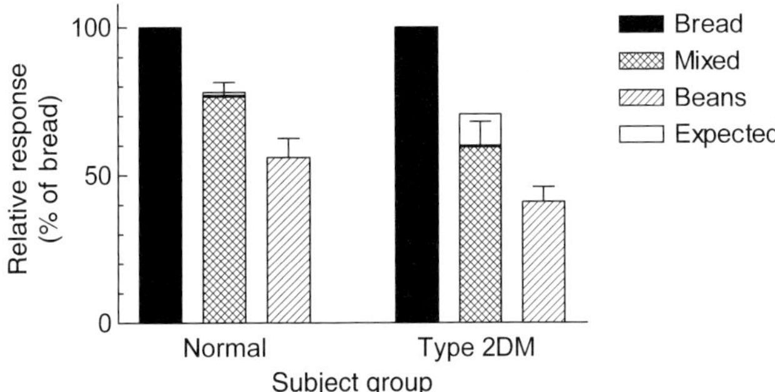


**Fig. 5.3.** Incremental area under the glucose response curves after test meals containing 50 g available carbohydrate (AC) from navy beans (beans) or 25 g AC from bread plus 25 g AC from beans (mixed) expressed as a percentage of that after 50 g AC from white bread (Bread) in normal subjects (Wolever *et al.*, 1985) or subjects with type 2 diabetes (Type 2DM; Jenkins *et al.*, 1984). The expected result for the mixed meal was taken to be the average of the means for bread alone and beans alone. Values are means ± SEM.

In subjects with type 1 diabetes, the situation was less clear. The incremental glycaemic response after beans was 84% of that after bread, much higher than the values of 56% and 41% seen in normal and type 2 diabetic subjects. Also, the response of the bread and beans mixed meal tended to be less than that of beans alone (Fig. 5.4). However, these results were confounded by differences in FBG at the start of the test, with fasting glucose before beans being 3 mmol/l less than before bread, and fasting glucose before the mixed meal being 1.5 mmol/l higher than before bread (Fig. 5.5). We have seen before (Chapter 2, this volume) that the IAUC after bread is inversely related to the fasting glucose level. Thus, the observed AUC after beans was greater than would have been expected if the fasting glucose before the meal had been the same as that before the bread meal; similarly, the observed AUC after the mixed meal was less than would be expected if the fasting glucose had been lower.

The effect of differences in fasting glucose can be corrected for by expressing the glycaemic response after each test meal as a percentage of estimated response after bread with the same fasting glucose level as the test meal. For example, Fig. 5.6 shows the results for the trials of white bread performed by one subject with type 1 diabetes who participated in the beans study; it shows a tight inverse correlation between AUC and

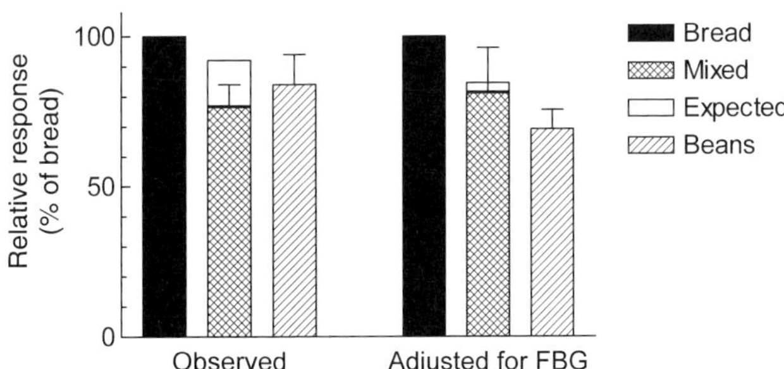


**Fig. 5.4.** Incremental area under the glucose response curves after test meals containing 50 g available carbohydrate (AC) from navy beans (beans) or 25 g AC from bread plus 25 g AC from beans (mixed) expressed as a percentage of that after 50 g AC from white bread (Bread) in subjects with type 1 diabetes (Jenkins *et al.*, 1984). The expected result for the mixed meal was taken to be the average of the means for bread alone and beans alone. Figure 5.5 shows the glycaemic responses for these meals. See text and Table 5.1 for explanation of how adjustment for fasting glucose (FBG) was done. Values are means ± SEM.

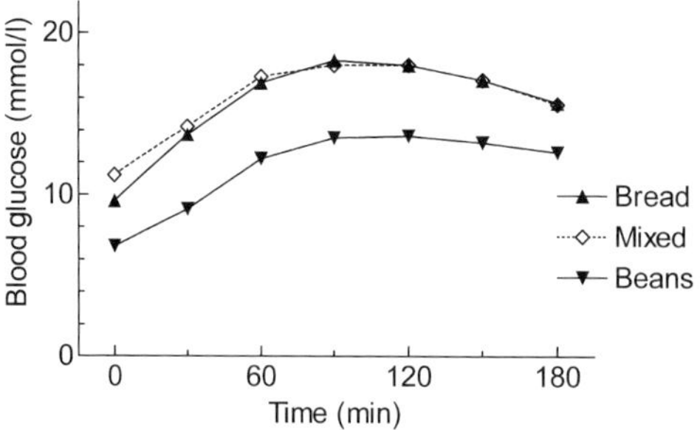


**Fig. 5.5.** Mean blood glucose responses elicited by test meals containing 50 g available carbohydrate (AC) from navy beans (beans) or 25 g AC from bread plus 25 g AC from beans (mixed) expressed as a percentage of that after 50 g AC from white bread (bread) in subjects with type 1 diabetes (data from Jenkins *et al.*, 1984; areas under the curves shown in Fig. 5.4). This illustrates the differences in fasting glucose before the different test meals (see text and Fig. 5.4).

fasting glucose. Using the regression equation, white bread AUC values can be estimated for the levels of fasting glucose observed for the test foods (Table 5.1) and the resulting values used to calculate the relative responses of the foods adjusted for differences in fasting glucose. The resulting mean adjusted response for beans alone is 69% that of bread. Therefore, the expected response for the mixed meal is $(100 + 69)/2 = 84.5$, a value very similar to the observed relative response adjusted for fasting glucose, 82% (Fig.

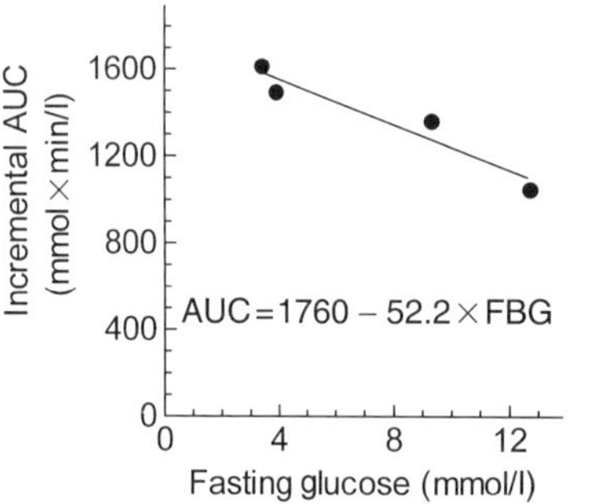


**Fig. 5.6.** Correlation between fasting blood glucose and incremental area under the curve (AUC) elicited by a 50 g available carbohydrate portion of white bread repeated four times by a subject who participated in the studies shown in Figs 5.4 and 5.5 (Jenkins *et al.*, 1984).

5.4). Thus, once adjusted for the effects of differences in fasting glucose, the results of the mixed meal tests in subjects with type 1 diabetes were consistent with those in normal and type 2 diabetic subjects. However, although these adjustments convinced us, it would have been better to repeat the experiment using methods to ensure that fasting glucose was within a narrow range on the morning of the tests.

## 5.2 Effects of Fat on Glycaemic Responses

It is generally accepted that adding fat to carbohydrate reduces postprandial glycaemic responses by delaying gastric emptying, and it has been suggested that the ability of fat to substantially change the glycaemic responses elicited by individual foods reduces the clinical utility of the GI (Beebe, 1999; Pi-Sunyer, 2002). The problem with this conclusion, however, is that most studies examining the effect of fat on metabolic responses used much larger amounts of fat than recommended, and only included a single level of fat, so that there is little information about the effect of varying fat across a normal range of intakes. In addition, it is not widely appreciated that the effect of fat on glycaemic responses varies substantially in different subjects and may be influenced by various factors including the subject's habitual diet (Morgan *et al.*, 1988a,b; Cunningham *et al.*, 1991), the nature of the fatty acids fed (Gatti *et al.*,1992) and the way in which the fat is incorporated into the test meal (Cunningham and Read, 1989). Finally, the results of studies in which fat is added to carbohydrate may not be applicable to recommended diets in which the energy content of different meals is constant. In this situation, energy from fat is substituted for energy from carbohydrate; thus, high-fat diets usually contain a reduced amount of carbohydrate.

### 5.2.1 Effects of fat added to fixed amount of carbohydrate

Figure 5.7 shows the results of a number of studies in which different amounts of fat were added to test meals containing predominantly carbohydrate

**Table 5.1.** Results of tests of beans, bread and a mixed meal of beans plus bread in one subject with type 1 diabetes illustrating how the relative responses were adjusted for differences in fasting glucose.

| | Beans alone | Beans and bread |
|---|---|---|
| Test food: observed FBG (mmol/l) | 3.9 | 12.5 |
| Test food: observed AUC (mmol × min/l) | 935 | 930 |
| White bread: observed FBG (mmol/l) | 12.7 | 12.7 |
| White bread: observed AUC (mmol × min/l) | 1047 | 1047 |
| Observed relative response of test food (%) | 89 | 89 |
| White bread: AUC adjusted for FBG (mmol × min/l) | 1556 | 1108 |
| Adjusted relative response (%) adjusted for FBG | 60 | 84 |

FBG = fasting blood glucose; AUC = incremental area under the blood glucose response curve.
Adjustment done using individual regression equation of AUC after white bread on FBG (Fig. 5.6). The regression equation is AUC = 1760 – 52.2 × FBG. For beans, FBG = 3.9, therefore the adjusted AUC for white bread = 1760 – 52.2 × 3.9 = 1760 – 204 = 1556. Thus, the adjusted relative response is 100 × 935/1556 = 60.

(Collier and O'Dea, 1983; Collier *et al.*, 1984; Jenkins *et al.*, 1984; Simpson *et al.*, 1985; Krotkiewski *et al.*, 1987; Welch *et al.*, 1987; Gannon *et al.*,1993; Murphy *et al.*, 1995; Owen and Wolever, 2003). The panel on the left of Fig. 5.7 shows the effect of fat on the incremental area under the blood glucose response curve while that on the right shows the effect of fat on the peak rise of blood glucose. The experimental designs of these studies differ with different amounts and types of fat and carbohydrate. Nevertheless, some sense appears to be achieved by plotting the incremental area under the glycaemic response curve or peak rise elicited by the high-fat meals expressed as a percentage of the response elicited by the low-fat meal on the grams fat added per gram of carbohydrate. Several points are apparent from Fig. 5.7. First, fat appears to have little or no effect on postprandial blood glucose in people with diabetes, but reduces glycaemic responses in normal subjects. This is an important clinical point which does not appear to be well known. I have often heard people with diabetes being advised to add sources of fat and protein to a carbohydrate snack, particularly a pre-bed snack, to help delay and prolong the rise in blood glucose. Certainly, current data suggest that fat has no such effect in people with diabetes.

Another important point about the effect of fat on glycaemic responses in normal subjects is

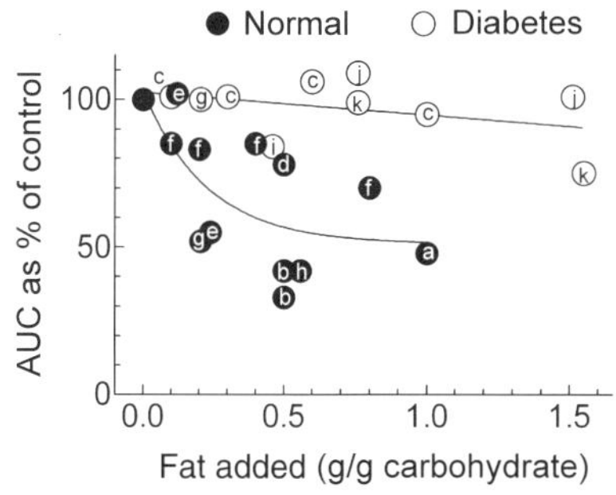


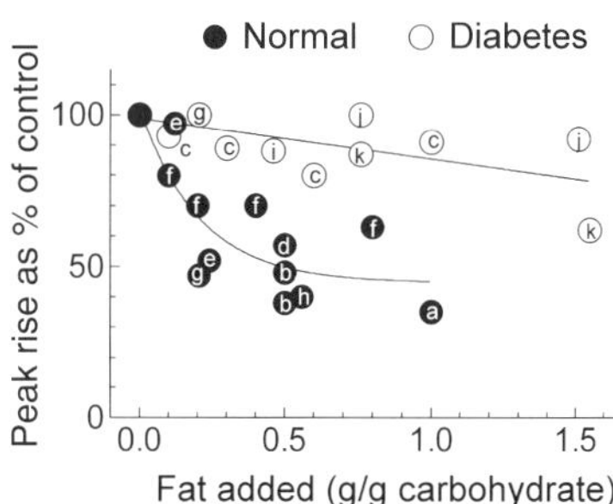


**Fig. 5.7.** Effects on incremental area under the curve (AUC, left) and peak rise (right) of adding various amounts of fat to carbohydrate in normal subjects and subjects with diabetes. Identification of points: a, Collier and O'Dea (1983) (butter added to boiled potato); b, Collier *et al.* (1984) (butter added to boiled potato or lentils); c, Gannon *et al.* (1993) (butter added to mashed potato); d, Krotkiewski *et al.* (1987) (butter added to boiled potato); e, Murphy *et al.* (1995) (cream, cheese and margarine increased in a mixed meal); f, Owen and Wolever (2003) (canola oil margarine added to bread); g, Simpson *et al.* (1985) (cream added to maize starch); h, Welch *et al.* (1987) (maize oil added to mashed potato); i, Jenkins *et al.* (1984) (butter added to bread); j, Rasmussen *et al.* (1996) (olive oil); k, Rasmussen *et al.* (1996) (butter).

that the shape of the dose–response curve may not be linear, with most of the effect occurring at relatively low levels of added fat (Fig. 5.7). Only two of the studies shown in Fig. 5.7 included a wide range of doses of fat, and one of these was in subjects with diabetes in whom fat had no effect. We studied the effect of adding 5, 10, 20 or 40 g fat as canola oil margarine to bread in normal subjects (Owen and Wolever, 2003), and obtained a generally smaller effect than most other studies shown on the figure. Nevertheless, the shape of the dose–response curve was similar to that for all of the studies, with a relatively large effect from adding a small amount of fat, with little further effect as the amount of fat added is increased. Most of the other studies on the figure used butter as the source of added fat. However, the difference in results cannot be explained by the type of fat used. Butter was the source of fat in study 'd' (Krotkiewski *et al.*, 1987), which obtained similar results to our study (study 'f'). However, unsaturated fat was used in studies 'e' (Murphy *et al.*, 1995) and 'h' (Welch *et al.*, 1987) which obtained the same results as most of the butter studies. One factor which might explain the difference is that we added fat to bread, whereas most other studies added fat to potato. However, Gatti *et al.* (1992) found that adding both maize oil and olive oil (35 g fat to 75 g carb) to bread reduced the incremental glycaemic response area by 70–80%. In studies with head-to-head comparisons of different types of fat, some have found that glycaemic responses are higher after saturated than unsaturated fat is added to carbohydrate (Gatti *et al.*, 1992; Dworatzek *et al.*, 2004) while others have found no difference (MacIntosh *et al.*, 2003).

The implication of the fact that the shape of the dose–response curve is in the form of an exponential decay is that the effect on glycaemic responses of varying fat across the normal (or usual, or recommended) range of intakes, approximately 20–45% of energy, is really rather small. The range corresponds roughly to about 0.2–0.4 g fat per gram of carbohydrate, across which range the regression line has only a small slope. This suggests that variation in fat across this range has little effect on glycaemic responses and, therefore, does not have any important confounding effect on the utility of the GI.

Using IAUC to show the effect of fat on glycaemic responses (Fig. 5.7, left) tends to underestimate the effect because fat usually delays the rise in blood glucose, but also delays the fall. Thus, fat reduces blood glucose concentrations for the first hour after eating, but increases them thereafter (Fig. 5.8). Thus, there can be a marked effect on the shape of the glycaemic response curve without much effect on the overall AUC. Figure 5.7 (right) shows the effect of fat on the peak rise of blood glucose; the effects tend to be larger than those for AUC, and also more consistent between the different studies.

### 5.2.2 Mechanism for the effect of fat on glycaemic responses

#### *5.2.2.1 Delayed gastric emptying*

It is generally considered that fat reduces glycaemic responses by delaying gastric emptying (Welch *et al.*, 1987). The delay in gastric emptying may be, at least in part, due to both acute and chronic effects of fat in stimulating gut hormones such as gastric inhibitory polypeptide (GIP) (Collier and O'Dea, 1983; Morgan *et al.*, 1988a,b) and glucagon-like peptide-1 (GLP-1) (Herrmann *et al.*, 1995; Drucker, 1998). However, ingested carbohydrate and protein also increase postprandial GIP and GLP-1 to a similar extent as fat (D'Alessio *et al.*, 1993; Elliott *et al.*, 1993; Herrmann *et al.*, 1995). Indeed the secretion of these gut hormones is regulated by a wide variety of intestinal endocrine and neurocrine peptides as well as nutrients

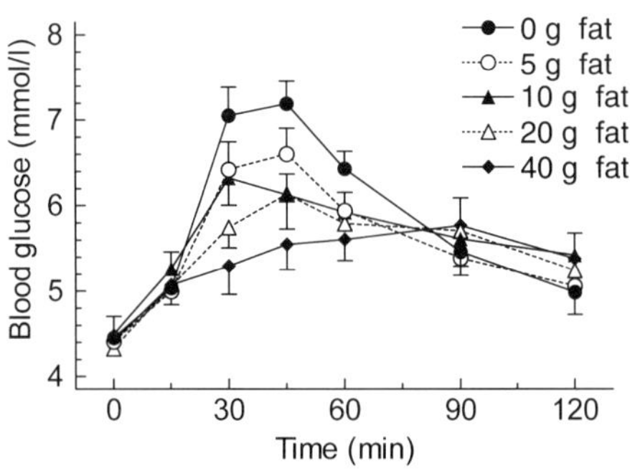


**Fig. 5.8.** Effect on glycaemic responses of normal subjects of adding various amounts of fat (as non-hydrogenated canola oil margarine) to 50 g available carbohydrate portions of white bread (Owen and Wolever, 2003). Values are means ± SEM.

and neurotransmitters (Brubaker, 1991; Roberge and Brubaker, 1991, 1993; Rocca and Brubaker, 1995). In addition, GLP-1 secretion is influenced by plasma long-chain (Ranganath *et al.*, 1999a,b) and short-chain (Reimer and McBurney, 1996), non-esterified or free fatty acids, glucose (Morgan *et al.*, 1988a) and amino acids (Herrmann *et al.*, 1995). Thus, the fact that adding fat to a meal delays gastric emptying is likely not a specific effect of fat, but is a general response to consuming additional nutrients. It is of interest that the responses of GIP and GLP-1 to oral carbohydrate and intravenous FFAs differ in lean and obese subjects (Ranganath *et al.*, 1996, 1999a). This type of effect might underlie the difference in the effect of fat on glycaemic responses in normal and diabetic subjects (Fig. 5.7).

Fat tends to reduce the initial rise of blood glucose after eating, but also, in some studies, delays the fall of blood glucose or creates a second peak (Normand *et al.*, 2001; Owen and Wolever, 2003) (Fig. 5.8). This pattern is compatible with delayed gastric emptying, but is delayed gastric emptying the only mechanism by which fat reduced glucose responses? Normand *et al.* (2001) showed that when 40 g fat was added to a $^{13}$C-labelled carbohydrate meal, the rate of appearance of dietary carbohydrate into the circulation was delayed, compatible with delayed gastric emptying. However, when 15 g fat was added to the meal blood glucose was reduced with no change in the rate of appearance of dietary glucose into the circulation. This is not compatible with delayed gastric emptying as an explanation for the reduced blood glucose response and suggests that another (unknown) mechanism must exist. It is possible to argue that the rate of appearance of dietary carbohydrate into the circulation may not change in the face of a reduced rate of absorption if less glucose was taken up by the liver; but this does not explain why blood glucose was reduced. However, it suggests a third mechanism by which fat may influence postprandial glucose metabolism, namely, altered hepatic uptake or release of glucose. Indeed, Normand *et al.* (2001) showed that the 40 g fat meal was associated with increased hepatic glucose output about 2–5 h after eating, contributing to a second peak of blood glucose, and corresponding in time with increased concentrations of plasma FFAs, a factor known to increase hepatic glucose output (Boden *et al.*, 1994; Lewis *et al.*, 1998).

#### *5.2.2.2 Increased hepatic glucose output*

We (Dworatzek *et al.*, 2004) and others (Gatti *et al.*, 1992) have found that different fat sources influence postprandial glucose responses differently, with plasma glucose after butter-containing meals being higher than after meals containing olive or maize/safflower oils, which are rich in monounsaturated and polyunsaturated fatty acids, respectively. It is possible that this might be due to an effect on hepatic glucose output based on differences in the route by which butter is absorbed compared to olive or maize oils. The process of fat absorption is well known; dietary fat is hydrolysed by pancreatic lipase to fatty acids and monoglycerides, which are absorbed into enterocytes in the small intestine. The absorbed fatty acids and monoglycerides are reassembled to triglycerides which are incorporated into chylomicrons, which in turn, are secreted by the enterocyte into the lymphatic circulation from which they enter the peripheral blood stream. However, not all the absorbed fatty acids are incorporated into chylomicrons; some enter the portal circulation as free fatty acids, and travel directly to the liver.

Studies in rats suggest that a significant proportion of fatty acids are absorbed via the portal vein, 29% for palmitic acid (C16:0), 19% for lauric acid (C12:0) and 83% for octanoic acid (C8:0) (Sigalet and Martin, 1999). The reason for these differences is not known, but they may be explained, at least in part, by differences in the affinity of specific fatty acids for intestinal fatty acid binding protein (FABP2), the protein involved in the transport of fatty acids from luminal membrane of the enterocyte to the endoplasmic reticulum for assembly into chylomicrons (Black, 1995). Human FABP2 has the highest binding affinity for long-chain dietary fatty acids, palmitic, stearic, oleic and linoleic acids, with the binding affinities tending to be lower as the chain length decreases (Richieri *et al.*, 2000). This is not entirely consistent with the absorption patterns of palmitic, lauric and octanoic acids found in the rat by Sigalet and Martin (1999). However, reduced incorporation of fatty acids into chylomicrons might explain why chylomicron triglyceride after consumption of butter was lower than after safflower and olive oils (Dworatzek *et al.*, 2004). Butter contains about 25% of its fat as short- and medium-chain fatty acids, compared to olive oil which contains about 75% oleic acid and safflower oil which has about 75% linoleic acid. Thus, the fatty acids in butter may be less likely to bind to FABP2 and transported to the sites of chylomicron synthesis, and more likely to be absorbed via the portal vein. High portal fatty acids, in turn, may increase hepatic glucose output and account for the higher plasma glucose response seen after butter.

#### 5.2.2.3 *Increased insulin secretion*

Yet another mechanism by which fat may influence postprandial blood glucose is by stimulating insulin secretion. Plasma insulin concentrations after adding fat to carbohydrate are not usually different from those elicited by the carbohydrate alone for 3–4 h after eating despite significantly lower plasma glucose concentrations (Ercan *et al.*, 1994; Normand *et al.*, 2001). This suggests that fat enhances the ability of glucose to stimulate insulin secretion. Collier *et al.* (1988) demonstrated this by showing an increased insulin and c-peptide response to intravenous glucose given 15 min after a high-fat meal. It was suggested that this was due to rising levels of GIP in response to fat ingestion. Acute rises of circulating FFAs are also known to increase insulin secretion from the β-cell directly (Prentki and Corkey, 1996; Carpentier *et al.*, 1999), but it is unlikely that this mechanism can explain the effect seen by Collier *et al.* (1988) because it is likely that serum FFAs would have been falling 15 min after ingestion of the test meal (Normand *et al.*, 2001). High-serum FFAs may have accounted for the increased plasma insulin concentrations occurring 3–7 h after a single high-fat meal, compared to a low-fat meal (Normand *et al.*, 2001). However, when Ercan *et al.* (1994) followed a high-fat breakfast by either a low-fat or a high-fat lunch, plasma insulin responses after lunch (i.e. 4–8 h after breakfast) were not increased despite markedly increased plasma FFA concentrations.

### 5.2.3 Isocaloric substitution of fat and carbohydrate

Studies in which fat is added to a fixed amount of carbohydrate are useful to understand the effects of fat on postprandial metabolism, but their results cannot be applied to practical diets because simply adding fat to carbohydrate markedly increases the energy content of a meal. Any theoretical benefit to be gained from the reduction in blood glucose seen with added fat would probably be offset by the increase in energy intake and resultant weight gain. Thus, any increases in fat intake which might be recommended would have to occur by isocaloric substitution of the added fat for either protein or carbohydrate. Thus, a number of studies have looked at the effect of isocaloric exchange of fat and carbohydrate on glycaemic responses.

Whitley *et al.* (1997) studied the effect of isocaloric variation in fat and carbohydrate on metabolic responses after normal subjects consumed four different meals. The meals contained a mixture of foods, and contained fat:carbohydrate:protein (% energy) as follows: 44:49:7, 65:28:7, 74:20:6 and 100:0:0. Glucose and insulin increased linearly with increasing carbohydrate and decreasing fat content, whereas postprandial chylomicrons and free fatty acids decreased. In accord with general concepts about fuel utilization (Flatt, 1995), carbohydrate oxidation decreased and fat oxidation increased as the fat content of the meal increased. In addition, carbohydrate balance decreased and fat balance increased as the fat content of the meals increased. Balance of a nutrient represents intake minus expenditure. Thus, with the 49% energy carbohydrate meal, some carbohydrate was stored (i.e. not oxidized) over the 5-h period of the study. However, the amount stored fell to zero with the 20% carbohydrate meal. By contrast, the amount of fat stored after each meal increased by 50% from 23 to 35 kJ/kg as the fat content of the meal increased from 44% to 74%.

We did a study to see if the fat content of a meal influenced the relative glycaemic effects of carbohydrate foods in subjects with type 2 diabetes (Wolever *et al.*, 1992a). Subjects consumed six different test meals containing the same amount of energy but varying in fat and carbohydrate content such that their composition of fat:carbohydrate:protein (% energy) was as follows: 55:29:16 (high fat), 35:49:16 (medium fat) and 16:69:15 (low fat). For each level of carbohydrate and fat, the carbohydrate source was either white bread or white spaghetti. Our results were consistent with those of Whitley *et al.* (1997) in that blood glucose and insulin responses increased linearly with increasing carbohydrate, while postprandial triglycerides and FFAs decreased. The novel aspect of this study was the demonstration that the glycaemic response elicited by spaghetti, expressed as a percentage of that elicited by bread, did not differ significantly ($F_{(2,30)} = 0.60$, $P > 0.25$) in the low- (74 ± 8%), medium- (62 ± 13%) and high-fat (55 ± 12%) meals, and these values were similar to our previously published GI value for spaghetti (tested alone, i.e. 2% energy as fat), 60 ± 10 (Jenkins *et al.*, 1983).

These studies both suggest that when fat is substituted on an isocaloric basis for carbohydrate, the reduced glycaemic responses of high-fat meals could be explained by the reduced carbohydrate intake as opposed to any effect of fat. This issue will be discussed in more detail below (Section 5.7).

## 5.3 Effects of Protein on Glycaemic Responses

There have been more systematic studies done on the effects of adding protein to carbohydrate than there have been on the effects of adding fat to carbohydrate. Several dose–response studies exist, and the effects of different kinds of protein and amino acids have been studied. The results of these studies show that it is not possible to generalize about the effects of protein on glycaemic responses because the effects vary considerably for different types of proteins and amino acids.

Figure 5.9 shows the effect of various doses of protein when added to carbohydrate on blood glucose (left) and insulin (right) responses in various subjects from three dose–response studies (Nuttall *et al.*, 1984; Spiller *et al.*, 1987; Westphal *et al.*, 1990) and two other studies (Jenkins *et al.*, 1984; Gulliford *et al.*, 1989). Study 'e' (Spiller *et al.*, 1987) shows a marked effect of protein on reducing glucose and increasing insulin responses; here a mixture of milk and soy proteins was added to a mixture of maltodextrin, fructose and lactose. Study 'd' (Nuttall *et al.*, 1984) shows a moderate effect of lean beef added to glucose on reducing glucose and a marked effect on increasing insulin in subjects with type 2 diabetes. However, a later study by the same group (study 'a', Westphal *et al.*, 1990) showed that adding lean beef to glucose had no effect on glucose and insulin responses in normal subjects. It is difficult to reconcile the differences between these three dose–response studies – if the difference between the two studies in normal subjects is due to a lack of effect of beef protein, then why did beef protein have marked effects on insulin secretion in subjects with type 2 diabetes, who should have impaired insulin secretion? The other two studies in Fig. 5.9 show no effect of protein on glucose responses.

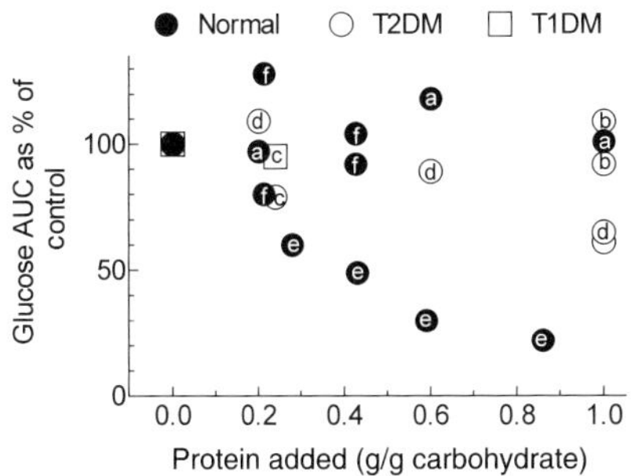


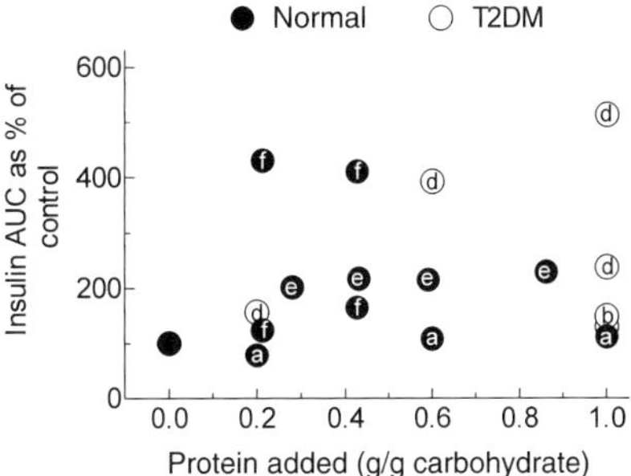


**Fig. 5.9.** Effects on incremental area under the curve (AUC) of glucose (left) and insulin (right) of adding various amounts of protein to carbohydrate in normal subjects and subjects with type 1 (T1DM) or type 2 (T2DM) diabetes. Identification of points: a, Westphal *et al.* (1990) (lean beef added to glucose); b, Gulliford *et al.* (1989) (tuna fish added to mashed potato or spaghetti); c, Jenkins *et al.* (1984) (skim cheese added to bread for T2DM subjects and peanut butter added to bread for T1DM subjects); d, Nuttall *et al.* (1984) (lean beef added to glucose); e, Spiller *et al.* (1987) (mixture of milk and soy proteins added to a mixture of maltodextrin, fructose and lactose); f, Liljeberg *et al.* (2001).

Table 5.2 shows the effect on mean glucose and insulin responses of different types of protein and amino acids in normal and diabetic subjects. In subjects with type 2 diabetes, Gannon *et al.* (1988) found that different protein sources added to glucose, all increased plasma insulin responses by two- to threefold compared to glucose alone. However, the effects on plasma glucose responses varied significantly ranging from no effect (egg white) to nearly a 40% reduction for cottage cheese. The results of van Loon *et al.* (2000) are even more varied. Most of the protein sources increased insulin responses by about 40–50%, but arginine tended to reduce plasma insulin, and pea hydrolysate and casein had very little effect. By contrast, the effects on plasma glucose were quite varied, and there was no relationship between plasma glucose and insulin responses. After arginine, both glucose and insulin tended to be reduced, whereas wheat hydrolysate raised both plasma glucose and insulin. Several treatments raised plasma insulin by over 40%, but the effects on glucose varied from a 73% reduction to a 12% increase. The authors concluded that the insulin responses were positively correlated with plasma leucine, phenylalanine and tyrosine concentrations.

Presumably, the reason why it is not possible to generalize about the effects of protein on glucose responses is that there are a number of potential mechanisms by which protein can affect glucose metabolism, and these not only operate in different directions (e.g. protein tends to increase both insulin and glucagon secretion, the former of which would reduce and the latter increase blood glucose concentrations) but also would be confounded by differences in the rates of digestion of proteins and the absorption and metabolism of the individual amino acids.

Amino acids stimulate insulin secretion (Floyd *et al.*, 1968), and this is believed to be the basis for the effect of protein in stimulating insulin secretion. Increased insulin secretion, therefore, is one mechanism by which protein influences postprandial glucose responses. However, the relationship between the changes in plasma insulin response and the changes in plasma glucose response induced by addition of protein to carbohydrate is not very close, indicating that other mechanisms are influencing the glycaemic response. Figure 5.10 plots

**Table 5.2.** Effect of different types of proteins and amino acids added to oral glucose on plasma glucose and insulin responses.

| Subjects[a] | Proteins/amino acids added to carbohydrate | RGR[b] | RIR[b] |
|---|---|---|---|
| T2DM | Beef | 90 | 218 |
| T2DM | Turkey | 80 | 202 |
| T2DM | Gelatin | 67 | 266 |
| T2DM | Egg white | 100 | 191 |
| T2DM | Cottage cheese | 62 | 355 |
| T2DM | Fish (sole) | 89 | 218 |
| T2DM | Soy | 65 | 210 |
| Normal 1 | Arginine | 85 | 70 |
| Normal 1 | Arginine + phenylalanine + leucine | 27 | 157 |
| Normal 1 | Arginine + phenylalanine + leucine + glutamine | 85 | 155 |
| Normal 1 | Whey hydrolysate | 53 | 143 |
| Normal 1 | Pea hydrolysate | 40 | 111 |
| Normal 1 | Wheat hydrolysate | 112 | 159 |
| Normal 1 | Casein | 68 | 109 |
| Normal 1 | Phenylalanine + leucine + wheat hydrolysate | 41 | 153 |
| Normal 1 | Arginine + phenylalanine + leucine + wheat hydrolysate | 46 | 142 |
| Normal 2 | Glycine | 47 | 103 |

[a]T2DM: type 2 diabetes: 25 g protein added to 50 g glucose (Gannon *et al.*, 1988).
[b]Mean incremental area under the glucose (RGR) and insulin (RIR) response curve over 0–2 h expressed as a % of that for carbohydrate alone.
Normal 1: normal subjects: 57 g protein/amino acid added to 57 g glucose plus 57 g maltodextrin (van Loon *et al.*, 2000).
Normal 2: normal subjects: 4.6 g glycine added to 25 g glucose (Gannon *et al.*, 2002).

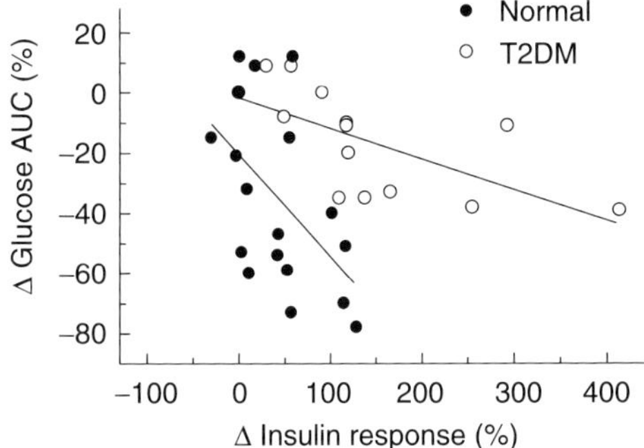


**Fig. 5.10.** Relationships between per cent changes in glucose and insulin responses elicited by adding protein to carbohydrate in normal subjects and subjects with type 2 diabetes. Data from Fig. 5.9 and Table 5.2. Correlation coefficients: normal subjects, $r = -0.528$ ($P = 0.024$); diabetes, $r = -0.654$ ($P = 0.011$). The significance of the difference between slopes for normal (−0.34) and diabetic subjects (−0.10) was $P = 0.069$.

changes in glucose response and insulin response for the data shown in Fig. 5.9 and Table 5.2. The correlation between change in insulin and change in glucose is significant in both in normal ($P = 0.024$) and diabetic ($P = 0.011$) subjects, but the variation in insulin responses only accounts for about 30–40% of the variation in glucose responses. In addition, the subjects with diabetes (open circles) tend to have a lower slope than normal subjects, indicating that for any given increase in insulin response, the magnitude of the reduction in glucose response is 70–75% less than that seen in normal subjects. This is consistent with our understanding of the pathogenesis of type 2 diabetes in which insulin resistance is a predominant feature.

Proteins which are slowly absorbed and do not raise plasma amino acids, therefore, would not stimulate insulin secretion. The relatively poor digestibility of egg white relative to cottage cheese has been proposed to explain why the latter raises insulin more than the former when added to glucose (Nuttall and Gannon, 1990). However, this does not explain why, for example, arginine failed to stimulate insulin secretion in normal subjects (van Loon *et al.*, 2000; Table 5.2), despite the fact that it raised plasma arginine levels, and arginine is a potent stimulus to insulin secretion when given intravenously (Floyd *et al.*, 1968). Some proteins might reduce plasma glucose responses by delaying gastric emptying, as it has been suggested for casein (Lang *et al.*, 1999a), or by stimulating a gut hormone which potentiates the effect of insulin on glucose removal from the circulation (Gannon *et al.*, 2002).

There are several mechanisms by which protein may raise plasma glucose including stimulation of glucagon secretion (Gannon *et al.*, 1988, 2002; Westphal *et al.*, 1990), the conversion of some amino acids to glucose (Kahn *et al.*, 1992; Tappy *et al.*, 1992; Gannon *et al.*, 2001a) and an effect of amino acids to increase insulin resistance (Tessari *et al.*, 1985; Boden and Tappy, 1990; Flakoll *et al.*, 1991; Pisters *et al.*, 1991). In this context, it is of interest that reduction of dietary protein from 12% to 0% energy reduced insulin requirements in subjects with type 1 diabetes by about 25%, and in normal subjects, reduced hepatic glucose output and fasting insulin by about 20%, and increased fasting glucagon by 24% (Larivière *et al.*, 1994). The acute blood glucose-raising effects of protein are most readily seen in subjects with type 1 diabetes, and several studies show that the addition of protein to test meals increases acute blood glucose responses. Adding 21 g protein to a meal containing 51 g carbohydrate and 10 g fat increased the glycaemic response AUC (0–3 h) by 63% (Simpson *et al.*, 1985); adding 9 g protein and 10 g fat to a meal containing 38 g carbohydrate, 10 g protein and 4 g fat increased the glycaemic response area (0–3 h) by 61% in children with type 1 diabetes (Wang *et al.*, 1991), and adding 51 g protein to a mixed meal containing 58 g carbohydrate, 25 g protein and 13 g fat increased the area under the glycaemic response curve (0–5 h) by about 20% (Peters and Davidson, 1993). In the latter study, over the period from 2.5 to 5 h, the area under the glucose curve was increased by 100% after the high-protein meal. Although consumption of protein alone tends to have no effect or reduce blood glucose concentrations postprandially in normal (Nuttall and Gannon, 1990) and type 2 diabetic subjects (Nuttall *et al.*, 1984; Gannon *et al.*, 2001a), it has been recently shown that the fall in blood glucose after consuming protein alone in normal subjects is directly related to the subject's insulin sensitivity. Subjects who were more insulin sensitive showed the largest falls in blood glucose after consuming a 75 g protein load (Brand-Miller *et al.*, 2000).

## 5.4 Effects of Combination of Fat and Protein on Glycaemic Responses

A number of studies have examined the effects of adding combinations of protein and fat to single carbohydrate foods, adding more protein and fat to mixed meals which already contain some protein and fat, or altering the source of protein in a mixed meal. The results of these studies are sometimes difficult to interpret because of possible unknown confounding effects of other meal components. Many of the effects are isolated observations of effects which are difficult to explain. In general, a combination of protein and fat tends to have larger effects on postprandial glucose than either alone, but this is not always the case and the dose–response effects are not known.

### 5.4.1 Studies in normal subjects

Pelletier *et al.* (1998) published the results of two experiments on the effect of cream cheese on glucose responses in normal subjects. In the first experiment, the control meal was bread, butter and jam (7 g protein, 11 g fat and 75 g carbohydrate); in the isocaloric test meal, 100 g 20% fat cream cheese was added, and the amount of butter reduced to compensate for the energy in the cheese (15 g protein, 8 g fat and 76 g carbohydrate). The incremental area under the glycaemic response curve over 0–2 h (recalculated from the data) was reduced by 64% with no difference in plasma insulin. In the second experiment, isocaloric meals containing 100, 200 or 300 g cream cheese were fed, all containing 75 g carbohydrate, with protein:fat contents in grams being 15:17, 24:13 and 32:11, respectively. This exchange of energy from fat and protein had no significant effect on postprandial glucose or insulin responses.

Lang *et al.* (1999a) studied the effects of varying the source of 65% of the protein in test meal lunches which contained either 430 or 860 kcal. The protein sources were casein, soy and gelatin. The lower energy lunches contained about 62–66 g carbohydrate, 24–25 g protein (15–16 g of which was manipulated) and 8 g fat. There was no difference in glucose, insulin, satiety or food intake between the different low-energy lunch meals. The higher energy lunches contained 126–133 g carbohydrate, 49–51 g protein (31–34 g of which was manipulated) and 15–16 g fat. The casein meal delayed glucose and insulin responses compared to soy protein but had no consistent effect on subjective satiety, and no effect on food intake.

### 5.4.2 Studies in subjects with diabetes

Simpson *et al.* (1985) showed that adding 21.4 g protein and 10.5 g fat to 51.2 g carbohydrate had no effect on glycaemic responses in subjects with type 2 diabetes, but markedly increased glycaemic responses in subjects with type 1 diabetes. This effect of protein or protein and fat increasing glucose response in subjects with type 1 diabetes has also been observed by Peters and Davidson (1993), Wang *et al.* (1991) and Rasmussen *et al.* (1990). Jenkins *et al.* (1984) showed that adding 25 g fat and 12 g protein had no effect on glycaemic responses in subjects with type 2 diabetes when given in the form of cheese and butter, but did have an effect when given in the form of peanut butter. Gulliford *et al.* (1989) found that adding 25 g protein as tuna fish to a test meal containing 25 g carbohydrate from potato or spaghetti did not affect blood glucose responses in six subjects with type 2 diabetes, but increased insulin responses by 25–50%. When 25 g fat as margarine was added to the meal already containing carbohydrate and protein, the glycaemic response tended to be reduced but there was no change in insulin response. The reduction in glucose when fat was added to the potato plus fish meal, 21%, was statistically significant; the reduction in glucose when fat was added to pasta plus fish was of similar magnitude (15%) but was not statistically significant. The authors, therefore, concluded that the difference in glycaemic response between potato and spaghetti is reduced when protein and fat are added. However, the authors were considering absolute differences, whereas the critical question is whether the differences in relative response were maintained when protein and fat were added. The mean area under the glycaemic response curve after spaghetti alone was 47% of that after potato alone, the response after pasta plus fish was 55% that of potato plus fish and the response after pasta plus fish plus margarine was 60% of that after potato plus fish plus margarine. With only six subjects, the CI about the differences found in this study are too wide to conclude that relative responses of 47%, 55% and 60% really differ from each other.

### 5.4.3 Interaction of GI with added protein and/or fat

A number of investigators have studied the interaction of GI with added protein and fat, the purpose being to see if the relative differences in glycaemic response between carbohydrate foods are affected by varying the amount of protein or fat present in the meal. A number of these studies have methodological problems which limit their usefulness.

#### *5.4.3.1 Studies concluding that the utility of GI is not affected by added fat and protein*

Perhaps the best study on the interaction between GI and added protein and fat is that by Bornet *et al.* (1987) who added ~20 g fat and 4–20 g protein to 50 g carbohydrate from six different carbohydrate foods in subjects with type 2 diabetes. The addition of fat and protein reduced the glycaemic responses, but did not have a significant effect on the relative glycaemic effect of the different foods. The mean glycaemic response of the six foods fed alone was 57% that of glucose, and when protein and fat were added, the mean glycaemic response was 45% that of glucose, and the difference of 12 ± 4 was significant ($P = 0.024$). However, there was a highly significant correlation between the mean RGR of the foods alone and the mean RGR of the foods plus fat and protein ($r = 0.94$, $P = 0.0048$; Fig. 5.11). Thus, there is no evidence from this study that fat and protein disrupt the ability of the GI to predict the relative glycaemic effects of mixed meals.

We (Wolever *et al.*, 1987) tested bread, rice, spaghetti and barley with and without ~10 g fat and ~8 g protein in the form of cheddar cheese in individuals with type 1 diabetes and in individuals with type 2 diabetes. In type 1 diabetes, adding cheese increased the mean glycaemic response relative to bread alone from 69% to 87% ($P < 0.05$), but the relationship between the responses with and without cheese was virtually perfect ($r = 1.000$). In type 2 diabetes, adding cheese had no significant effect on the mean RGR (increased from 69% to 72%), and the correlation was very good between the glycaemic responses with and without added cheese ($r = 0.994$).

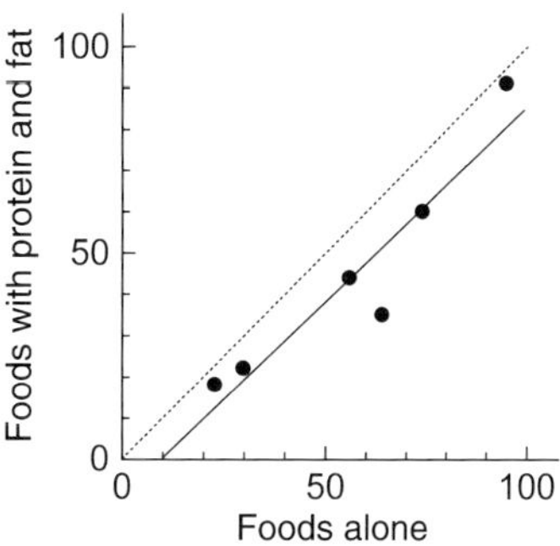


**Fig. 5.11.** Relationship between relative glucose responses of six carbohydrate foods alone or the same foods with added protein and fat. Dotted line is the line of identity, solid line is the regression line ($r = 0.94$, $P = 0.0048$). Data from Bornet *et al.* (1987).

Hermansen *et al.* (1987) compared the effects of spaghetti and potato consumed as part of a mixed meal by subjects with type 1 diabetes. Each meal contained 48 g carbohydrate, 18 g fat and 23–26 g protein. As expected from the GI of the individual foods, the incremental glycaemic response elicited by spaghetti Bolognese was only about 50% of the elicited by potato in Bolognese sauce.

Parillo *et al.* (1985) fed 50 g carbohydrate portions of pasta, bread or potatoes in mixed meals containing 27 g added fat and 31 g added protein to subjects with type 2 diabetes. The IAUC from 0 to 2 h and from 0 to 5 h after the bread meal was 37% ($P < 0.05$) and 68% ($P < 0.02$), respectively, higher than after the pasta meal. Potato elicited a response 44% higher than pasta ($P < 0.05$) over 0–2 h and 49% (ns) higher than pasta over 0–5 h. These differences are similar to the relative GI values of the individual foods (bread = 71; new potato = 62; spaghetti = 41).

Le Floch *et al.* (1992) measured glucose and insulin responses elicited by 50 g glucose or a 50 g carbohydrate portion of rice alone or with 32 g protein and 20 g fat in 30 subjects with type 2 diabetes. The mixed meals elicited lower glucose responses than the carbohydrates alone (rice 38%, glucose 32%), but adding fat and protein did not affect the RGR of rice. Rice alone elicited a glycaemic response 47% that of glucose alone, and the response elicited by the rice mixed meal was also 47% that of the glucose-mixed meal. However, adding fat and protein increased the insulin responses, with the 72% increase in insulin after the rice-mixed meal (compared to rice alone) being significantly greater than that for the glucose-mixed meal (138%, $P < 0.05$). Thus, the authors concluded that the GI of isolated carbohydrate foods predicted their relative responses in mixed meals. However, the insulin secretagogue effect of fat and protein varied according to the source of carbohydrate in the meal.

Miller *et al.* (2003) determined the GI of two different varieties of dates consumed alone, and mixed with yogurt, as traditionally consumed in Arabic countries. The amount of yogurt added (125 g) contained 4.5 g fat and 4.9 g protein. The GI of Rutab dates, 47 ± 5, was significantly greater than that of commercial dates, 36 ± 3. The GI of the commercial dates was, therefore, 23% less than that of Rutab dates. When Rutab and commercial dates were mixed with yogurt, the glycaemic responses relative to glucose tended to be less than those for the dates alone; Rutab dates plus yogurt, 37%; commercial dates plus yogurt mixture, 29%. However, the difference in response between the date/yogurt mixtures, (37−29)/37 = 22%, is almost exactly the same difference as that between the GI of the dates alone, 23%.

#### 5.4.3.2 Studies concluding that the utility of the GI is reduced by protein and fat

Calle-Pascual *et al.* (1987) studied the glycaemic responses elicited by rice, potato or lentils with different amounts of protein or fat in normal subjects. All meals contained 50 g carbohydrate. The four macronutrient distributions were as follows (% energy from carbohydrate:fat:protein): 60:30:10, 60:10:30, 40:40:20 and 40:20:40. This is a very well-conceived study. The results showed that the areas under the glycaemic response curves were similar despite the fact that the foods had different GIs, and the authors' conclusion implies that the GI of individual foods does not apply in a mixed meal setting. The main methodological problem in this study is that the authors calculated total AUC, rather than incremental. Inspection of the results suggests that the results support the utility of the GI in the face of different levels of fat and protein. In this study, IAUC accounted for only about 10% of the TAUC (based on multiplying the fasting glucose of about 75 mg/dl by 180 min = 13,500 out of a total area of about 15,000; Fig. 5.12). The grams of protein in the different test meals varied from 8 to 50 g and the amount of fat from 4 to 22 g. It is of interest that this range of differences had no effect on TAUC or IAUC, and the ranking of glycaemic responses (i.e. rice > potato > lentils) was the same for all the different macronutrient compositions. It is not possible to tell if the IAUC values for the different foods differed significantly, but it would seem likely that they would, since blood glucose 30 min after lentils was always significantly less than that after the other two foods. It is also not possible to say if these results could be predicted by the GI of the individual foods because the authors did not determine the GI of the individual foods.

Gulliford *et al.* (1988) determined the glycaemic responses elicited by 25 g carbohydrate from

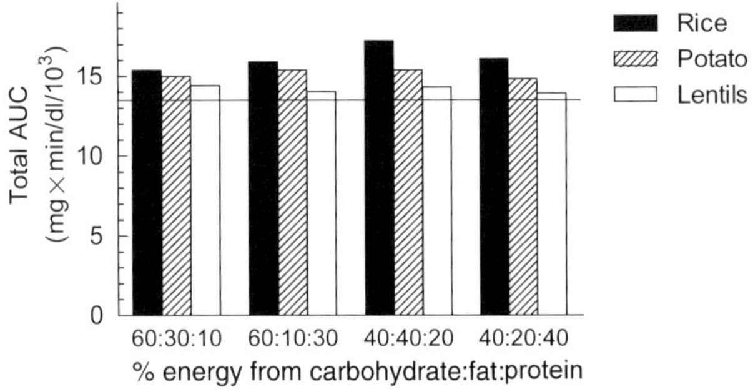


**Fig. 5.12.** Effect of varying the amounts of protein and fat of isocaloric test meals based on three different carbohydrate foods on total area under the blood glucose response curve (AUC) of normal subjects (Calle-Pascual *et al.*, 1987). The horizontal solid line represents the estimated total AUC contributed by the fasting level. The height of the bars above this line, therefore, represents the estimated incremental glycaemic responses of the different test meals.

potato and spaghetti alone and with the addition of 25 g protein or 25 g protein plus 25 g fat in subjects with type 2 diabetes. They concluded that the co-ingestion of protein and fat reduced the difference between the glycaemic responses of the two carbohydrates, implying that the GI was not useful for predicting the glycaemic responses of mixed meals. The data for IAUC are shown in Table 5.3. There are two methodological problems which make this conclusion weak. One problem is that there is no demonstration that the reduction in the difference between spaghetti and potato was statistically significant. However, the main problem is that the conclusion is based on the absolute differences in glycaemic response, whereas the GI predicts the relative differences in response, i.e. the response of one meal as a percentage of that of the other. It appears that the difference in response between potato and spaghetti fed alone, 235 mmol × min/l, is greater than the differences when the foods were fed with protein, 182 mmol × min/l, and with protein and fat, 130 mmol × min/l (Table 5.3). However, such an effect is to be expected because adding protein and fat tended to reduce the glycaemic responses of the meals (Table 5.3). If spaghetti elicited a response 50% that of potato (e.g. 50 vs 100 units), then if, for example, the addition of protein and fat causes a 40% reduction in response, both the potato and spaghetti responses fall by 40% (to 60 and 30, respectively), and the difference between the spaghetti and potato responses will also be reduced by 40%, in this case from 50 (i.e. 100 minus 50) to 30 (i.e. 60 minus 30). Table 5.3 shows that the overall mean response of spaghetti was 53% that of potato. Figure 5.13 shows the glycaemic responses of the spaghetti meals under the different conditions (alone and with protein and fat) which would be expected if they were 53% that of potato. In all cases, the expected response is <1 SEM of the observed response. Therefore, this study does not have nearly enough power (with only six subjects) to show that the utility of the GI is affected by added fat and protein. In my view, the results are consistent with the conclusion that adding large amounts of protein and fat do not affect the utility of the GI.

## 5.5 Calculation of Meal or Diet GI

In the following discussion, the term 'mixed meal' will mean a mixture of several foods including more than one food rich in carbohydrate, to which is added at least one other food which contains predominantly fat or protein (e.g. meats, eggs, butter, cheese, oils, etc.). It is evident from the discussion earlier in this chapter that the glycaemic response elicited by a mixed meal depends on many factors. The GI merely reflects the biological impact of the available carbohydrate in the meal; clearly, the glycaemic response may be affected by the amount of carbohydrate, the amount and nature of the fat and protein consumed with the carbohydrate, and possibly other meal-related factors. Thus, it is naïve to believe that the GI is the only or even the major determinant of the postprandial glycaemic response. Since protein and fat affect glycaemic responses, the GI of a mixed meal should not be measured like the GI of a food. For example, if it is found that a certain mixed meal containing 50 g available carbohydrate elicits a glycaemic response 50% that of 50 g glucose, it is not right to say that the GI of the meal is 50. The GI is a property

**Table 5.3.** Incremental areas under the glycaemic response curve in subjects with type 2 diabetes after consuming test meals of potato and spaghetti alone, or with added protein or added protein plus fat (from Gulliford *et al.*, 1989).

| | Potato (mmol × min/l) | Spaghetti (mmol × min/l) | Difference (mmol × min/l) | RGR[a] (%) |
|---|---|---|---|---|
| 25 g carbohydrate (CHO) | 442 ± 43 | 207 ± 62 | 235 | 47 |
| 25 g CHO + 25 g protein | 408 ± 69 | 226 ± 81 | 182 | 55 |
| 25 g CHO + 25 g protein + 25 g fat | 323 ± 60 | 193 ± 55 | 130 | 60 |
| Mean of all conditions | 391 | 209 | | 53 |

[a]Relative glycaemic response = mean response of spaghetti as % of that for potato.

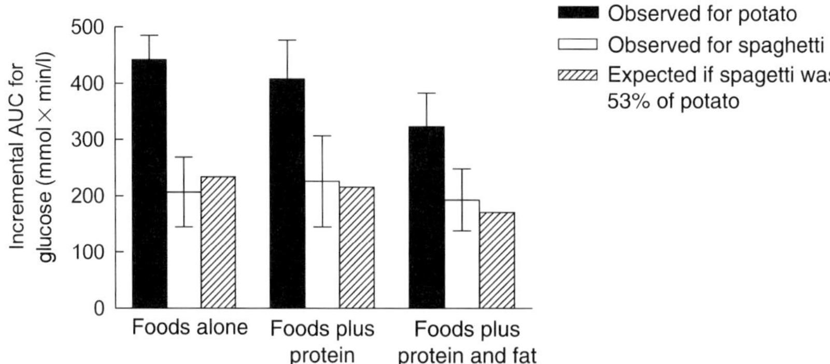


**Fig. 5.13.** Effect on the incremental area under the blood glucose response curve (AUC) of adding protein alone or protein plus fat to potato or spaghetti in subjects with type 2 diabetes (Gulliford *et al.*, 1988). The authors concluded that the effect on glycaemic responses of adding fat and protein to potato differed from that when protein and fat were added to spaghetti. However, this conclusion is not warranted if one considered the hatched bars which show what the response would be the spaghetti meals elicited responses 53% of those of the potato tests meals (based on difference in GI between spaghetti and potato). The observed responses (open bars) are within 1 SEM of expected.

of carbohydrate-rich foods consumed alone. Therefore, the GI of a meal is, properly, a calculated value which reflects the glycaemic impact of the mixture of carbohydrate foods in the meal or diet. The value obtained is independent of the amount of carbohydrate in the meal and ignores the effects of fat and protein. Thus, to see if GI alone predicts the glycaemic response elicited by different mixed meals relative to each other, the different meals should have the same nutrient (i.e. protein, fat and carbohydrate) composition. It may be possible to take differences in amount of carbohydrate, fat and protein into consideration (see Section 5.7 below), but different types of protein and fat may have different effects on glycaemic responses (e.g. Villaume *et al.*, 1986). In addition, the accuracy of the GI for predicting mixed meal glycaemic responses can only be assessed fairly if accurate GI values of the individual carbohydrate foods in the meal are known, and the correct methodology is used, with particular attention to using the appropriate method of calculating the AUC (IAUC), taking all of the carbohydrate foods in the meal into account, and considering only available carbohydrate in the calculations (Wolever and Jenkins, 1986).

The correct way to calculate the GI of a meal or diet is shown in Table 5.4. Here we consider a meal containing three carbohydrate foods, A, B and C, with GI values of $GI_a$, $GI_b$ and $GI_c$ and containing $g_a$, $g_b$ and $g_c$ grams of available carbohydrate, respectively. The total amount of available carbohydrate in the meal is $G = g_a + g_b + g_c$. The proportions of meal available carbohydrate contributed by each food, $P_a = g_a/G$, $P_b = g_b/G$ and $P_c = g_c/G$, are multiplied by the respective

**Table 5.4.** Method of calculating meal GI ($GI_M$).

| Food | Food GI | Available carbohydrate | Proportion of carbohydrate | Meal GI |
|---|---|---|---|---|
| A | $GI_a$ | $g_a$ | $P_a = g_a/G$ | $M_a = P_a \times GI_a$ |
| B | $GI_b$ | $g_b$ | $P_b = g_b/G$ | $M_b = P_b \times GI_b$ |
| C | $GI_c$ | $g_c$ | $P_c = g_c/G$ | $M_c = P_c \times GI_c$ |
| Sum | | $G$ | 1.0 | $GI_M$ |

See text (Section 5.5) for explanation.

food GI value as follows: $M_a = P_a \times GI_a$, $M_b = P_b \times GI_b$ and $M_c = P_c \times GI_c$. The sum of the resulting values is the meal GI, i.e. $GI_M = M_a + M_b + M_c$.

Table 5.5 shows an example of the method of calculating meal GI from a recent study in the literature (Schäfer *et al.*, 2003). The authors did not include any GI calculations in their paper, but it is possible to use the data given to see how well the GI predicts the results obtained. It is a useful example, because it illustrates the importance of needing to know the correct GI value for the individual foods used. The authors fed three traditional German meals: split peas, sausages and vegetables; potato, pork, vegetables and gravy; or a mixture of peas and potatoes with sausages and vegetables. The authors did not determine the GI of any of the individual foods fed in the test meals, and there is no indication as to how the potatoes were cooked and served. These issues are important because the reported GI values of potatoes vary widely from <50 to >110 which may be related to both the variety and cooking methods used (Foster-Powell *et al.*, 2002). The GI value ascribed to potato affects the calculated meal GI (Table 5.5) and hence the predictive value of the GI. If the meal GI worked perfectly, meal GI would be proportional to the observed glycaemic response; if this were the case, the regression line of observed glycaemic response on meal GI would pass through the origin and the correlation coefficient would be 1. The average GI for boiled new potatoes is 62 (Foster-Powell *et al.*, 2002). Using this GI value for potato (Table 5.5, top; Fig. 5.14, top), there is a good correlation between the meal GI values and observed mean glycaemic responses for the three meals, but the slope of the regression line (solid line) is considerably greater than that of the regression line forced through the origin (dotted line). Nevertheless, the error bars of the observed responses overlap the regression line, and hence are not significantly different from it. However, the fit is not very good, and meal GI is not proportional to observed response. The mean GI for baked russet potatoes is 85 (Foster-Powell *et al.*, 2002). If 85 is taken to be the GI of the potato used by Schäfer *et al.* (2003) (Table 5.5, bottom), then the regression line falls almost exactly on top of the dotted lines going through the origin (Fig. 5.14, bottom). This would indicate that the observed glycaemic responses were almost exactly proportional to that predicted by the GI. Whether one of these GI values for potato is correct, or if it should be some other value, is not known.

**Table 5.5.** Example meal GI calculation (values are rounded).

| | | Meal 1 | | | Meal 2 | | | Meal 3 | | |
|---|---|---|---|---|---|---|---|---|---|---|
| | Food GI | CHO (g) | CHO Prop | Meal GI | CHO (g) | CHO Prop | Meal GI | CHO (g) | CHO Prop | Meal GI |
| Potato | 62* | 0.0 | 0.000 | 0.0 | 11.8 | 0.295 | 18.3 | 35.5 | 0.853 | 52.9 |
| Split pea | 32 | 37.1 | 0.914 | 29.2 | 24.7 | 0.618 | 19.8 | 0.0 | 0.000 | 0.0 |
| Carrot | 92 | 2.4 | 0.059 | 5.4 | 2.4 | 0.060 | 5.5 | 3.6 | 0.086 | 8.0 |
| Celery | 92 | 1.1 | 0.027 | 2.5 | 1.1 | 0.028 | 2.6 | 1.7 | 0.041 | 3.8 |
| Cream | 46 | 0.0 | 0.000 | 0.0 | 0.0 | 0.000 | 0.0 | 0.8 | 0.019 | 0.9 |
| Total | | 40.6 | | 37.2 | 40.0 | | 46.2 | 41.6 | | 65.5 |
| Potato | 85* | 0.0 | 0.000 | 0.0 | 11.8 | 0.295 | 25.1 | 35.5 | 0.853 | 72.5 |
| Split pea | 32 | 37.1 | 0.914 | 29.2 | 24.7 | 0.618 | 19.8 | 0.0 | 0.000 | 0.0 |
| Carrot | 92 | 2.4 | 0.059 | 5.4 | 2.4 | 0.060 | 5.5 | 3.6 | 0.086 | 8.0 |
| Celery | 92 | 1.1 | 0.027 | 2.5 | 1.1 | 0.028 | 2.5 | 1.7 | 0.041 | 3.8 |
| Cream | 46 | 0.0 | 0.000 | 0.0 | 0.0 | 0.000 | 0.0 | 0.8 | 0.019 | 0.9 |
| Total | | 40.6 | | 37.2 | 40.0 | | 52.9 | 41.6 | | 85.1 |

Data from Schäfer *et al.* (2003). GI value for celery was guessed.
*Investigators did not test GI values of individual foods, nor specify how potato was cooked or served. Reported GI values for potato vary from about <50 to >110; the top half shows the meal GI values if potatoes are taken to be new potatoes (GI = 62); the bottom shows the meal GI if the potatoes are taken to be baked russett potatoes (GI = 85) (Foster-Powell *et al.*, 2002).

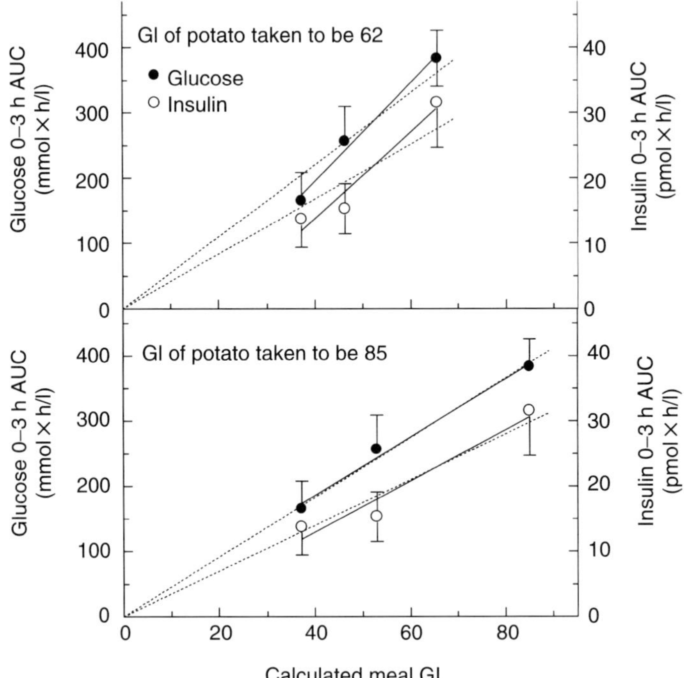


**Fig. 5.14.** Relationship between calculated meal GI and observed glycaemic responses in study by Schäfer *et al.* (2003) showing the importance of knowing the GI of the individual foods fed in the test meals. Meal GI calculations shown in Table 5.5. Potatoes were a component of the meals, but the type of potatoes and how they were prepared is not indicated. Top: meal GI calculated assuming potato to have a GI of 62 (boiled new potatoes). Bottom: meal GI calculated assuming potato to have a GI of 85 (baked russet potato).

## 5.6 Different Meals with the Same Nutrient Composition

There are at least 14 studies in which the blood glucose responses elicited by different meals of approximately the same macronutrient composition were determined in the same group of subjects, and for which data are included, and sufficient detail of methods given to allow calculation of the GI of the meals and the incremental areas under the glycaemic response curves. Amongst these 14 studies, 18 different groups of subjects (5 groups of normal subjects, 12 groups of subjects with type 2 diabetes, and 1 group with type 1 diabetes) were fed between two and six different test meals for a total of 121 paired comparisons. The studies fall into three groups: five studies in which the authors concluded that the glycaemic responses of the meals were not predicted by the GI, three in which the authors concluded that the glycaemic responses of the meals were predicted by the GI and six in which the GI was not considered (Table 5.6).

The fact that there are more studies against the GI than in favour of it (5 vs 3) suggests that the weight of evidence is against the utility of the GI. However, the total number of paired meal comparisons in the three positive studies, 55, is nearly three times as many as in the five negative studies, 19 (Table 5.6). In addition, the adequacy of the data presented and the quality of the methods used in the studies must be considered. The negative studies were less well designed than the positive ones to test the hypothesis that the GI has utility in a mixed meal setting. For example, the negative studies tested only two to four different test meals (average three) compared to five to six different meals in the positive studies; thus, there

**Table 5.6.** Characteristics of studies on the utility of the GI in predicting glycaemic responses.

| | Summary of study conclusions related to GI | | | |
|---|---|---|---|---|
| | All studies | Anti-GI | Pro-GI | GI not mentioned |
| No. of studies | 14 | 5 | 3 | 6 |
| No. of subject groups | 18 | 6 | 4 | 8 |
| No. (range) test meals per group | 4.0 (2–6) | 3.0 (2–4) | 5.5 (5–6) | 3.9 (3–5) |
| Total no. of different test meals | 72 | 18 | 22 | 32 |
| No. of paired comparisons | 122 | 19 | 55 | 48 |
| No. of PD +ve comparisons[a] | 82 | 18 | 37 | 27 |
| No. (%) correct ranked predictions | 78 (95%) | 17 (94%) | 35 (95%) | 26 (96%) |
| No. of PD −ve comparisons[a] | 40 | 1 | 18 | 21 |
| No. (%) correct ranked predictions | 26 (65%) | 1 (100%) | 10 (56%) | 15 (71%) |
| Ratio GIa/GIb[b] | 0.69 ± 0.02 | 0.63 ± 0.04 | 0.62 ± 0.04 | 0.78 ± 0.03 |
| Ratio GRa/GRb[b] | 0.69 ± 0.02 | 0.78 ± 0.04 | 0.61 ± 0.04 | 0.70 ± 0.05 |
| | ns | $P = 0.005$ | ns | $P = 0.03$ |

[a]Number meal pairs for which the difference in GI is greater than the predictive difference (PD). PD is the difference in GI which, theoretically, will predict the ranking of the glycaemic responses of two mixed meals with 95% probability (Wolever *et al.*, 1989).
[b]Ratios: means of ratios GIa/GIb and GRa/GRb were GIb and GRb are the GI and glycaemic response, respectively, of the test meal in each study with the highest calculated GI and GIa and GRa are the respective values of the other test meals (see Section 5.6.5 for further explanation). Details of studies are given in Table 5.8.

was more power in the positive studies to examine correlations between expected and observed responses.

What does a conclusion that the GI has no clinical utility in the context of a mixed meal really mean? It is usually accepted that the conclusion means that the GI really does not work in principle. However, the same conclusion could come about because the authors did not have accurate information about the GI of the individual foods in the mixed meals or used inappropriate methods. The latter are serious problems but their implications are very different from those of the former. The fact that many investigators, including our laboratory, have shown that the glycaemic responses of mixed meals can be predicted by the GI suggests that the concept is useful. In the analyses which follow, I have applied a uniform approach to calculating the GI of mixed meals (using, where possible, the values given in the manuscript) and the AUC of the mixed meals (using, where possible, the values for IAUC given in the manuscript). However, before examining the results, the question must be asked as to what criteria can be applied to support or refute the hypothesis that the GI has clinical utility in the context of mixed meals?

### 5.6.1 What criteria should be used to determine whether the GI has utility?

The ideal test of whether the GI has clinical utility would be to see if an experimental diet designed to differ only in GI produced differences in hard endpoints, such as risk of retinopathy, or myocardial infarction or death. Such studies have not been done. Thus, in the absence of 'hard' endpoints, one has to make do with surrogate endpoints, that is, variables which are believed to be related to the risk of disease, complications or death such as blood lipids or markers of blood glucose control. A number of studies examining how differences in diet GI influence a variety of surrogate endpoints have been done, and they will be discussed later in the book. However, when discussing the utility of the GI in the mixed meal setting, what is usually meant is the question as to whether the GI can predict the acute blood glucose response elicited by a meal. The answer to this question may or may not have anything at all to do with long-term outcomes, and I agree with the recommendation of Coulston *et al.* (1984b) that dietary recommendations should not be based on the results of acute test meal studies.

However, the question of whether the GI can predict acute glycaemic responses is very appropriate and interesting, and may have clinical relevance in some situations (e.g. in calculating pre-meal insulin doses for people with type 1 diabetes). Therefore, we need to ask the questions: What can the GI predict? What is meant by 'predict'?

What can the GI predict? The GI is a measure of the blood glucose raising potential of the carbohydrates in foods, relative to that of the same amount of carbohydrate as glucose taken by the same subject. Thus, it can be used to predict the relative IAUC of different meals taken by the same subject or group of subjects. It is not to be expected that the GI alone could predict absolute or relative blood glucose *concentrations* after meals, or to predict the glycaemic responses of one group of subjects relative to that of a different group.

Upon what criteria should conclusions regarding the clinical utility of the GI in mixed meals be based? It is interesting to compare the criteria used in the three studies concluding that the GI predicts the glycaemic responses of mixed meals, with those used in the five studies concluding that the GI does not predict the glycaemic responses of mixed meals. The three positive studies based their conclusions on the presence of a statistically significant correlation between the calculated GI of the different meals and the observed mean glycaemic responses. However, the negative studies based their conclusions on the lack of a statistically or biologically significant difference between the glycaemic responses elicited by different test meals. In addition, the five negative studies used what I consider to be incorrect methods; thus, a detailed commentary on each of these five studies follows.

### 5.6.2 Studies concluding against the utility of the GI

Coulston *et al.* (1984a) fed four different test meals to subjects with type 2 diabetes and concluded that their results were '. . . totally disparate from what would have been predicted by previously published values for the glycaemic index of the foods studied'. We (Wolever and Jenkins, 1986) pointed out that this conclusion was not justified because it was based on incorrect methodology. The method of calculating meal GI did not take into consideration all the carbohydrate foods in the meals, and the conclusions were based on TAUC rather than IAUC. In addition, the GI value Coulston used for baked potato was that for new boiled potato determined by us, which is considerably lower than the estimated value obtained for baked potato in the Stanford laboratory on several previous occasions, and thus, we thought it very reasonable to use the GI for baked potato than for boiled new potato. Our reanalysis of their data (Wolever and Jenkins, 1986) is illustrated in Fig. 5.15, and it shows that the meal GI was almost perfectly proportional to the observed mean glycaemic responses. The Stanford group is aware of this reanalysis of their data; indeed I presented it at the annual meeting of the American Diabetes Association in 1985 in their \presence. The group has had 20 years to point out any scientific or logical flaw in our treatment of their data, and has not done so; I can only assume they can find no fault with it.

Behme and Dupre (1989) fed mixed test meals including corn flakes or All Bran to 11 healthy women, and concluded that the differences observed were less than would be predicted by the GI. However, they did not take into consideration all the foods in the test meal in calculating diet GI. My own reanalysis of these data (Wolever, 1990c) suggested that the predictive ability of the GI was almost perfect; the GI of the All Bran meal was 72% that of the corn flakes meal, and the mean glycaemic response it elicited was 71% that of the corn flakes meal.

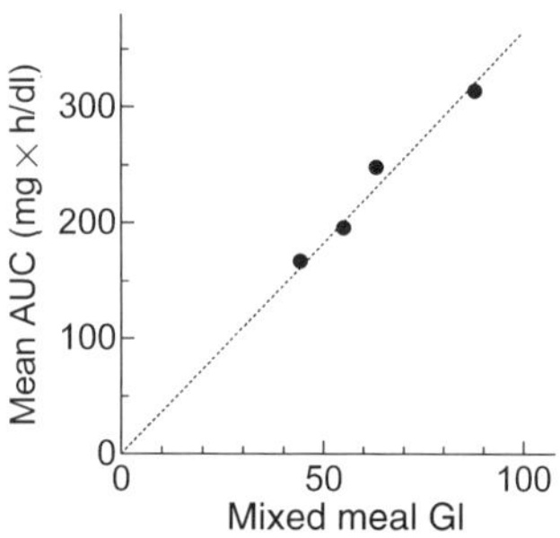


**Fig. 5.15.** Reanalysis (Wolever and Jenkins, 1986) of data from Coulston *et al.* (1984a) who concluded that the observed glycaemic responses of mixed meals were totally disparate from what would be predicted from the GI of the individual foods. Dotted line is the regression line forced through the origin.

Coulston *et al.* (1987) fed three different meals to six normal subjects and nine with type 2 diabetes. They based their conclusion on TAUC rather than IAUC, but indicated that the incremental glucose responses 'were similar' in both subject groups. In the subjects with diabetes, the mean AUC's were ranked correctly by the GI, but the differences in observed response were about half that predicted by the meal GI values the authors calculated. However, white rice comprised 60% of the carbohydrate in the high-GI meal, and Coulston *et al.* ascribed a GI to it of 72. This value is based on the GI of polished rice tested by us in the UK (Jenkins *et al.*, 1981a). There are many varieties of rice with very variable GI values, but the average GI for polished white rice is about 58 (Foster-Powell *et al.*, 2002). Coulston *et al.* (1987) did not specify which kind of rice they used. However in the 1970s, two studies from the Stanford laboratory (Crapo *et al.*, 1977, 1981) found Uncle Ben's Converted rice to elicit glycaemic responses 58% and 72% that of white bread. Thus, the average response was 65% of bread, or a GI of about 46. We confirmed the difference in GI between polished and parboiled long-grain white rices (Wolever *et al.*, 1986a), finding GI values of 59 and 48, respectively. In the Coulston *et al.* (1987) paper, if we take the GI of rice to be 46 (assuming they used parboiled rice as before) then the GI of the high-GI meal falls from 71 to 55, and thus, the GI of the low-GI meal, 34, is 62% that of the high-GI meal, rather than 48%. The former number is better prediction of the observed glycaemic response of the low-GI meal, which, in the diabetic subjects was 74% that of the high-GI meal (Fig. 5.16).

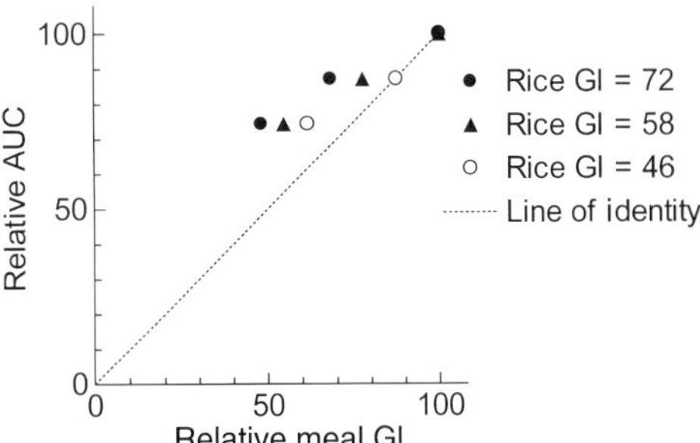


**Fig. 5.16.** Relative AUC plotted against relative meal GI (relative to the test meal with the highest GI and glycaemic response) for three mixed meals, some of which contained rice, consumed by subjects with type 2 diabetes (Coulston *et al.*, 1987). The graph illustrates the effect of using different GI values for rice on the results for relative meal GI.

The normal subject's glycaemic responses to the three meals given by Coulston *et al.* (1987) are shown in Fig. 5.17. It is clear that the pattern of glycaemic responses tends to differ, consistently with high-, medium- and low-GI meals, and the peak rise and AUC over the first hour is lowest after the low-GI meal. However, the IAUC measured over the entire time period is actually lowest for the high-GI meal. There are two confounding issues here; one is that blood was not sampled frequently enough over the first hour in the normal subjects to capture an accurate picture of the glycaemic response. In addition, these test meals were fed to the subjects at noon, after a standard breakfast. We have previously demonstrated that the difference in glycaemic response between different foods tested at mid-day after a standard breakfast is about half that seen when exactly the same foods are fed in the morning after an overnight fast (Wolever and Bolognesi, 1996c; Fig. 5.18).

Hollenbeck *et al.* (1988) fed high, intermediate and low-GI breakfast, lunch and dinner meals to subjects with type 2 diabetes. The three different breakfast meals elicited similar glycaemic responses, but blood glucose after lunch and dinner was substantially less after the low-GI meals than the others. They reported no significant difference in IAUC, but it is not clear if they calculated the increments from the fasting plasma glucose or from the plasma glucose concentration at the start of each meal (and it is not clear which is

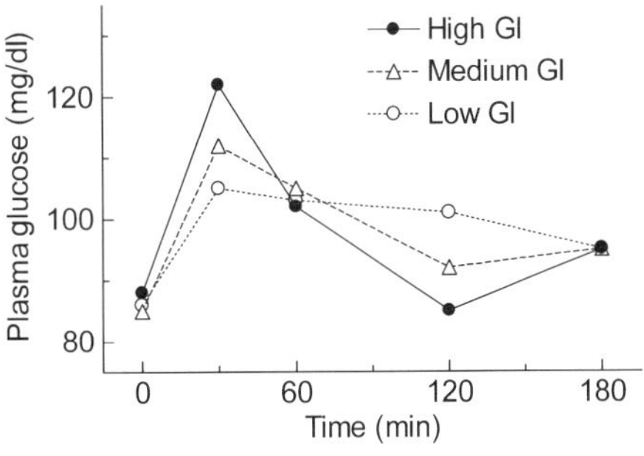


**Fig. 5.17.** Glycaemic responses of six normal subjects elicited by mixed meals with high, medium and low GI (Coulston *et al.*, 1987).

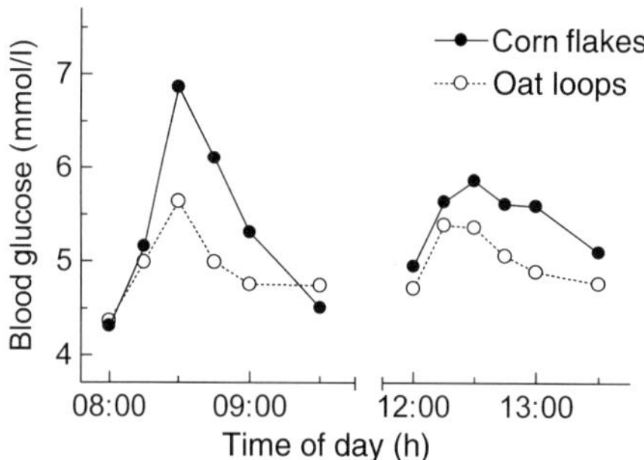


**Fig. 5.18.** Mean glycaemic responses of a group of normal subjects elicited by equal carbohydrate portions of corn flakes or oat loops cereals. Left: cereals were taken in the morning after an overnight fast. Right: the same cereals were taken by the same subjects 4 h after a standard breakfast was consumed (Wolever and Bolognesi, 1996c).

most appropriate). Nevertheless, the overall increments they report were correctly ranked by the GI. In addition, they found that the day-long plasma glucose concentration on the high-GI diet, 209 mg/dl, was significantly higher than that on the low-GI diet, 192 mg/dl. However, they concluded that '... day long plasma glucose response did not vary substantially when patients with NIDDM consumed meals of widely different glycemic potency, providing further evidence that there is relatively little clinical benefit to be gained by designing meals based on the published glyemic index.... ' In other words, the conclusion was based on the authors' opinion about what constitutes a clinically important difference in blood glucose. Not only this is not relevant to the question of whether the GI can predict glycaemic responses, but also, one might ask how do these authors know whether a difference of day-long plasma glucose of 17 mg/dl (0.94 mmol/l) is clinically important? There is accumulating evidence that such small differences in average blood glucose could, indeed, be important. For example, cardiovascular risk increases continuously as blood glucose increases within the normal range (Coutinho *et al.*, 1999). In addition, data in experimental animals to suggest that a sustained increase in mean plasma glucose of less than 1 mmol/l can have marked effects on β-cell function via glucose toxicity (Leahy *et al.*, 1987, 1988).

In the fifth study against the GI, Laine *et al.* (1987) fed three different test meals to groups of normal subjects and subjects with type 2 diabetes in the morning after overnight fasts. The meals varied in GI from 66 to 33 and also varied in protein (27–50 g) although the amounts of available carbohydrate (88–91 g) and fat (26–28 g) were similar. All three meals had the same combination of diabetic exchanges. The peak postprandial glucose differed significantly between meals in both normal and diabetic subjects, but the differences in IAUC, some of which were substantial in magnitude, did not reach statistical significance (Table 5.7).

The authors concluded that '... diabetic exchange lists more accurately predict postprandial

**Table 5.7.** Test meal composition and mean glycaemic responses in study by Laine *et al.* (1987).

| | High-GI meal | Medium-GI meal | Low-GI meal |
|---|---|---|---|
| Carbohydrate[a] (g) | 91.1 | 88.0 | 89.6 |
| Fat (g) | 27.4 | 25.7 | 27.7 |
| Protein (g) | 30.1 | 26.5 | 50.4 |
| GI[b] | 65.9 | 48.0 | 33.1 |
| *Peak glucose (mg/dl)* | | | |
| Diabetic subjects | 296[cd] | 305[d] | 274[c] |
| Normal subjects | 136[d] | 134[cd] | 124[c] |
| *Incremental AUC (mg × min/dl)* | | | |
| Diabetic subjects | 17,100 | 16,240 | 15,520 |
| Normal subjects | 3,370 | 3,000 | 1,880 |

[a]Available carbohydrate (total minus dietary fibre).
[b]Glycaemic index recalculated.
[cd]Means with a different letter superscript differ significantly ($P < 0.05$).

responses to carbohydrate-containing foods eaten as part of a mixed meal than does the GI of foods'. However, I believe this conclusion is faulty for three reasons:

**1.** The exchange lists did not predict the glycaemic responses. The number of exchanges in each meal was the same, so if exchanges were accurate predictors of glycaemic responses, the glycaemic responses observed should have been the same, but they were not; there were significant differences in peak glucose concentrations.
**2.** The study was poorly designed to test the predictive ability of the exchange lists because the number of exchanges was the same for all treatments. It is impossible to prove the null hypothesis (i.e. prove that different treatments elicit the same response). It is only possible to show that the difference between treatments is less than a certain value; that value can be made smaller and smaller by doing a larger and more powerful study, but it cannot be proven that different treatment produce *identical* results. Since, experimentally it is easier to reject the null hypothesis (i.e. prove that different treatments elicit different responses), a much better study design to test the predictive ability of exchange lists would entail giving test meals with different numbers of exchanges and show that the responses elicited differed.
**3.** The conclusion was presumably based on the lack of significant difference between the AUC values elicited by the different meals. However, failure to reject the null hypothesis (i.e. the failure to find statistically significant differences between mean responses) does not prove the null hypothesis (i.e. prove that the responses are all equal). In fact, the study was likely not powerful enough to detect a difference in glycaemic response between the test meals in the normal subjects. This leads to a brief discussion of statistical power.

### 5.6.3 Statistical power

There are two types of errors associated with statistical comparisons. A type I error is concluding that a difference does exist when, really, there is no difference, or, more strictly, rejecting the null hypothesis when, in fact, the null hypothesis is true. A type II error is concluding that a difference does not exist when, really, there is a difference, or, more strictly, failing to reject the null hypothesis when, in fact, the null hypothesis is false (Motulsky, 1995). Usually, scientists are more interested in detecting differences and are most concerned with type I errors. The *P*-values cited in most papers represent the probability of making a type I error. In other words, when it is stated that the response elicited by treatment A differed significantly from that elicited by treatment B ($P < 0.05$), what is meant is that there is less than a 5% chance that A really elicits the same response as B. However, failing to find a significant difference between the responses elicited by treatments A and B does not necessarily mean that the responses are the same.

Statistical power, as applied to glycaemic responses, is illustrated in Figs 5.19–5.21. Figure 5.19 represents the theoretical distribution of the mean glycaemic response elicited by test meal B in eight normal subjects, assuming that such responses are normally distributed (I believe this assumption to be valid as discussed in Chapter 2, and illustrated in Fig. 2.11). The mean is set at 80 with a SD of 20, with the value for SD being based on the fact that the mean

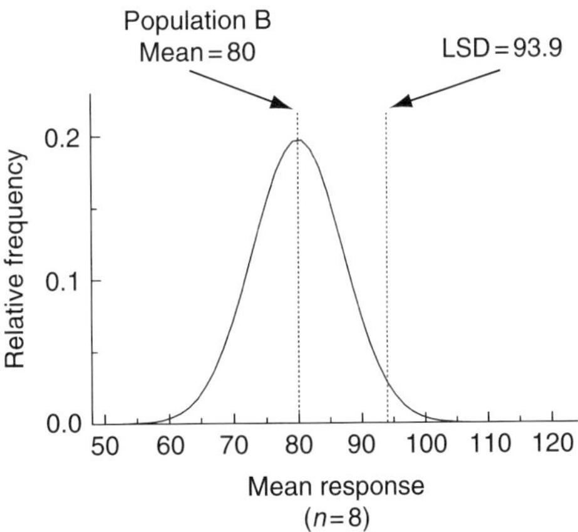


**Fig. 5.19.** Distribution of means of eight randomly selected values from population B with a mean of 80 and SD of 20 (population B represents the distribution mean glycaemic responses elicited by meal B – see text). LSD = least significant difference = 1.96 × SEM greater than the mean for meal B (based on a two-tailed *P*-value of $P \leq 0.05$). There is a 2.5% chance that the mean of eight randomly selected values drawn from population B is ≥93.8.

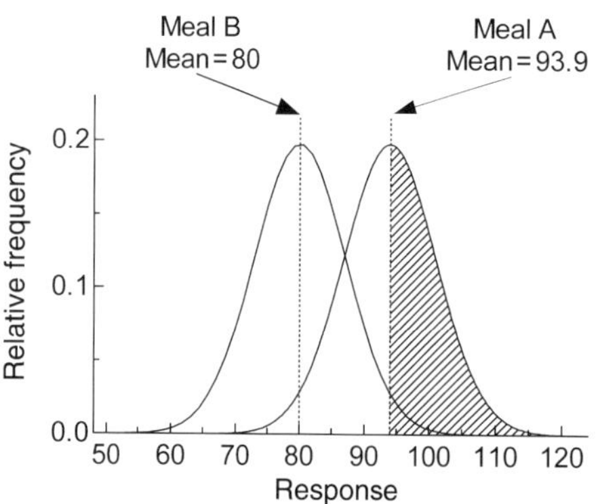


**Fig. 5.20.** Distributions of means of eight randomly selected values from populations B (meal B) and A (meal A) with means of 80 and 93.8, respectively, and SD of 20. The mean for A (93.8) is equal to the LSD (Fig. 5.19), i.e. if the observed mean of eight values selected from population A ≥93.8 then it would be concluded that A is significantly different from B. However, even though A really has a mean value different from B, there is a 50% chance that the observed mean for A would be <LSD. The shaded area represents power, i.e. the chance that a difference will be detected. Thus, if the actual mean for meal A is 93.8, then there is a 50% chance that the observed mean of eight values from A will be found to be significantly greater than that for B.

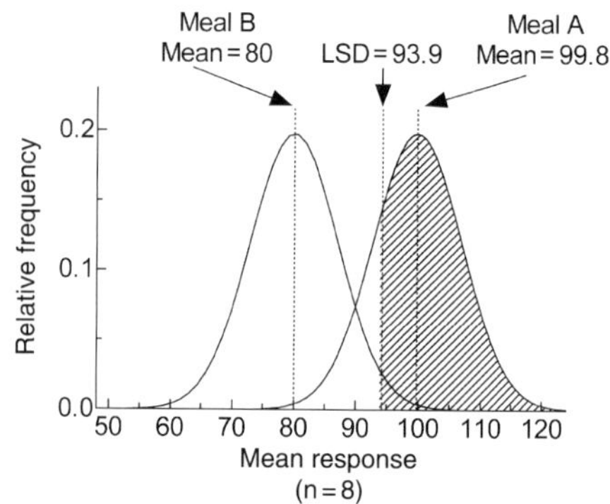


**Fig. 5.21.** Distributions of means of eight randomly selected values drawn from populations B (meal B) and A (meal A) with means of 80 and 99.8, respectively, and SD of 20. The mean for A (99.8) is such that 80% of the means of eight randomly selected values from population A are greater than 93.9. Thus, there is an 80% chance that the mean of eight randomly selected values from population A will be greater than or equal to the LSD (least significant difference) for population B (93.9, see Fig. 5.19), i.e. power (shaded area) = 80%.

within-subject CV of glycaemic responses of normal subjects is about 25% (Chapter 2, this volume). A common criterion for declaring statistical significance is a two-tailed *P*-value of ≤0.05. This is achieved if an observed value is least 1.96 × SEM greater or less than the mean for B, because 5% of the area under the normal distribution curve is outside these limits. Thus the least significant difference (LSD) is $1.96 \times \text{SD}/\sqrt{n}$ which, in this case, is a value of $80 + 1.96 \times 20/\sqrt{8} = 93.8$ (Fig. 5.19). Thus, if we tested meals A and B in eight normal subjects and observed a mean response of 80 for meal B and ≥93.8 for meal A, we would conclude that the glycaemic response elicited by meal A was significantly greater than that for meal B.

However, if the true mean response of A equals 93.8 (Fig. 5.20), it can be seen that only 50% of the population of A mean responses are greater than the LSD. Thus, if the true mean for A is equal to the LSD, then there is only a 50% chance of finding A to be significantly greater than B. The statistical power of an experiment is the probability it has of detecting a difference which really exists. So in this case, the power is 50%. When designing experiments, it is usually considered prudent to have a power of at least 80%, or in other words, an 80% chance of finding a difference that really exists. To have 80% power to detect a difference between A and B, without changing the SD or the number of subjects tested, then the mean for A has to be increased such that 80% of the area under the distribution curve for the A is greater than the LSD line; this moves the mean for A about 0.84 × SEM above the LSD, or 2.80 × SEM above the mean for B (Fig. 5.21). Another way to increase power is to reduce the variability of the distributions, which can be achieved by increasing the number of subjects studied, but I will not discuss this in detail.

Returning now to the results of the normal subjects studied by Laine *et al.* (1987); since the low-GI meal had a GI about 50% that of the high-GI meal, the *expected* reduction in glycaemic response is 50%. The authors report their study had 80% power to detect 1.3 times the LSD, and the LSD for the normal subjects was reported to be 1570. Thus, a difference of 1.3 × 1570 = 2040 could have been detected. Since, the high-GI meal elicited a response of 3370, for adequate power, the response elicited by the low-GI meal would have to be 3370−2040 = 1330, which is 61% less than the response of the high-GI meal, a considerably greater difference than that expected. What is the power of the study to detect a 50% reduction in glycemic response? The expected difference is 50% of 3370 = 1685. The LSD is 1570. Assuming the LSD is 1.96 × SEM from the mean, then the SEM is estimated to be 1570/1.96 = 801. Thus, the actual mean response of the low-GI meal is expected to be (1685−1570)/801 = 0.14 × SEM greater than the LSD; 56% of the area under the normal distribution is more than 0.14 × SEM less than the mean. Thus, I estimate the power of this study to detect a 50% difference in glycaemic response in the normal subjects was only 56%. Thus, the fact that no significant difference existed in AUC in the normal subjects does not mean that no difference existed, and in fact, the above analysis suggests there is a 44% chance that a 50% difference in response really does exist. Indeed, the observed mean response of the low-GI meal in the normal subjects was 56% of that for the high-GI meal, which (given the magnitude of variation) is quite similar to the value of 50% expected by the GI.

However, for the diabetic subjects studied by Laine *et al.* (1987), the GI did not perform as well, with the low-GI meal eliciting a response only about 9% less than that of the high-GI meal, compared to the 50% difference expected. I cannot explain this, and it is the best evidence against the GI that I know of. Nevertheless, the GI correctly ranked the glycaemic responses of the three meals in the subjects with diabetes. In addition, the fact that different meals with identical numbers of exchanges elicited significantly different peak glycaemic responses in the subjects with diabetes does not support the conclusion that exchange lists accurate predict glycaemic responses. Thus, I believe that the results of subjects with diabetes are more consistent with the conclusion that the GI predicts glycaemic responses better than the exchange lists, than the opposite conclusion drawn by the authors.

Having discussed the approaches which I believe are inappropriate for determining whether the GI predicts mixed meal glycaemic responses, what approaches do I think are appropriate? There are two approaches: a qualitative approach and a quantitative approach; these have been mentioned above, but will be discussed in more detail below, and illustrated using data from the literature.

### 5.6.4 Qualitative approach to prediction

The qualitative approach deals with the ranking of glycaemic responses – answering the question will meal B elicit a higher or lower glycaemic response than meal A? When considering this question, it must be keep in mind that an experiment, such as measuring glycaemic responses, only takes a small sample of all the possible results which exist in the entire population. Glycaemic responses within-individuals vary from day to day, and the distribution of the responses appears to be normally distributed (Fig. 2.11). Thus, if the glycaemic responses elicited by the same meal on different days is measured in the same person under standard conditions, the results will vary from day to day. This is illustrated in Fig. 5.22 which shows a normal distribution of values with a mean of 80 and SD of 20. Point '1' represents the result of a single test which is approximately 1 SD below the mean, and point '2' represents the result on another test in the same individual which is approximately 1 SD above the mean.

Figure 5.23 shows the distributions of glycaemic responses for two test meals, A and B, in an individual subject, assuming that the variation of responses for meal A is equal to that for meal B. The mean response for meal A is 120 while the

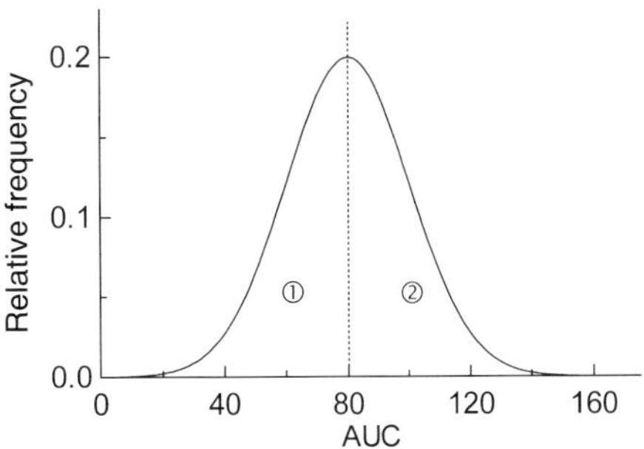


**Fig. 5.22.** Normal distribution of values representing glycaemic responses (AUC) of an individual elicited by a test meal with mean of 80 and SD of 20. Points 1 and 2 represent values −1 and +1 SD from the mean.

mean for B is 80. Therefore, most of the time, we would expect meal A to elicit a higher glycaemic response than meal B. However, on some occasions, meal B will be found to elicit a higher response than meal A. Consider point '*a*' which is a response for meal B which is about 1.5 SD below the mean, and point '*b*,' which is a response for meal B which is about 1.5 SD above the mean. The response at point '*a*' is less than that at point '*b*', even though the mean response for A is greater than B. What is the chance that meal A will elicit a response less than meal B, i.e. $(a-b) < 0$? This can be computed from the difference between the means of A and B, i.e. 40, and the SD of the differences. If we assume that the SD of A = SD of B = 20, then the SD of the values $(a-b) = 20 \times \sqrt{2} = 28.3$. This is shown in Fig. 5.24, the dotted line is a difference of 0. The proportion of the total area to the left of the dotted line represents the probability that meal A will elicit a response less than meal B. In this example, the dotted line is 40/28.3 = 1.41 SD below the mean. The cumulative area under the normal curve <1.41 SD below the mean is 0.079. This means that, for meals A and B, with mean responses of 120 and 80, respectively, and SD = 20, there is about an 8% chance (i.e. about 1/13) that meal A will be observed to elicit a lower response than meal B when tested once each in a single individual. Conversely, there is a 92% chance that meal A will elicit a response greater than meal B.

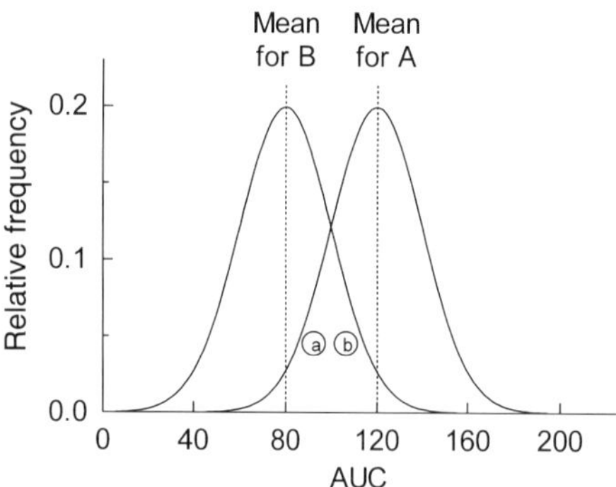


**Fig. 5.23.** Normal distribution of values representing glycaemic responses (AUC) of an individual elicited by two test meals with means of 80 and 120 and SD of 20. Point 'a' represents a value $-1.5 \times$ SD less than the mean for A, and point 'b' represents a value $+1.5 \times$ SD from the mean for B.

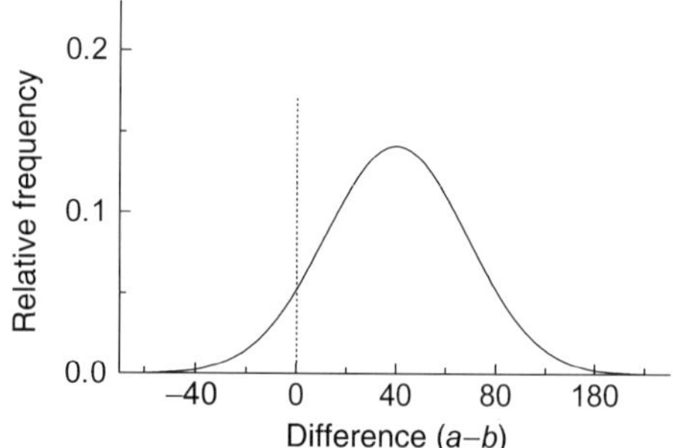


**Fig. 5.24.** Distribution of differences (*a*–*b*), where *a* and *b* are randomly selected values from the populations A and B which have means of 80 and 120, respectively, and SDs of 20. The resulting distribution has a mean of 40 and a SD of $20/\sqrt{2} = 28.3$.

The chance that meal A will elicit a greater response than meal B depends on three factors: the magnitude of day-to-day variation of glycaemic responses within subjects, the number of subjects tested and the magnitude of the expected difference. Figure 5.25A shows the same hypothetical distributions of glycaemic responses of meals A and B as shown in Fig. 5.23. The means for A and B are 80 and 120 and the SDs are 20. Figure 5.25D shows the distributions of the differences between A and B as shown in Fig. 5.24, with a mean of 40 and SD of 28.3, about 8% of AUC is <0, thus, the probability that A is greater than B is about 92%. Figure 5.25B shows the effect of reducing the variability of the glycaemic responses from a CV of 25% to 15% (e.g. this could represent doing the measurement in a subject with type 2 diabetes instead of a subject without diabetes, or using the average response in four subjects instead of 1). Figure 5.25E shows the distribution of these differences, and in this case, the probability that A is greater than B is 99%. Figure 5.25C shows the effect of a larger difference between the means for A and B. Increasing the mean difference to 60, without changing the SD (SD = 20), results in a distribution of differences shown in Fig. 5.25F where the chance that A is greater than B is 98%.

Wolever *et al.* (1989) derived the so-called 'predictive difference' in GI, which was defined as the difference in GI between two meals such that there would be a 95% probability that the meal with the greater GI would elicit the greater

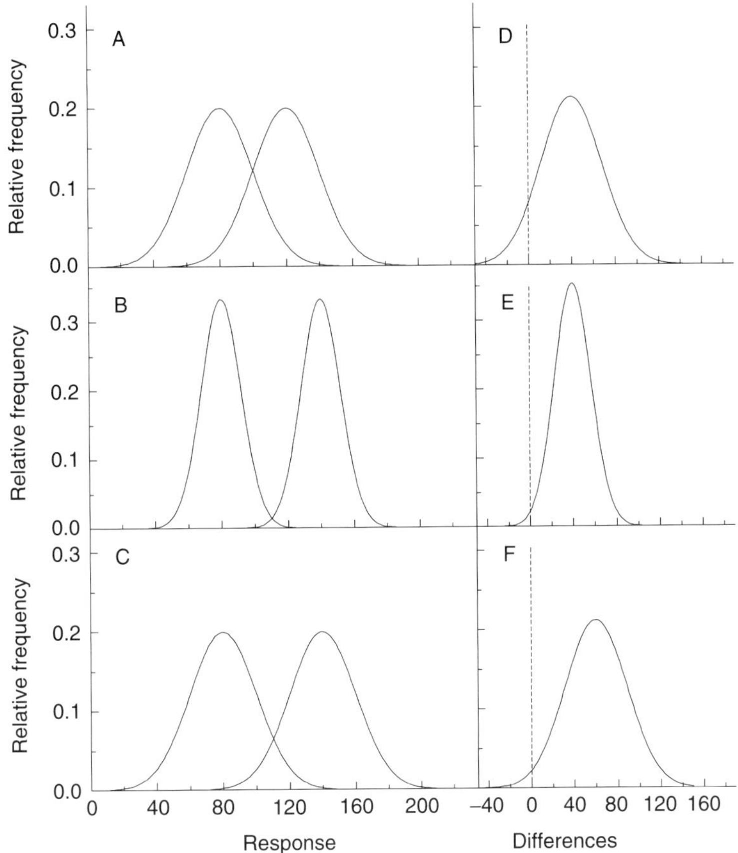


**Fig. 5.25.** Theoretical effect of altering within-subject variation and mean difference on the distribution of differences in glycaemic response between two meals. A and D: distribution of theoretical glycaemic responses of an individual elicited by two test meals with means of 80 and 120 and SD of 20, and the distribution of differences in responses between the test meals. B and E: effect of reducing SD from 20 to 12. C and F: effect of increasing mean difference from 40 to 60.

glycaemic response when both meals were tested by a single subject or a group of subjects. The formula is as follows:

$$\mathrm{PD} = (1.645 \times s_{\mathrm{w}} \times \sqrt{2})\sqrt{n}$$

where PD is the predictive difference, $s_{\mathrm{w}}$ is the within-subject variation of GI values and $n$ is the number of subjects studied. The values of $s_{\mathrm{w}}$ for subjects with type 1 and type 2 diabetes, respectively, were estimated to be 15.3 and 10.6. Based on the relative within-subject coefficients of variation of repeated tests of bread or glucose in normal subjects, the value for $s_{\mathrm{w}}$ in normal subjects is estimated to be 13.2. Thus, for example, the PD in GI for $n = 10$ subjects with type 2 diabetes is $(1.645 \times 10.6 \times 1.41)/3.16 = 7.8$. If the GI could accurately predict the ranking of glycaemic responses, we would expect that for 95% of meal pairs with a GI difference greater than the PD, the meal with the greater GI would elicit a greater mean glycaemic response (i.e. a successful prediction). In addition, if the difference in GI was less than the PD, then the meal with the greater GI would elicit the greater glycaemic response only about 50% of the time.

Table 5.8 shows the calculated meal GI values and IAUC results for the 14 studies summarized on Table 5.6. I have not included the results for normal subjects by Coulston *et al.* (1987) because there are several methodological problems making the interpretation of the results complex (see paragraph 4, Section 5.6.2). There are a total of 122 paired meal comparisons; for 82 of these the difference in GI is >PD and for 40 the difference

**Table 5.8.** Details of studies on the utility of the glycaemic index (GI) in mixed meals.

| Studies against GI | | | Studies in favour of GI | | | GI not mentioned | | |
|---|---|---|---|---|---|---|---|---|
| Subjects (PD)* | GI | AUC | Subjects (PD) | GI | AUC | Subjects (PD) | GI | AUC |
| 8 T2DM[a] | 88.1 | 313 | 9 Normal[f] | 100 | 100 | 8 T2DM[i] | 60.9 | 106 |
| (8.7) | 63.4 | 247 | (10.2) | 58 | 56 | (8.7) | 59.6 | 105 |
| | 55.2 | 195 | | 56 | 61 | | 53.2 | 47 |
| | 44.3 | 166 | | 55 | 67 | 8 T2DM[j] | 82.1 | 302 |
| 9 T2DM[b] | 70.2 | 647 | | 47 | 59 | (8.7) | 75.3 | 243 |
| (8.2) | 55.5 | 672 | | 38 | 45 | | 66.9 | 207 |
| | 38.8 | 510 | 10 T2DM[f] | 100 | 100 | | 62.6 | 207 |
| 11 Normal[c] | 67.7 | 124 | (7.8) | 58 | 50 | 5 T2DM[k] | 61 | 5,879 |
| (9.3) | 48.7 | 88 | | 56 | 67 | (11.0) | 57 | 3,965 |
| 13 Normal[d] | 65.9 | 3,370 | | 55 | 67 | | 47 | 4,199 |
| (8.5) | 48.0 | 3,000 | | 47 | 59 | 10 Normal[l] | 77.5 | 5,310 |
| | 33.1 | 1,880 | | 38 | 24 | (9.7) | 69.0 | 4,010 |
| 12 T2DM[d] | 65.9 | 17,100 | 8 Normal[g] | 69 | 66 | | 61.6 | 2,140 |
| (7.1) | 48.0 | 16,200 | (10.8) | 69 | 86 | | 60.5 | 2,340 |
| | 33.1 | 15,520 | | 65 | 73 | | 41.1 | 1,190 |
| 12 T2DM[e] | 71 | 558 | | 60 | 60 | 12 T1DM[l] | 77.5 | 21,700 |
| (7.1) | 48 | 533 | | 40 | 52 | (9.6) | 69.0 | 19,900 |
| | 34 | 520 | | 38 | 40 | | 61.6 | 18,200 |
| | | | 6 T2DM[h] | 68.9 | 1,281 | | 60.5 | 20,400 |
| | | | (10.0) | 61.7 | 1,117 | | 41.1 | 9,770 |
| | | | | 54.1 | 947 | 10 T2DM[l] | 77.5 | 20,000 |
| | | | | 46.4 | 713 | (7.8) | 69.0 | 20,000 |
| | | | | 33.3 | 563 | | 61.6 | 15,400 |
| | | | | | | | 60.5 | 18,600 |
| | | | | | | | 41.1 | 10,800 |
| | | | | | | 9 T2DM[m] | 80.9 | 381 |
| | | | | | | (8.2) | 51.6 | 257 |
| | | | | | | | 37.2 | 164 |
| | | | | | | 12 T2DM[n] | 57.9 | 2,245 |
| | | | | | | (7.1) | 53.1 | 2,030 |
| | | | | | | | 51.9 | 2,008 |

*PD = predictive difference (see Section 5.6.4).
AUC = incremental area under the glycaemic response curve.
[a]Coulston *et al.* (1984a) re-analysed by Wolever and Jenkins (1986). AUC units = mg × h/dl.
[b]Hollenbeck *et al.* (1988). AUC units = mg × h/dl.
[c]Behme and Dupre (1989) re-analysed by Wolever (1990c). AUC units = mmol × min/l.
[d]Laine *et al.* (1987). AUC units = mg × min/dl.
[e]Coulston *et al.* (1987). AUC units = mg × h/dl.
[f]Indar-Brown *et al.* (1992). AUC units = % of response after 50 g glucose.
[g]Chew *et al.* (1988). AUC units = % of response after 50 g glucose.
[h]Collier *et al.* (1986). AUC units = mmol × min/l.
[i]Colagiuri *et al.* (1986). AUC units = mg × h/dl.
[j]Nuttall *et al.* (1983) re-analysed by Wolever *et al.* (1985). AUC units = mg × h/dl.
[k]Parsons (1984). AUC units = mg × min/dl.
[l]Bantle *et al.* (1983) re-analysed by Wolever *et al.* (1985). AUC units = mg × h/dl.
[m]Schäfer *et al.* (2003). AUC units = mmol × min/l.
[n]Hollenbeck *et al.* (1985) re-analysed by Wolever (1985). AUC units = mg × h/dl.

in GI is <PD. The GI correctly predicted the ranked glycaemic response in 78 of the 82 (95%) cases where difference in GI was >PD, a proportion which is highly significantly different from 50% ($P = 10^{-10}$). In addition, there was no significant difference in the proportion of correct predictions for studies concluding that the GI had no clinical utility, compared to those which supported the GI or those which did not mention the GI. This suggests that the conclusions of the negative studies are not supported by the data. For the 40 comparisons in which the difference in GI was <PD, the GI correctly ranked the glycaemic response in 26 cases (65%), which is not significantly different from 50% ($P = 0.17$).

### 5.6.5 Quantitative approach to prediction

The quantitative approach to using the GI to predict glycaemic responses is based on the hypothesis that GIa/GIb = GRa/GRb, where GIa and GIb are the calculated GI values of meals A and B and GRa and GRb are the mean values for incremental area under the glucose response curve elicited by meals A and B. This hypothesis implies that the relative difference in GI is equal to the relative difference in glycaemic response. There would be two ways to test this, one being comparing the mean ratios of GIa/GIb and GRa/GRb for a number of different test meals. The other method would be to use correlation analysis to assess the relationship between the ratios for several meals. If the hypothesis were true, we would expect to see that GIa/GIb equals GRa/GRb. In addition, the correlation between the GI ratios and the GR ratios would be significant and the regression equation would have a slope of 1 and a *y*-intercept of 0. As indicated above, the accuracy of such comparisons depends not only on whether the hypothesis is true, but also on the methodology (e.g. accuracy of the GI values ascribed to the individual foods used and the methods used to determine glycaemic response).

Table 5.6 summarizes the means of the ratios of GIa/GIb and GRa/GRb where GIb is taken to be the test meal in each study with the highest GI and GRb is the glycaemic response of the test meal with the highest GI. Thus, in a study with four test meals, three ratios of GIa/GIb and three ratios of GRa/GRb were compared. Amongst the studies with conclusions against the GI, the average of the RGR, 0.78, was significantly greater than the relative GI values, 0.63. Figure 5.26 (left) shows this as the slope being significantly less than 1, with the line of identity falling outside the 95% CI of the regression. Thus, amongst these studies, the difference in glycaemic response was less than that predicted by GI. Amongst the studies with conclusions in favour of the GI, the average of the RGR, 0.61, was virtually identical to that of the GI values, 0.62. Figure 5.26 (centre) shows that the slope of the regression line of relative GR on relative GI for these studies is not significantly different from 1, with the line of identity falling within the 95% CI of the regression. This

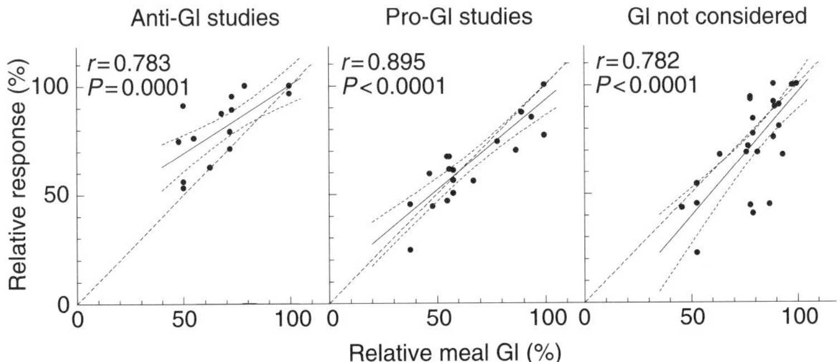


**Fig. 5.26.** Correlations between relative mixed meal GI and relative glycaemic response for studies concluding against the utility of the GI in mixed meals (left), those concluding in favour of the GI (centre) and those in which GI was not considered (right). Dashed lines = lines of identity. Solid line and dotted lines = regression line with 95% confidence intervals. See text, Section 5.6.5 for further explanation.

indicates that amongst these studies GI accurately predicted the RGR. Amongst the studies which do not mention GI, the mean relative GR, 0.70, was significantly less than the mean relative GI, 0.78, and the slope of the regression line is greater than 1, although not significantly so, with the line of identity falling within the 95% CI for the regression (Fig. 5.26, right). Thus, amongst these studies the GI underestimated the difference in glycaemic response. For all 14 studies, including 54 different test meal comparisons, the mean GI ratio, 0.69 ± 0.02, was the same as the mean GR ratio, 0.69 ± 0.03, and the regression of RGR on relative GI is not significantly different from the line of identity (Fig. 5.27).

## 5.7 Different Meals with Different Nutrient Composition

Can the glycaemic responses of meals of varying nutrient composition be predicted? There are few studies looking at this issue, possibly because there are so many variables involved that it is considered too complex. Nevertheless two studies have tested the hypothesis that carbohydrate source and amount predict glucose and insulin responses of single mixed meals of varying composition (Wolever and Bolognesi, 1996b; Flint *et al.*, 2004).

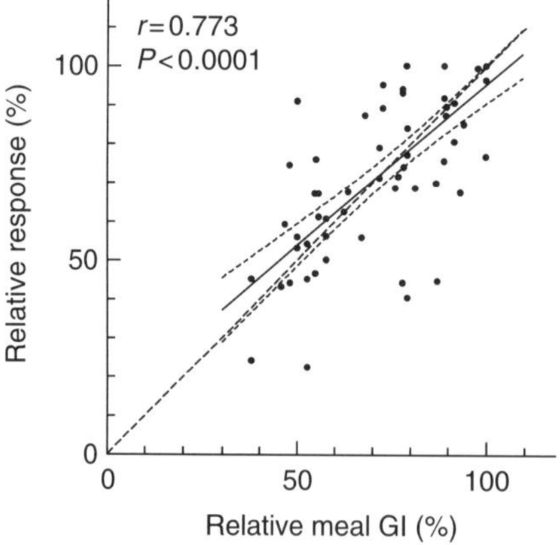


**Fig. 5.27.** Correlations between relative mixed meal GI and relative glycaemic response for all studies shown in Fig. 5.26. Dashed lines = lines of identity. Solid line and dotted lines = regression line with 95% confidence intervals. See text, Section 5.6.5 for further explanation.

We (Wolever and Bolognesi, 1996b) set out to test the hypothesis that the major determinant of postprandial glucose and insulin responses elicited by normal meals varying in energy, carbohydrate, protein and fat was the source (i.e. GI) and amount of carbohydrate they contained. There were two questions which needed answering in order to design the study – what is the range of variation in protein, fat and carbohydrate in normal meals and how do variations in amount and GI of dietary carbohydrate interact to influence glucose and insulin responses? The later question was addressed by performing a preliminary study to develop an equation describing glycaemic responses as a function of grams of carbohydrate and GI of carbohydrate (Wolever and Bolognesi, 1996a). The results of this study are discussed in Chapter 4, and shown in Fig. 4.1. The former question, 'What is a normal meal?', was very difficult to answer, and we do not know how representative the test meals we chose were. In designing the test meals, we also needed to choose foods for which we had previously determined the GI and to develop meals with a range of GI values. We decided to test cheese omelette with bread, margarine, eggs and cheese, spaghetti with tomato, cheese and lentils, maize flakes with bread, milk and margarine, oatmeal with bread, milk and margarine, and barley with tomato and cheese sauce. These meals varied in energy from 395 to 610 kcal, fat from 8 to 24 g (15–47% energy), protein from 12 to 25 g (11–20% energy), available carbohydrate from 38 to 104 g (33–69% energy) and GI from 43 to 99 (31 to 71 on the glucose scale) (Table 5.9). For these meals, neither GI nor carbohydrate were significantly related to the mean glucose and insulin AUC values, but the predicted responses, based on GI and amount of available carbohydrate were significantly related to the glucose and insulin responses, explaining over 90% of their variation (Fig. 5.28). There was no association between the fat and protein contents of the meals and their glycaemic or insulinaemic responses. Thus, we concluded that the amount and source of dietary carbohydrate are the main determinants of postprandial glucose and insulin responses.

Flint *et al.* (2004) came to a very different conclusion! They measured glucose and insulin responses elicited by 13 different meals in 18–21 normal subjects. The meals were designed '... to resemble typical European breakfast meals....'

**Table 5.9.** Composition of mixed meals tested by Wolever and Bolognesi (1996b).

| Test meal | Energy (kcal) | $CH_2O$[a] (g) | Protein (g) | Fat (g) | Meal GI[b] | Predicted[c] | |
|---|---|---|---|---|---|---|---|
| | | | | | | Glucose | Insulin |
| Omelette | 468 | 38 (33%) | 24 (20%) | 24 (47%) | 84 | 76 | 59 |
| Spaghetti | 529 | 87 (66%) | 25 (19%) | 9 (15%) | 59 | 83 | 71 |
| Corn flakes | 610 | 104 (68%) | 18 (12%) | 13 (20%) | 99 | 139 | 149 |
| Oatmeal | 453 | 62 (55%) | 12 (11%) | 17 (34%) | 85 | 99 | 87 |
| Barley | 395 | 68 (69%) | 12 (13%) | 8 (18%) | 43 | 59 | 43 |

Values in brackets are % of energy.
[a]Available carbohydrate defined as total carbohydrate minus dietary fibre.
[b]GI values given are based on bread scale (i.e. bread = 100); multiply by 0.71 to convert to glucose scale.
[c]Predicted responses relative to those elicited by 50 g available carbohydrate from white bread, calculated as follows: glucose $= 1.5 \times GI \times (1-e^{-0.018g}) + 13$; insulin $= 2.9 \times (0.6 \times GI + 0.003 \times GI^2) \times (1-e^{-0.0078g}) + 5$, where GI is meal glycaemic index and g is grams of available carbohydrate in the meal.

All of them contained 50 g available carbohydrate, but they varied in protein (5–28 g; 6–22% energy), fat (3–42 g; 11–55% energy) and energy (271–715 kcal); thus carbohydrate contributed 30–75% energy. All subjects took a reference test of white bread and the glucose and insulin responses of the test meals were expressed as a percentage of those of the reference food and termed 'glycaemic index' (GI) and 'insulinaemic index' (II). There was no significant association between the predicted and measured GI values of the meals ($P$ = 0.88; Fig. 5.29), nor between observed GI and II ($P$ = 0.40), but there was a significant inverse correlation between measured GI and the grams of fat in the meals ($P < 0.001$). Even if the five meals with less than 55% energy from carbohydrate were excluded, there was still no significant correlation between measured and predicted GI values ($P$ = 0.16; Fig. 5.29). The authors concluded, therefore, that carbohydrates do not play the most important role in determining the glucose and insulin responses of mixed meals.

Wolever and Bolognesi (1996b) concluded that carbohydrate is the most important determinant of postprandial glucose and insulin responses and that variations in protein and fat had little effect, whereas Flint *et al.* (2004) concluded that carbohydrates do not play the most important role, but rather fat, protein and/or energy content

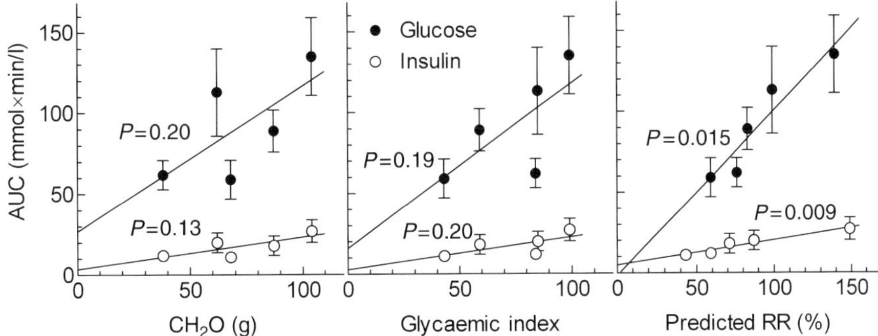


**Fig. 5.28.** Determinants of mean ± SEM postprandial glucose and insulin responses, expressed as incremental areas under the curve (AUC), of five mixed meals taken by normal subjects. The composition of the meals is shown in Table 5.8. Relationships between glucose and insulin responses and amount of available carbohydrate ($CH_2O$, left), meal GI (centre) and predicted relative response (RR, right) calculated from amount and GI of available carbohydrate (Table 5.9). Lines represent regression equations extrapolated to $x = 0$ but not forced through the origin. None of the $y$-intercepts is significantly different from 0.

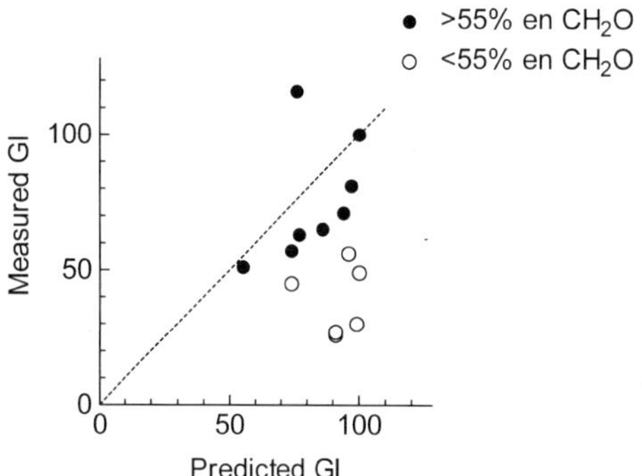


**Fig. 5.29.** Relationship between means of predicted GI and measured GI for 14 different test meals containing 50 g available carbohydrate tested by normal subjects (redrawn from Flint *et al.*, 2004).

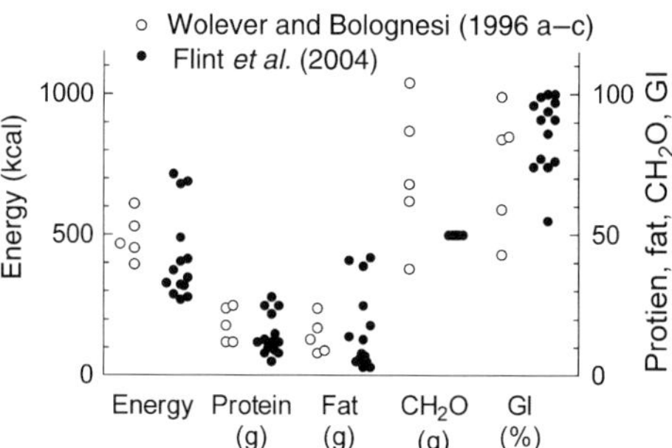


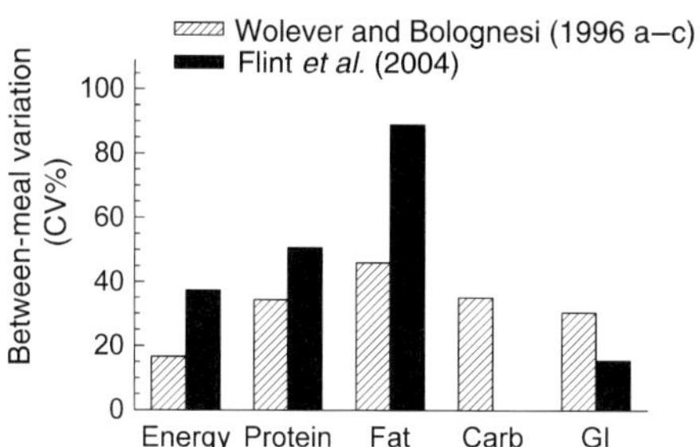


**Fig. 5.30.** Variation of contents of energy, fat, protein, available carbohydrate and GI of test meals fed by Wolever and Bolognesi (1996b) and Flint *et al.* (2004) in studies to determine which factors determined postprandial glucose and insulin responses. Top: individual values for the five meals from Wolever and Bolognesi (1996b) and the 14 meals from Flint *et al.* (2004). Bottom: between-meal variation expressed as coefficient of variation (CV = 100 × SD/mean).

have more important effects. How can these divergent conclusions be reconciled? We strongly criticized the methods of Flint *et al.* (2004) (Brand Miller and Wolever, 2005) because of doubts about the selection of correct GI values for the foods in the test meals, the fact that they only measured the glycaemic response elicited by the reference food one time in each individual which does not conform to FAO/WHO recommendations (Food and Agriculture Organization of the United Nations, 1998) on GI methodology, that they used venous plasma rather than capillary blood which increases variation of the results, and the narrow range of GI values tested. Here, however, I would like to emphasize the latter point – the range of intakes of energy, fat, protein, carbohydrate and GI in the various meals (Fig. 5.30). If one wants to determine if variation in a factor is related to variation in response, then the factor must be varied over a range large enough to elicit differences in response and hence, be able to draw a valid conclusion. If the test involves varying several factors, each of which are known to have an effect on the response, then, for a fair comparison, the degree of variation of the different factors should be similar.

The different test meals of Flint *et al.* (2004) had more variability of energy, fat and protein contents than those of Wolever and Bolognesi (1996b) (Fig. 5.30, top), but less variation in carbohydrate. In fact, the amount of carbohydrate did not vary at all in Flint *et al.* (2004); thus, it is difficult to see how their conclusion can be valid that variation in carbohydrate does not play an important role in mixed meal glycaemic responses; indeed if there is no variation in the amount of carbohydrate, then it cannot play a role! Figure 5.30, bottom, shows the between-meal coefficient of variation of energy, protein, fat, available carbohydrate and GI. It can be seen that, in the test meals designed by Wolever and Bolognesi (1996b), the variations in fat, protein, available carbohydrate content and GI across the different meals were approximately equivalent, with CVs varying from about 35–45%. By contrast, for the meals designed by Flint *et al.* (2004), the variation in amount of available carbohydrate was 0, the variation in protein was over three times the variation in GI (51% vs 16%) and the variation in fat, CV = 89%, was over 5.5 times greater than that for GI! Thus, since we know that fat and protein influence glycaemic responses, and since the amounts of protein and fat in the different meals varied three to five times more than did the GI of the different meals, it is not surprising that GI was not important in determining the glycaemic responses of this set of meals. By contrast, in the meals designed by Wolever and Bolognesi (1996b), the variations in protein, fat, carbohydrate and GI, expressed as CV, were similar; in that situation, the amount and GI of dietary carbohydrate was a more important determinant of glycaemic responses than protein and fat.

Thus, I believe sense can be made of this by concluding that protein, fat, amount of available carbohydrate and GI all have independent effects on glucose and insulin responses, but that these effects can only be seen if there is a reasonable amount of variation in their intakes.

## 5.8 Effect of Low-GI Diet on 24-h Glucose Profile

The technology now exists to measure blood glucose in free-living subjects continuously for up to 3 days using small metre that monitors glucose in interstitial fluid via a needle inserted into the tissues of the abdominal wall. Frost's group has shown that a low-GI diet reduces mean 24-h glucose concentration in normal and type 2 diabetic subjects. In the subjects with diabetes (Brynes *et al.*, 2003), the reduction in mean 24-h glucose appeared to be due to both a reduction in fasting glucose and a reduction in postprandial glucose rises. However, in the normal subjects (Brynes *et al.*, 2005), the reduction in 24-h glucose concentration was due to a reduction in fasting and postabsorptive glucose concentrations with no reduction in the peak levels achieved. Thus, the postprandial rises in glucose on the low-GI diet were higher than those on the high-GI diet, despite a lower GI (52 vs 60) and reduced glycaemic load (26 vs 33). This is not consistent with the proposed effect of a low-GI diet to reduce postprandial glucose responses. Both these studies could be criticized as being non-randomized studies in a single group of subjects with the measurements being done before and after a low-GI diet. Indeed, the glucose profile on the baseline diet in the normal subjects looks rather unusual, with the glucose profile fluctuating only between 5.0 and 6.0 mmol/l at baseline, compared to 4.0–6.0 mmol/l after the low-GI diet for 2 weeks.

## 5.9 Conclusions

Fat and protein have effects on glycaemic responses which are independent of those produced by carbohydrates and occur by different mechanisms. The effects of mixtures of carbohydrate foods on glycaemic responses are the same in normal and diabetic subjects and are predictable based on the foods' GI values and the relative proportion of available carbohydrate they contribute to the meal. The effects of fat and protein are inconsistent and have not been systematically studied. However, it appears that the ability of fat to reduce glycaemic responses is reduced in subjects with diabetes compared to subjects without diabetes. Most studies concluding that the GI does not predict glycaemic responses in mixed meals employed study designs with inadequate power to detect differences in glycaemic response or used inappropriate or faulty methods. When analysed using appropriate methods, virtually all studies show that the relative glycaemic impact of mixed meals is predicted by the amount of available carbohydrate they contain and GI. Protein, fat, amount of available carbohydrate and GI all have independent effects on glucose and insulin responses, but these effects can only be detected if there is sufficient amount of variation in their intakes.

# 6
# Measuring Diet GI

Diet GI is calculated from the GI values of the individual foods in a diet, and can be thought of as a measure of the quality of the carbohydrate in the diet, independent of the amount consumed. The validity of the results of studies on the relationship between GI and measures of human health and disease depends on the validity of the estimate of diet GI. This is so for any nutrient, biological marker or risk factor. Therefore, before we look at the results of studies related to the role of GI in human health and disease, it is worthwhile looking at how diet GI is assessed, whether the methods used are valid and how well the different methods agree. If valid methods exist, then we can ask questions such as: What is a 'normal' diet GI? How large a difference in GI is required to be physiologically meaningful?

Diet GI is determined by extending the calculations done for meal GI, that is:

$$\left\{\sum_{x}^{n=1} \mathrm{GI}_n \times g_n\right\}/G$$

where for $x$ foods in the diet, $\mathrm{GI}_n$ is the GI of the $n$th food, $g_n$ is the grams of available carbohydrate consumed from the $n$th food and $G$ is the amount of available carbohydrate in the entire diet (Wolever *et al.*, 1994b). It can be readily appreciated, then, that the accuracy of the diet GI calculation depends on the accuracy of the estimates of the amount of available carbohydrate consumed and the accuracy of the diet GI values for every food in the diet.

## 6.1 Assessing Available Carbohydrate Intake

It is well known that measuring nutrient intake is very difficult because of the inaccuracies involved in measuring what kinds and exactly how much food people eat (Barrett-Connor, 1991; Beaton, 1994; Beaton *et al.*, 1997). A detailed treatment of this topic is beyond the scope of this book. However, briefly, the three major ways of estimating food intake are methods involving direct observations, dietary recalls or records and food frequency questionnaires (FFQ).

### 6.1.1 Direct observations

Direct observations of subjects while eating can provide a very accurate measure of what they are eating, but the results may not be applicable to real life because subjects are often constrained to an experimental laboratory, and may or may not be consuming preweighed diets. Under such conditions, subjects are not following their normal routines and may not eat as they normally do. Also, such methods are very expensive and, thus, only can be applied to relatively small groups of subjects. Other related methods include duplicate collection of the diet in which the subject collects duplicate portions of everything consumed and returns it to the laboratory for analysis, or the subject takes a photograph of each meal before it is consumed. Although these kinds of procedures can be much more accurate methods than simply having the subject record what they eat, they rely on the subject actually remembering to collect a duplicate portion or to photograph everything consumed. In addition, it is expensive to carry out these procedures and to analyse the results obtained.

### 6.1.2 Food records or recalls

With these methods subjects are asked to recall the foods they ate the previous day or to write down the foods they eat while eating them for a period of one or more days. One difficulty with these methods is that people may not remember to include all the foods they eat, or may not bother to eat them so they do not have to write them down. In addition, the description of the type of food or the amount consumed may be inaccurate or incomplete. People often underestimate the amount of food they eat, and this is called under-reporting. The problem of under-reporting of energy intake is well known (Black *et al.*, 1993; Martin *et al.*, 1996; Sawaya *et al.*, 1996), and this obviously influences the accuracy of estimates of absolute nutrient intakes. Under-reporting of energy intake has been found to be greater in females than males, and positively associated with % body fat, attempted weight loss in past 12 months, being above self-reported ideal weight and amount of weight gained in last 10 years (Novotny *et al.*, 2003). The effect of under-reporting of energy on the estimates of nutrient intakes when expressed as a per cent of energy or in amounts per 1000 kcal may be less than when they are expressed in grams or milligrams, but there is still likely to be an effect since it seems unlikely that people will under-report everything they eat to exactly the same extent (Poppitt *et al.*, 1998). The effect of under-reporting on the estimate of diet GI has not been studied and, therefore, is unknown. The accuracy of portion size estimation can be improved by providing subjects with a scale on which to weigh everything consumed, but this not only increases the expense of collecting the dietary information, but increases the difficulty involved which, in turn, may reduce the ability or willingness to comply.

### 6.1.3 Food frequency questionnaires

In FFQ, subjects indicate how often they consume a specific list of foods or groups of foods. The FFQ can be used to obtain information about food intake over almost any period of time from last week to last year. However, their accuracy depends on whether most of the foods people eat are included in the list of foods asked about. If the population studied eat foods which are not included on the FFQ, it will not capture the nutrients in those foods and nutrient intakes will be underestimated. Thus, FFQ need to be developed and validated for different populations. In addition, single questions on the FFQ often include several foods (e.g. breads); this may work well for some nutrients but not others. For example, different kinds of breads have similar amounts of fat, but might have quite different GI values. Thus, this question would accurately capture fat intake from bread, but not GI. The advantages of FFQ are that they are easy to administer and can capture food intake over long periods of time (e.g. 1 year).

Validity is a measure of how close to the 'true' result the measured result is. Thus, the validity of an FFQ is a measure of how accurately it measures food intake. There are several components to validity, including reproducibility, accuracy and precision. Therefore, to assess the validity of an FFQ, it is administered twice and the results from the FFQ are compared to multiple food records collected by the same subjects. The results of one administration of the FFQ are compared with those of the other administrations of the FFQ to determine the reproducibility. The difference between the mean values of nutrient intakes assessed by food records and FFQ is a measure of the bias, or systematic error. The correlation between the estimates of nutrient intakes in each subject based on food records and FFQ indicates how well the FFQ distinguishes between individuals who have high and low intakes of nutrients (Willett and Lenart, 1998). The correlation between nutrient intakes assessed by food records and FFQ is often considered to be a measure of the validity of the FFQ. FFQ currently used were often originally designed to assess dietary fat intake (Block *et al.*, 1986; Kristal *et al.*,

1997). It is of interest that the validity of the FFQ varies in different populations and may vary for different nutrients (Block *et al.*, 1990; Kristal *et al.*, 1997; Willett and Lenart, 1998; Mayer-Davis *et al.*, 1999).

There is no published information of which I am aware indicating the validity of any FFQ for determining diet GI. Some of the published validation studies of FFQ do not even indicate the validity of the instrument for determining dietary carbohydrate intake (Block *et al.*, 1986; Kristal *et al.*, 1997). However, many FFQ validation studies do include carbohydrate; they show that the performance of the FFQ for determining carbohydrate intake varies from being the same as to being considerably less good than that for determining fat intake.

Figures 6.1 and 6.2 illustrate studies in which the validity for carbohydrate is similar to that for fat intakes. Figure 6.1 shows data from Block *et al.* (1990) in which the validity of the FFQ was assessed in groups of women in a feasibility study designed to teach women to maintain a low-fat diet. One group of women maintained their usual diets and the other group was taught a low-fat diet. It is of interest that the validity of the FFQ for measuring carbohydrate intake in grams was reported, but not for measuring carbohydrate as a percentage of energy. Figure 6.2 shows data from Rimm *et al.* (1992) on the validity of the FFQ used in the Male Health Professional Study and illustrates a number of points. First, the validity of the FFQ appears to improve if subjects are familiar with it, i.e. the correlation coefficients between nutrients assessed by FFQ and food records are larger on the second administration of the FFQ compared to the first. In addition, the validity appears to be improved when nutrient intakes are adjusted for energy. In this study, when intakes were not adjusted for energy, both the validity and reproducibility of the FFQ were somewhat better for fat than carbohydrate. However, when adjusted for energy the validity for carbohydrate was better than for fat.

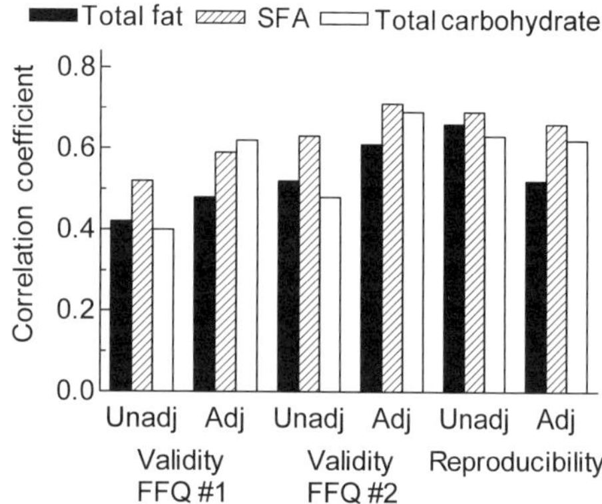


**Fig. 6.2.** Validity of a food frequency questionnaire (FFQ) for measuring fat and carbohydrate intakes (Rimm *et al.*, 1992). The FFQ was administered twice. Results are shown before (unadj) and after (adj) adjustment for energy intake.

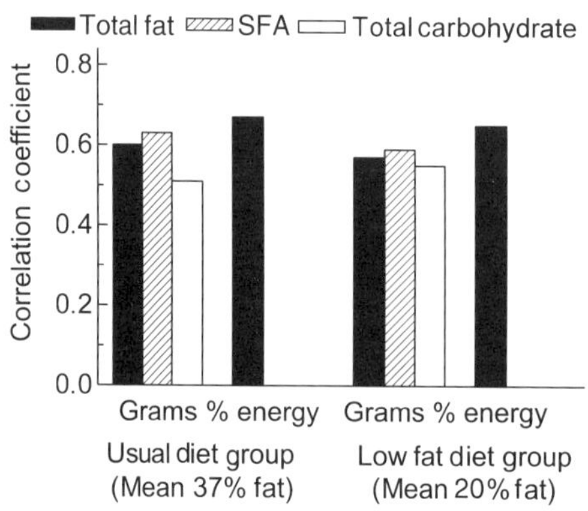


**Fig. 6.1.** Validity of a food frequency questionnaire for measuring fat and carbohydrate intakes (Block *et al.*, 1990).

Figures 6.3 and 6.4 show data from Mayer-Davis *et al.* (1999) which illustrates not only that the validity of FFQ vary in different populations based on ethnicity and education level, but also that the effect of these variables differs for carbohydrate and fat. Figure 6.3 shows the validity and reproducibility of the FFQ used in the Insulin Resistance Atherosclerosis Study (IRAS). It can be seen that ethnicity influences the validity of the FFQ for carbohydrate intake (range of *r*-values is 0.12–0.66) to a much greater extent than it does for total fat (0.37–0.61). For reproducibility, the range of *r*-values in different ethnic groups is similar for carbohydrate (0.35–0.66) and fat (0.42–0.88), but the direction of the effects differs – for example, compared to urban non-Hispanic whites, the reproducibility of the FFQ for fat intake in rural non-Hispanic whites tended to be better, but that for carbohydrate was worse. Figure 6.4 shows that the validity of the FFQ for measuring fat intake

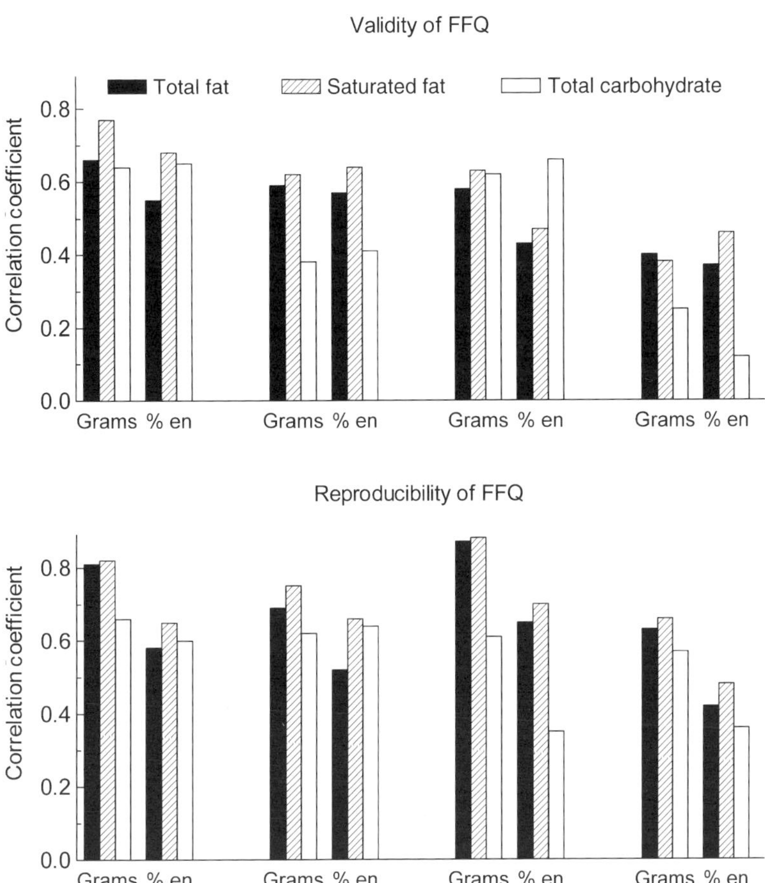


**Fig. 6.3.** Validity and reproducibility of the food frequency questionnaire (FFQ) used in the IRAS study by ethnicity (Mayer-Davis *et al.*, 1999). NHW, non-Hispanic white; AA, African American; Hisp, Hispanic.

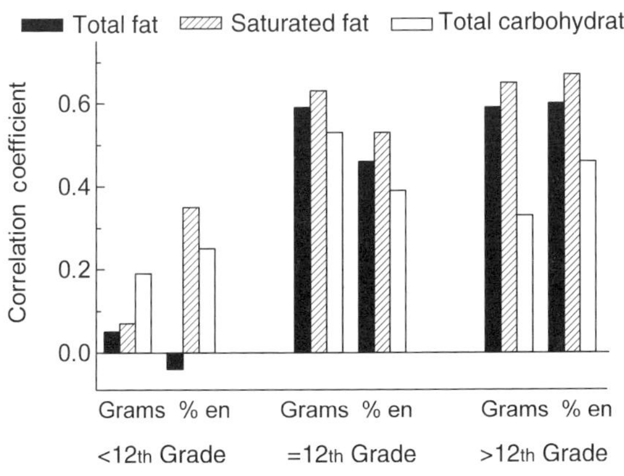


**Fig. 6.4.** Validity of the food frequency questionnaire used in the IRAS study by level of education (Mayer-Davis *et al.*, 1999).

varies differently by education level than that for carbohydrate. For example, there is only a modest difference in the validity of the FFQ for measuring carbohydrate intake in subjects with less than 12th grade education ($r \approx 0.25$) compared to those with more than 12th grade education ($r \approx 0.35$), but the validity for measuring fat intake markedly improved from 0.00 to 0.60.

Willett and Lenart (1998) provide a much more complete review of the reproducibility and validity of FFQ than I can here. However, the examples given here illustrate that the validity of an FFQ for measuring carbohydrate intake cannot be taken for granted. In their papers on the effect of GI and GL on risk for diabetes and heart disease, Willett's group cites studies showing that performance of the FFQ for determining the intakes of individual foods has been validated (e.g. Liu *et al.*, 2001). This does not necessarily mean that the instrument is valid for measuring diet GI. There could be a number of potential effects of using an invalid instrument on the results of epidemiological studies. If the FFQ produced a biased (i.e. incorrect) estimate of diet GI, then this could result in spurious and invalid correlations between diet and GI and health outcomes. If the FFQ was invalid because of a low correlation between diet GI assessed by FFQ and diet GI assessed by food records, this may result in the failure to detect correlations between diet GI and health outcomes which really exist. For these reasons, and in light of the fact that the validity of any FFQ for measuring diet GI has not been demonstrated, the results of studies demonstrating, or failing to demonstrate links between health outcomes and diet GI or GL assessed by FFQ must be interpreted with caution.

## 6.2 Assigning GI Values to Foods

The quality of the information obtained from studies utilizing data from databases can only be as good as the quality of the information in the database. If the information in the database is faulty, then the results of studies done using the database will also be wrong. Nowhere is this more critical than for studies involving assessment of the GI (and glycaemic load) values of diets. Diet GI values are derived using the type of calculation described above whereby the daily diet GI equals the sum of the products of the GI value of each food consumed during the day times, the grams of available carbohydrate in each respective food divided by the total amount of available carbohydrate in the day. To accomplish such calculations, the GI values of all the foods in the diet, or a pooled GI value for the foods represented by a question on an FFQ, must be added to the nutrient database being used. The question then becomes where do such GI values come from, and how reliable are they?

Ideally, the GI of each food in the diet would actually be measured. In addition, since methods of cooking or processing, or different varieties of food (e.g. rice, potatoes) may influence their GI values, these factors would, ideally, be taken into account. However, in practice, such vigilance is virtually impossible. Thus, investigators rely on published GI values. The task of finding published GI values has been greatly facilitated by the compilation of international tables of GI values (Foster-Powell and Brand Miller, 1995; Foster-Powell *et al.*, 2002). However, these tables often contain more than one GI value for the same or similar food and these values vary. For example, in the 2002 tables (Foster-Powell *et al.*, 2002) under the heading 'rye breads', there are two food items; number 84 is for 'rye-kernel (pumpernickel) bread', and there are six values ranging from 41 to 62 with an average of 50, and item 85 is 'whole-meal rye bread' and there are four values ranging from 41 to 66, with an average of 58. Next, there is a heading 'specialty rye breads' under which there are eight food items (numbers 86 through 94) with 11 individual values ranging from 48 to 86 and an average of 64. In examining these data, it is not clear why certain breads were put into certain categories, for example, items 88 and 94, under specialty rye breads, are labelled as being whole meal or whole grain breads, and perhaps should be included under items 84 or 85. This leads me to question whether other foods are categorized correctly, or even if there should be any categories at all? If I were trying to ascribe a GI value for rye bread in my database, which GI value should I use? Investigators from Denmark recently (Flint *et al.*, 2004) took the approach which many would likely take, which is to use the average for all ten of these items (item numbers 84–94). Use of the average would be the correct approach if the variation in GI values (from 41 to 86) was due to random error. However, if the variation in GI values in the tables was due to true differences between foods or to methodological differences, then use of the average value is not appropriate, and the particular food item in the GI table which represents the food in the diets or meals being assessed should be chosen after accounting for methodological differences.

In order to determine the magnitude of random error associated with determining the GI values of foods, we conducted an interlaboratory GI study (Wolever *et al.*, 2003a). Each laboratory determined the GI of four foods provided from a central location and local white bread in 8–10 subjects. The laboratories used the same methodology with respect to portion size, cooking procedures, subject selection and preparation, use of repeated measures of the reference food (glucose), type of blood sampling and schedule of blood sampling. All data were submitted to a central location for calculation of AUC and GI. Since the variation between labs for white bread GI was no different than that for the centrally provided foods, the data for bread were included in the calculation. The pooled SD of the mean GI values for five foods from five laboratories (interlab SD) was approximately 9 (GI of glucose = 100; for GI values based on bread, the interlab SD = 9 $\times$ 1.4 $\approx$ 12.5).

Table 6.1 shows the mean and SD of GI values for 62 groups of similar foods reported in the international GI tables (Foster-Powell *et al.*,

**Table 6.1.** Analysis of variance of GI values of 62 types of foods reported in international tables of GI.

| Category | Group | *n* | Mean GI | SD of GI | Variance ratio* | *P*** |
|---|---|---|---|---|---|---|
| Breads | Gluten-free | 5 | 75.8 | 4.7 | 0.27 | 0.924 |
| Dairy | Pudding | 8 | 36.4 | 5.2 | 0.33 | 0.943 |
| Breakfast cereals | RTE rice | 5 | 87.0 | 5.4 | 0.36 | 0.866 |
| Fruit | Apple | 10 | 36.8 | 5.7 | 0.40 | 0.926 |
| Sugars | Fructose | 6 | 18.7 | 6.2 | 0.48 | 0.815 |
| Beverages | Dairy drinks | 6 | 37.5 | 6.2 | 0.48 | 0.815 |
| Dairy | Soy | 5 | 37.6 | 6.2 | 0.48 | 0.787 |
| Dairy | Yogurt | 13 | 26.8 | 6.4 | 0.51 | 0.888 |
| Breakfast cereals | RTE wheat | 17 | 71.6 | 6.9 | 0.59 | 0.857 |
| Fruit | Pear | 7 | 37.7 | 7.3 | 0.65 | 0.707 |
| Fruit | Mango | 5 | 48.4 | 7.7 | 0.73 | 0.610 |
| Beverages | Juices | 16 | 46.4 | 7.9 | 0.78 | 0.690 |
| Breakfast cereals | RTE maize | 14 | 77.7 | 8.7 | 0.92 | 0.555 |
| Fruit | Orange | 9 | 45.3 | 8.9 | 0.98 | 0.492 |
| Meal replacer | Meal replacer | 20 | 33.8 | 8.9 | 0.98 | 0.524 |
| Vegetables | Maize | 8 | 52.5 | 9.0 | 1.00 | 0.471 |
| Potato | Mashed | 9 | 81.8 | 9.4 | 1.09 | 0.424 |
| Breakfast cereals | RTE muesli | 9 | 52.2 | 9.4 | 1.09 | 0.420 |
| Legumes | Lentils | 10 | 30.1 | 9.9 | 1.20 | 0.358 |
| Legumes | Butter | 6 | 34.7 | 9.9 | 1.20 | 0.354 |
| Snack | Nut | 5 | 19.6 | 10.0 | 1.23 | 0.340 |
| Legumes | Dried peas | 5 | 30.8 | 10.2 | 1.29 | 0.315 |
| Breakfast bars | Breakfast bars | 8 | 65.8 | 10.4 | 1.33 | 0.300 |
| Beverages | From powder | 13 | 43.8 | 10.6 | 1.39 | 0.265 |
| Cookies | Cookies | 45 | 57.4 | 10.7 | 1.41 | 0.230 |
| Crackers | Crackers | 20 | 68.9 | 10.7 | 1.42 | 0.241 |
| Breakfast cereals | Oats | 19 | 61.5 | 10.7 | 1.42 | 0.241 |
| Fruit | Banana | 11 | 52.9 | 10.9 | 1.47 | 0.236 |
| Noodles | Spaghetti | 33 | 44.9 | 11.2 | 1.55 | 0.176 |
| Noodles | Pasta | 15 | 50.5 | 11.2 | 1.56 | 0.195 |
| Legumes | Chickpeas | 6 | 32.3 | 11.9 | 1.74 | 0.177 |
| Breads | Wheat | 70 | 65.7 | 12.1 | 1.81 | 0.092 |
| Sugars | Glucose | 15 | 93.7 | 12.2 | 1.83 | 0.121 |

*Continued*

**Table 6.1.** *Continued.*

| Category | Group | *n* | Mean GI | SD of GI | Variance ratio* | *P*** |
|---|---|---|---|---|---|---|
| Legumes | Haricot | 7 | 35.4 | 12.6 | 1.95 | 0.128 |
| Breads | Rye | 22 | 58.0 | 12.6 | 1.96 | 0.086 |
| Grains | Wheat | 15 | 50.3 | 12.8 | 2.01 | 0.088 |
| Breads | Barley | 16 | 53.1 | 12.8 | 2.02 | 0.086 |
| Bakery | Breakfast | 10 | 76.7 | 13.0 | 2.08 | 0.092 |
| Fruit | Apricot | 7 | 47.6 | 13.1 | 2.11 | 0.102 |
| Breakfast cereals | RTE bran | 15 | 51.7 | 13.4 | 2.22 | 0.062 |
| Breads | Unleavened | 6 | 73.0 | 13.5 | 2.25 | 0.091 |
| Snack | Chocolate | 15 | 46.9 | 13.5 | 2.25 | 0.059 |
| Fruit | Peach | 7 | 47.6 | 13.7 | 2.33 | 0.076 |
| Breakfast cereals | RTE | 34 | 68.9 | 14.3 | 2.54 | 0.025 |
| Dairy | Milk | 12 | 27.8 | 14.4 | 2.56 | 0.041 |
| Beverages | Soft drinks | 6 | 67.2 | 14.7 | 2.66 | 0.055 |
| Bakery | Muffins | 12 | 60.6 | 15.1 | 2.80 | 0.028 |
| Dairy | Ice cream | 11 | 50.3 | 15.2 | 2.84 | 0.029 |
| Grains | Barley | 13 | 41.5 | 15.2 | 2.85 | 0.025 |
| Bakery | Cakes | 10 | 57.6 | 15.5 | 2.95 | 0.026 |
| Mixed | Mixed | 26 | 49.4 | 15.6 | 3.02 | 0.012 |
| Sugars | Honey | 11 | 54.5 | 16.2 | 3.26 | 0.016 |
| Sugars | Sucrose | 10 | 68.7 | 16.3 | 3.26 | 0.017 |
| Legumes | Kidney | 11 | 34.6 | 17.0 | 3.58 | 0.010 |
| Breakfast cereals | Cooked | 13 | 61.4 | 17.9 | 3.97 | 0.005 |
| Potato | Sweet | 8 | 52.3 | 18.8 | 4.34 | 0.006 |
| Noodles | Noodles | 10 | 53.5 | 19.3 | 4.58 | 0.004 |
| Grains | Maize | 5 | 75.6 | 20.3 | 5.08 | 0.006 |
| Potato | Whole | 29 | 67.9 | 20.4 | 5.11 | 0.001 |
| Grains | Rice | 87 | 61.3 | 21.2 | 5.52 | 0.000 |
| Snack | Fruit | 8 | 63.5 | 25.7 | 8.17 | 0.000 |
| Dairy | Misc | 8 | 51.0 | 26.3 | 8.55 | 0.000 |

RTE = ready-to-eat.
*Variance ($SD^2$) of GI values (glucose = 100) in the international tables (Foster-Powell *et al.*, 2002) divided by the pooled interlab variance from interlab GI study (Wolever *et al.*, 2003a).
**Probability that the variance of GI values from international tables is greater than pooled interlab variance from interlab GI study.

2002). The items in the table are ranked by the SD. I grouped foods together according to what seemed to me to be similar types of foods and often combining several items from the GI tables which did not necessarily seem to be distinguishable on the basis of their GI values. The column headed '*n*' represents the number of individual mean GI values reported in the table. For example, considering the first item in Table 6.1, gluten-free bread; there are three numbered items for gluten-free bread in the tables (items 76, 77 and 78) but there are actually five mean GI values. 'mean' represents the mean of the five GI values and 'SD' represents the SD of these five GI values reported for gluten-free bread. Although pooled SD was not calculated, this approach seems reasonable since it is the mean GI value which is being used in nutrient databases. In some cases, such as gluten-free bread, the food group in Table 6.1 is the same as that in the international GI tables (Foster-Powell *et al.*, 2002), but in others, such as ready-to-eat (RTE) wheat cereals, different foods were grouped together. Readers may not agree with my grouping of foods, on the grounds that readily identifiable different foods are grouped together. Nevertheless, in some cases, such as RTE wheat cereals, the difference between their GI values is quite small.

Column 5 of Table 6.1 is headed 'variance ratio', which is the variance ($SD^2$) of the different GI values for that food reported in the international GI tables (Foster-Powell *et al.*, 2002) divided by the estimate of error variance provided by the interlab GI study (pooled interlab SD$^2$), and the '$P$'-value is the probability that the variance of the GI values for the food is greater than that from the interlab GI study, i.e. the probability that there is significant heterogeneity amongst the GI values for that food. For example, there are 29 GI values for potato in the GI tables (these do not include mashed potato or sweet potato which are separate items in Table 6.1), and there is highly significant heterogeneity amongst these values ($P < 0.001$). This implies that there are either true methodological differences or real differences in GI values for potatoes, and therefore, it is not appropriate to use a mean GI value for potato to represent the GI value for potato in an FFQ, food record or test meal.

Just because the variance ratio is not statistically significant does not mean that the GI values for the foods do not vary. For example, for the 22 rye breads the SD is 12.6 and the significance of the variance ratio is 0.086, is not statistically significant. This means that there is an 0.086 probability that the variation in GI values of those rye breads is due to random error (i.e. homogeneous values), and conversely, therefore, there is $1 - 0.086 \approx 0.91$ probability that the GI values of those rye breads are really different (i.e. heterogeneous). There are 12 items on Table 6.1 with a SD between 12 and 14. Summing the value $(1-P)$ for the 12 items gives a total of 10.9. This suggests that, for 11 of these 12 items, the GI values are heterogeneous, i.e. the variance in GI is due to real differences between foods or methodological differences. Figure 6.5 shows the distribution of interlab SD values for the 62 groups of foods shown in Table 6.1. The total height of the bars indicates the number of foods within each range of interlab SD. The open bars represent the number of foods whose GI values are homogeneous, and the filled in bars represent the number of foods whose GI values are heterogeneous. This probability analysis suggests that the total number of foods with heterogeneous GI values is 45, or about 70% of the total. If this is so, simply taking the average GI value for a food from the international table of GI values (Foster-Powell *et al.*, 2002) is unlikely to be the appropriate approach to ascribing GI values to foods in a nutrient database.

It is of interest to note that some of the foods with the most highly variable GI values are starchy staples such as rice, potato, maize, noodles

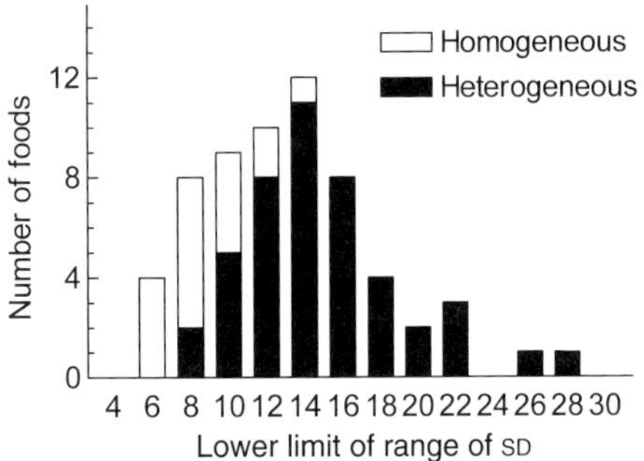


**Fig. 6.5.** Distribution of SD of GI values for the 62 groups of similar foods shown in Table 6.1. The shaded portion of each bar shows the sum of the probabilities that the heterogeneity of the GI values within each food group is statistically significant.

and cooked breakfast cereals. It is known that varietal differences in starch structure and differences in cooking and processing can affect the glycaemic responses of these types of foods (Wolever *et al.*, 1986a, 1994a; Panlasigui *et al.*, 1991; Brand Miller *et al.*, 1992; Soh and Brand-Miller, 1999; Larsen *et al.*, 2000; Fernandes *et al.*, 2005). Another interesting observation is that the GI values for sucrose are significantly heterogeneous, and the SD of the GI values for glucose, 12.2, is considerably higher than the pooled interlab SD from the interlab GI study (Wolever *et al.*, 2003a). Since these are simple sugars, the high variation in their GI values is presumably due to important methodological differences, which presumably may also be reflected in the GI values for other foods. On the other hand, some foods whose GI values might be expected to vary considerably, such as apples ($n = 10$), RTE wheat cereals of various kinds ($n = 17$), yogurt of various kinds ($n = 13$) and some other fruits (pear, mango, orange) are quite homogeneous.

## 6.3 Distribution of Diet GI Values in Individuals

We (Wolever *et al.*, 1994b) recommended that the unit of calculation for diet GI be a single day, and that, therefore, the weekly diet GI would be the average of the diet GI values calculated for each day. If there were large variations in the amount of carbohydrate consumed from day to day, this would yield a somewhat different weekly GI than if the unit of calculation was the week's diet. However, the advantage of calculating diet GI on a daily basis was that it allows estimation of the effects of day-to-day variation in diet GI on various metabolic parameters (Wolever *et al.*, 1999).

Some papers report mean GI values and others report medians. For normally distributed data, the mean equals the median, and since many types of biological data are normally distributed, the mean is usually reported. The median is considered better for distributions which are skewed. This raises the question as to what is the distribution of individual diet GI values in a population. Individual data on diet GI from a large number of normal subjects following typical western diets are not available in published form to allow the distribution of the values to be assessed. We reported that the GI values of 342 individuals with type 2 diabetes, calculated from two 3-day diet records, was normally distributed (Wolever *et al.*, 1994b) (Fig. 6.6, top).

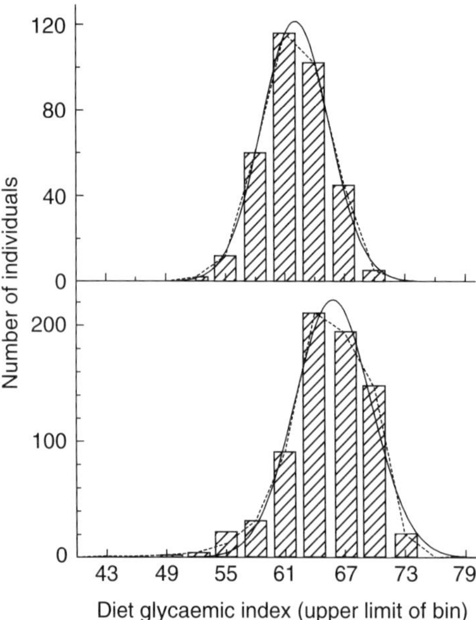


**Fig. 6.6.** Distribution of GI values: top, in 342 individuals with type 2 diabetes assessed by 3-day food record (Wolever *et al.*, 1994b); and bottom, in over 700 Ojibway-Cree individuals from a remote community in northern Ontario assessed by 24-h recall (Wolever *et al.*, 1997b). Solid lines represent normal distributions with the same mean and SD. Dashed lines show the observed distributions.

More recently, we determined diet GI using a 24-h dietary recall method in a population survey of over 700 Ojibway-Cree individuals living in a remote community of northern Ontario, Canada (Wolever *et al.*, 1997b). These values tend to be skewed to the left (Fig. 6.6, bottom) but the distribution is not significantly different from normal. The reason for the tendency of the latter distribution to be skewed is not clear, but could be related to the difference in methods used to collect dietary information (6 days as opposed to 1 day of food records in each subject), or to the fact that the mean diet GI of the Ojibway-Cree population was higher than that of the diabetic population, and approached a value of 70, which is about the maximum diet GI value it is possible to have. A diet GI over 70 would mean that the diet contains very few dairy products, fruits, sugar and sweetened drinks (all of which have GI values less than 70), and that dietary carbohydrate consists primarily of bread, other foods made of wheat flour (GI of 71), from foods such as refined breakfast cereals and instant potato (GI 75–85). Thus, if most people have a GI near the upper limit of possible values, the tail of the distribution has to be longer at the lower end of values.

A recently published study of 572 healthy adults in central Massachusetts from whom multiple 7-day diet records were collected confirms that the diet GI values of individuals is normally distributed (Ma *et al.*, 2005).

## 6.4 Assessment of Diet GI by FFQ

### 6.4.1 Population GI values assessed by FFQ

Diet GI values assessed by FFQ are shown in Table 6.2 and Fig. 6.7. Mean values in different populations range from about 50 to 60 with 80% of the population having values within about 5–6 of the mean. It is not known whether the differences in mean GI between different studies are due to differences in the database used or due to true differences in the population. However, in one study (Schulz *et al.*, 2005), it was shown that diet GI was significantly higher in men than women and significantly higher in Hispanics than non-Hispanic whites (Fig. 6.8).

**Table 6.2.** Values of diet GI assessed by food frequency questionnaire.

| Population (ID[a]) | Quintiles of GI 1 | 2 | 3 | 4 | 5 | Reference |
|---|---|---|---|---|---|---|
| Women's Health Study | | | | | | |
| US (40–65 year, $n = 65{,}173$) (a) | 44.7 | 48.4 | 50.2 | 52.1 | 55.3 | Salmerón *et al.* (1997b) |
| US (>45 year, $n = 38{,}876$) (b) | 49 | 51 | 53 | 54 | 57 | Higginbotham *et al.* (2004) |
| US (30–55 year, $n = 88{,}802$)[b] (c) | 46.2 | 49.7 | 52.5 | 54.7 | 57.5 | Michaud *et al.* (2002) |
| US (24–44 year, $n = 91{,}249$)[b] (d) | 50.5 | 53.0 | 54.5 | 56.1 | 58.3 | Schulze *et al.* (2004) |
| Male Health Professionals Study | | | | | | |
| US (40–75 year, $n = 42{,}759$) (e) | 46.2 | 49.5 | 51.6 | 53.5 | 56.3 | Salmerón *et al.* (1997a) |
| Other studies | | | | | | |
| US White (45–64 year, $n = 11{,}478$) (f) | 49.1 | 52.9 | 54.8 | 56.6 | 59.2 | Stevens *et al.* (2002) |
| US African (45–64 year, $n = 4{,}211$) (g) | 50.9 | 55.1 | 56.9 | 58.6 | 61.5 | Stevens *et al.* (2002) |
| US Adults (26–82 year, $n = 2{,}834$)[b] (h) | 51.1 | 54.0 | 55.4 | 57.5 | 59.6 | McKeown *et al.* (2004) |
| US Children (8 year, $n = 111$) (i) | | | 58 | | | Scaglioni *et al.* (2004) |
| IRAS Population (40–69 year, $n = 1071$) (j) | 52.9 | 56.1 | 57.9 | 59.8 | 63.1 | Schulz *et al.* (2005) |
| Italian (25–79 year, $n = 478$)[c] (k) | – | – | 53.1 | – | – | Tavani *et al.* (2003) |
| Italian female (20–74 year, $n = 2{,}588$)[c] (l) | – | 50.6 | 52.8 | 54.9 | – | Augustin *et al.* (2001) |
| Italian (19–74 year, $n = 4{,}154$)[c] (m) | – | 51.3 | 53.4 | 55.4 | – | Franceschi *et al.* (2001) |
| Italian female (22–75 year, $n = 753$)[c,d] (n) | – | 51.1 | 53.6 | 55.8 | – | Augustin *et al.* (2003b) |
| Italian adults (<77 year, $n = 3{,}322$)[c] (o) | – | 51.6 | 53.9 | 56.1 | – | Augustin *et al.* (2003c) |
| Swiss female (22–75 year, $n = 753$)[c,d] (p) | – | 57.2 | 59.5 | 61.4 | – | Augustin *et al.* (2003b) |

Values are means unless otherwise indicated.
[a]ID = Identification of studies on Fig. 6.7.
[b]Medians.
[c]Mean of extremes.
[d]753 = Total for Swiss and Italian.

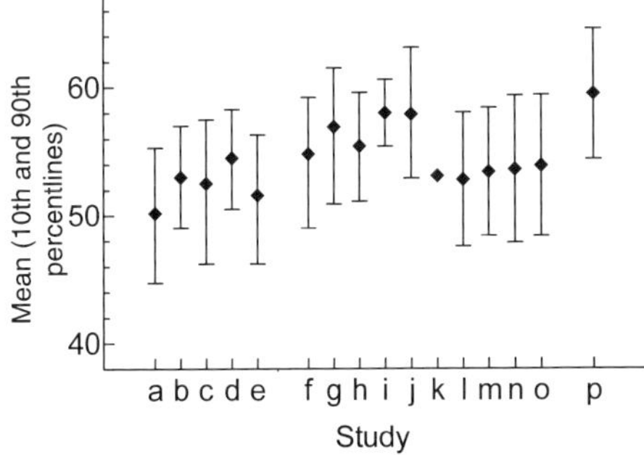


**Fig. 6.7.** Diet GI values assessed by food frequency questionnaire. Symbols represent means or medians and the ends of the error bars represent the 10th and 90th percentiles. The studies (a–o) are identified on Table 6.2, which also includes further details about the populations studied.

### 6.4.2 Validity of FFQ for assessing diet GI

Since the validity of the FFQ for assessing diet GI is not known, we attempted to assess this recently in Trinidad and Tobago in 156 individuals (Malik, 2003). Males and females between the ages of 20 and 65 who were healthy and not following any special diet for medical purposes were randomly selected from an area of Trinidad and Tobago which is representative of the country's population. An FFQ was developed based on a validated semi-quantitative FFQ developed by the Epidemiology Program of the Cancer Center of Hawaii, University of Hawaii (Kolonel *et al.*, 2000; Stram *et al.*, 2000). The food items on the FFQ were modified based on the foods consumed by individuals participating in a previous non-random dietary survey by 24-h recall (Wolever *et al.*, 2002a). Subjects completed a 7-day food record

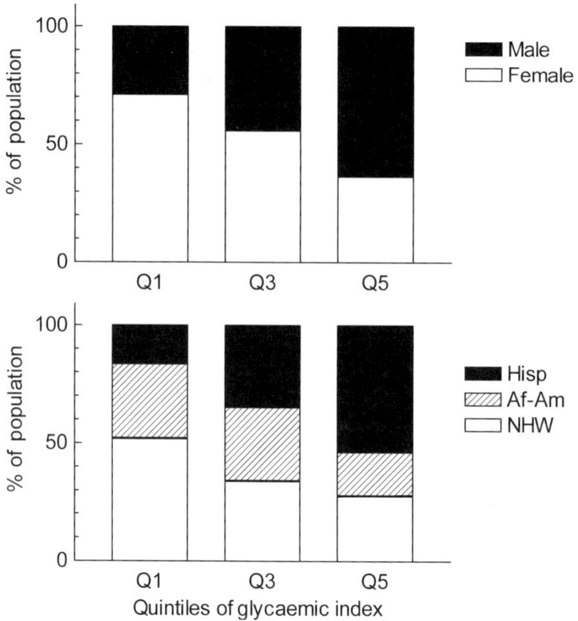


**Fig. 6.8.** Distribution of diet GI values in the Insulin Resistance Atherosclerosis Study population by gender and ethnicity (Liese *et al.*, 2005).

and the FFQ in random order. The correlation between carbohydrate (grams, $r = 0.35$; % energy, $r = 0.45$) and fat (grams, $r = 0.51$; % energy, $r = 0.48$) intakes assessed by 7-day food record and FFQ were within the ranges seen in other validation studies (e.g. Figs 6.1–6.4), but that for GI was very poor ($r = 0.25$). If this result were true, it would cast doubt upon the validity of the FFQ for assessing diet GI. Unfortunately, however, the study has a number of flaws. The 7-day food record assessed dietary intake at the time of the study, while the FFQ assessed dietary intake over the previous 12 months. The study was conducted between May and August when the diet (as assessed by 7-day food record) may be different from that during the other months of the year (included in the FFQ assessment) due to differences in food availability. Thus, for the results of this study to be reliable, the food records should have been collected at various times throughout the year. Nevertheless, these results suggest that it cannot be taken for granted that the FFQ is a valid instrument for assessing diet GI, and that a proper validation study needs to be done.

## 6.5 Assessing Diet GI by Food Records

Mean values for diet GI assessed by food records in various selected studies are shown in Fig. 6.9. Again, it is not possible to know if the differences between studies are due to differences in the database or to true differences between the populations. However, within studies there are a number of significant differences between different populations in the same study, for example, in a remote community of Ojibway-Cree in northern Ontario men had a higher diet GI than women, as did older individuals compared to younger (Wolever *et al.*, 1997a). Men with type 2 diabetes (T2DM) in Canada had a significantly higher diet GI than women (Wolever *et al.*, 1994b), as did men with type 1 diabetes (T1DM) in Europe (Toeller *et al.*, 2001) (the paper did not indicate if the latter difference was statistically significant, though it appears to be so), and healthy men in the USA (Ma *et al.*, 2005). There were also significant differences in diet GI between African and South Asian males in Trinidad (Wolever *et al.*, 2002a)

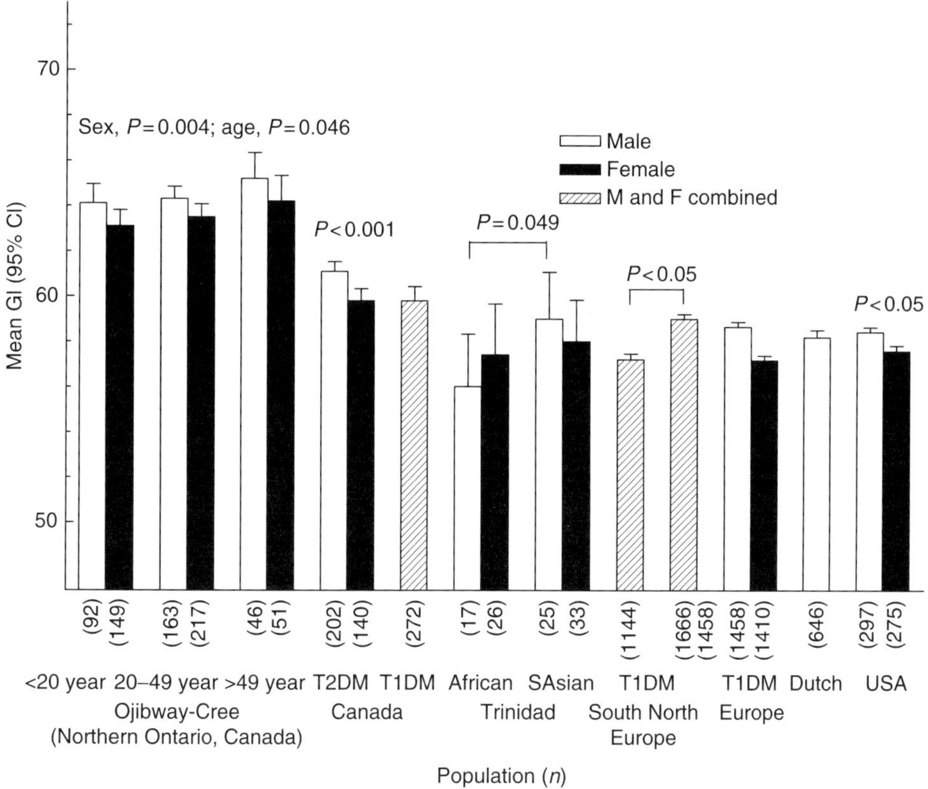


**Fig. 6.9.** Diet GI values assessed by food records in selected studies (means and 95% confidence intervals). Numbers of individuals shown in brackets below the bars. Ojibway-Cree (Wolever *et al.*, 1997a); T2DM (type 2 diabetes mellitus) Canada (Wolever *et al.*, 1994b); T1DM (type 1 diabetes mellitus) Canada (Wolever *et al.*, 1999); Trinidad (Wolever *et al.*, 2002a); North and South Europe T1DM (Buyken *et al.*, 2001); T1DM Europe (Toeller *et al.*, 2001); Dutch (van Dam *et al.*, 2000); USA (Ma *et al.*, 2005).

and between individuals with T1DM living in northern compared to southern Europe (Buyken *et al.*, 2001).

It is of interest to note that mean diet GI values derived from food records (Fig. 6.9; range 56–65) tend to be greater than those derived from FFQ (Fig. 6.7; range 50–60). Part of this is due to the very high diet GI in the Ojibway-Cree, a special population which forms a disproportionately large part of the food record data. Nevertheless, even when these subjects are excluded, the mean diet GI in the other populations assessed by food records was about 58, compared to about 53 in the FFQ populations. This is a large difference, compared to differences between populations assessed using the same method. It could be due to real differences in diet GI between the populations studied, or to different databases, or to methodological bias.

## 6.6 Conclusions

The validity of measuring diet GI depends on several factors, all of which are problematic for most investigators. It is well known that it is difficult to measure energy and nutrient intakes accurately and precisely by any method. This is a problem because knowledge of carbohydrate intake is necessary to calculate diet GI and glycaemic load. Assigning GI values to foods in nutrient databases is problematic because the GI values for foods can be influenced by methods used to measure the GI, and by food variety, cooking, processing, etc. The international GI tables (Foster-Powell *et al.*, 2002) list more than one GI value for most common foods, and these values can vary considerably. Thus, it is difficult to know which value to choose. However, the variation in GI values for most foods published in international GI tables probably represents real variation rather than random error; thus, it is not appropriate to take the average value for similar foods. Measuring diet GI using FFQ has not been validated, but would appear to lack precision because of the grouping together of foods which may have different GI values in a single question. Diet GI values measured using food records are normally distributed, but appear to be larger than those measured by FFQ. It is not known if this difference represents methodological bias, differences in the assignment of GI values in the database or real differences between the populations studied. Research on the methodology of measuring diet GI is urgently needed.

# 7

# Glycaemic Index and Health

The factors which influence the extent to which the available carbohydrate in foods raises post-prandial blood glucose include differences in the rate and extent to which carbohydrates are digested and absorbed in the gastrointestinal tract, and differences in the metabolism of different monosaccharides. Thus, the physiological and metabolic effects of these factors go far beyond merely influencing glycaemic responses; indeed, recent research indicate that differences in the GI of dietary carbohydrates, independent of the amount of carbohydrate, influence a wide variety of physiological processes which are relevant not only to the prevention and treatment of disease but also to the functioning and performance of healthy individuals. This chapter will review, briefly, the effects of GI in health, and the next chapter the effects of GI in the prevention and treatment of disease. However, it is recognized that the distinction between health and disease is somewhat artificial, for example, body weight regulation is discussed in this chapter, but it has a huge implication for the prevention of disease. By the same token, prevention and treatment of diabetes is discussed in the next chapter, but preventative measures are practised in people who do not yet have the disorder, and, according to current thinking, many people with diabetes would consider themselves, and be considered by many health professionals, to be 'healthy' in that there is no reason they cannot do all the things that someone without diabetes can do.

Lack of space and lack of expert knowledge do not permit a full discussion of any of the processes discussed below. My purpose here is merely to illustrate how GI has a broad implication for the functioning and performance of the healthy human body.

## 7.1 GI and Athletic Performance

The ability to perform physical activity depends on the muscle being able to obtain an adequate supply of substrate for oxidation, or, in lay terms, fuel. The fuels available to muscles are fat and glucose, and these are supplied from stores within the muscle and from blood FFA and glucose. For mild activity, the muscle uses mostly fat as fuel. As the intensity of activity becomes more vigorous, the muscle draws more and more on glucose. Very intensive exercise can only be sustained as long as a supply of glucose is available to exercising muscle. Exhaustion occurs when muscle glycogen is depleted, and at this stage the intensity of exercise must diminish (Burke *et al.*, 2004). A high-carbohydrate diet is associated with increased stores of muscle glycogen, and thus, endurance is longer if the athlete eats a high-carbohydrate diet before the event than if (s)he eats a low-carbohydrate diet (Bergstrom *et al.*, 1967). There are two ways in which the GI affects athletic performance. One is the effect of a pre-event snack on endurance and the other is the effect of the diet on the recovery of muscle glycogen after vigorous exercise.

A number of studies have looked at the effect of high- or low-GI snacks consumed before exercise on performance or endurance during exercise in trained athletes. Two studies showed that a low-GI snack significantly prolonged time to exhaustion compared to a high-GI snack containing the same amount of carbohydrate. In one study (Thomas *et al.*, 1991), subjects ate the snack 60 min before starting to cycle at 65–70% of maximum oxygen uptake until exhausted, which occurred at 97 min for potato and 117 min for lentils. In the other study (DeMarco *et al.*, 1999), subjects ate the snack 30 min before starting to cycle at 70% maximum oxygen uptake. They cycled at that intensity for 2 h then increased to 100% maximum oxygen uptake until exhausted (130 min for high GI and 207 min for low GI). These results appear to be contradicted by two other studies which looked at the effect of pre-exercise snacks on work output during a 15-min performance cycle which was done after 50 min of exercise at 67% of maximum oxygen uptake (Sparks *et al.*, 1998) or 120 min at 70% of maximum oxygen uptake (Febbraio and Stewart, 1996). Despite differences in blood glucose, there was no effect of GI on work output, but also no effect of consuming carbohydrate compared to a placebo pre-exercise snack. The apparent contradiction is possibly explained by differences in protocol and the fact that different endpoints were measured.

Two studies have shown an effect of diet GI on muscle glycogen. In one study, low- and high-GI diets were consumed for 30 days by moderately active young men undergoing their normal activities (Kiens and Richter, 1996). Both muscle glycogen and muscle triglyceride content were significantly lower after the low-GI diet than the high-GI diet. In the other study, trained cyclists undertook an exercise trial to deplete muscle glycogen, followed by a high- or low-GI diet for the next 24 h. Muscle glycogen increased to a significantly greater extent after the high-GI diet compared to the low-GI diet (Burke *et al.*, 1993).

In summary, low-GI foods taken before prolonged vigorous exercise appear to increase endurance, although they may not enhance work output. On the other hand, high-GI foods appear to be most useful for recovery after prolonged vigorous activity, because they enhance muscle glycogen content.

## 7.2 GI and Cognitive Function

Glucose is the major fuel for the brain. Traditionally it was thought that concentration of interstitial glucose was the same in all parts of the brain, and that the ability to transport glucose exceeded the demand of the brain for glucose. According to this view, the only time when glucose would be limiting to brain function would be during hypoglycaemia when the very low levels of glucose in the blood would limit transport into the brain. However, this view is not consistent with recent research which shows that increased mental activity creates a demand for increased glucose consumption by the specific region of the brain involved, and that the ability to carry on increased cognitive activity can be influenced by the supply of glucose to the affected region of the brain. Reducing the supply of glucose results in poorer cognitive performance (reviewed by Benton and Nabb, 2003). This leads to the hypothesis that manoeuvres which increase the supply of glucose to the brain, such as eating a carbohydrate-rich meal, will improve cognitive function. This hypothesis is supported by many studies, such as, for example, those showing that eating a breakfast cereal for breakfast improve school performance in children (reviewed by Benton and Parker, 1998).

However, rises in blood glucose are not the only mechanism by which breakfast can improve cognitive function. In young normal subjects, ingestion of protein alone, fat alone or carbohydrate alone had different effects on brain function (Fischer *et al.*, 2001). In elderly subjects, ingestion of protein or fat alone had similar effects on enhancing memory in elderly subjects as consuming carbohydrate, but specific effects on other aspects of cognition (Kaplan *et al.*, 2001). Indeed, chronic elevation of blood glucose tends to be associated with impaired cognition, such that subjects with diabetes have poorer cognitive function that matched controls without diabetes. In elderly subjects without diabetes, higher blood glucose concentrations and an increased glycaemic response to a standard meal are also associated with reduced short-term memory (reviewed by Greenwood, 2003).

These considerations have led some investigators to study the effects of different carbohydrates on cognitive function, and all of the studies to date suggest that carbohydrates which elicit low glycaemic responses have different effects than those with high responses. Benton *et al.* (2003) compared verbal memory in normal subjects after breakfast meals consisting of biscuits containing a low or high amount of slowly available glucose (SAG). The high-SAG meal elicited a lower glycaemic response than the low-SAG meal. Memory scores were similar at 30 and 90 min after eating, but were significantly higher (i.e. more words remembered) 150 and 210 min after the low-GI than the high-GI meal. Similar effects were seen in rats.

Kaplan *et al.* (2000) studied the effect on blood glucose responses and memory of consuming 50 g available carbohydrate portions of glucose, instant potato and pearled barley in a group of 20 elderly subjects. The mean net incremental areas under the glucose response curve elicited by glucose, instant potato, pearled barley and water alone, $325 \pm 34$, $270 \pm 21$, $85 \pm 11$ and $-11 \pm 7$ mmol $\times$ min/l, respectively, were all significantly different from each other. The carbohydrate meals were found to improve memory, relative to water, only in subjects with β-cell function (assessed by HOMA) below the median value in the 20 subjects studied. In these subjects, the improvement in memory was independent of glycaemic response, and in fact, tended to be greater after barley than glucose or potato.

Greenwood *et al.* (2003) showed that in 19 subjects with type 2 diabetes, memory was significantly related to glycaemic control, with more words and paragraphs able to be recalled in subjects with good glycaemic control. In contrast to subjects without diabetes, Greenwood *et al.* (2003) found that, in people with type 2 diabetes, consumption of a high-GI carbohydrate meal significantly impaired memory relative to consuming water alone.

Thus, there is evidence that low-GI starchy foods may improve postprandial cognitive performance when compared to high-GI foods, at least in some subject groups. Since the effect of carbohydrates on brain function varies with the time of day and other factors (Kanarek, 1997), the interaction between these factors and food GI will have to be studied. It is not known whether there are any long-term effects of diet on cognitive function.

## 7.3 GI and Weight Management

Obesity is a major public health concern because of its rising prevalence (Mokdad *et al.*, 2001) and its association with increased mortality and morbidity from cardiovascular disease, hypertension, stoke, diabetes and cancer (World Health Organization, 1998) and excess burden of respiratory symptoms, low back pain and difficulties in physical functioning (Lean *et al.*, 1998). Obesity, and especially central adiposity as determined by an increased waist circumference (Després *et al.*, 2001), is associated with IGT, insulin resistance and hyperinsulinaemia (DeFronzo and Ferrannini, 1991).

### 7.3.1 Pathogenesis of obesity

Fundamentally, obesity is caused by energy intake being greater than energy expenditure. However, obesity is a complex problem because both genetic and environmental factors interact to determine both energy intake and energy expenditure (Montague and O'Rahilly, 2000). It is clear that reduced energy expenditure is a very important factor, as illustrated, for example, by studies showing that the prevalence of obesity in children is directly related to the hours of television watched (Crespo *et al.*, 2001). However, excess energy intake is also likely important. Traditionally it has been considered that high-fat diets promote obesity because the adipose tissue mass has to increase to allow for increased fat oxidation (Flatt, 1995) and because high-fat foods are energy dense and promote passive overconsumption (Stubbs *et al.*, 1995). The association of high fat intake with obesity (Romieu *et al.*, 1988) is an important reason why nutrition recommendations over the past 20 years have focused on reducing fat intake. However, the wisdom of this is now questioned (Willett, 1998), at least in part because the prevalence of overweight in the USA continues to increase despite decreasing fat intake, the so-called 'American Paradox' (Heini and Weinsier, 1997). Overconsumption of low-fat products (Shide and Rolls, 1995) has been proposed as an explanation for the 'American Paradox', as well as under-reporting of fat intake and clustering of obesity-promoting lifestyles in subgroups of the population (Astrup, 1998). Nevertheless, current reports suggesting increased sugar intake in the USA (Guthrie and Morton, 2000), an inverse relationship between the satiating effects of foods and their blood glucose- and insulin-raising potential (Ludwig, 2000), and an association between consumption of sugar-sweetened drinks and obesity in children (Ludwig *et al.*, 2001), have implicated high carbohydrate intake and hyperinsulinaemia in the promotion of obesity.

An important question is whether insulin is a cause of obesity or merely an effect (Ravussin and Swinburn, 1996; Sims, 1996). It is known that overfeeding and weight gain cause hyperinsulinaemia, but it remains to be determined if the reverse is true, that hyperinsulinaemia leads to obesity. The 'thrifty gene' hypothesis (Neel, 1962) suggested that individuals predisposed to obesity and diabetes differ metabolically from those who are not, and that hyperinsulinaemia may precede obesity (Neel, 1982). From this arose the concept that hyperinsulinaemia increases the efficiency of fat storage, and plays a crucial role in the development of obesity. Studies in adults from several ethnic groups tend to contradict this, in that hyperinsulinaemic or insulin-resistant subjects tend to gain less weight compared to insulin-sensitive subjects with low plasma insulin (Swinburn *et al.*, 1991a; Valdez *et al.*, 1994; Hoag *et al.*, 1995; Schwartz *et al.*, 1995). In addition, treatment of diabetes with the insulin sensitizer, pioglitazone for 2 years was associated with reduced insulin resistance and plasma insulin concentrations and improved glycaemic control compared to treatment with the insulin secretogog gliclazide, nevertheless, subjects on pioglitazone gained more weight than those on gliclazide (Tan *et al.*, 2005). This is consistent with the finding that plasma lipoprotein lipase (LPL) activity and adipose tissue LPL mRNA levels were higher in insulin-sensitive than insulin-resistant subjects (Maheux *et al.*, 1997). These studies suggest that insulin resistance and hyperinsulinaemia are secondary to obesity, and that the hyperinsulinaemia of obesity may protect against further weight gain. However, in Pima Indian children studied initially at ages 5–9 and followed up 9 years later, high fasting plasma insulin was associated with increased weight gain in both boys and girls (Odeleye *et al.*, 1997).

Hyperinsulinaemia is proposed to be a pathogenic factor in obesity by its lipogenic actions (Cusin *et al.*, 1992). After a mixed meal, insulin promotes fat storage and causes preferential oxidation of carbohydrate over fat (Flatt, 1995). Insulin increases LPL activity in adipose tissue but decreases it in skeletal muscle (Eckel *et al.*, 1995) thus decreasing fat oxidation in muscle and increasing fat storage in adipose tissue. In addition, high-GI foods with high insulin responses have been suggested to be less satiating than low-GI foods, thus promoting overeating and obesity (Ludwig, 2000). Against this, however, are data showing that insulin can gain access to the brain through a specialized transport system (Schwartz *et al.*, 1991) where it suppresses appetite and food intake (Brief and Davis, 1984; Foster *et al.*, 1991; Woods *et al.*, 1996) and may increase energy expenditure (Berne *et al.*, 1992). Intravenous infusions of glucose and/or insulin in humans or animals have been shown to increase food intake in some studies (Rodin *et al.*, 1985; Koopmans *et al.*, 1998), decrease it in some (Woods *et al.*, 1984) and have little or no effect in others (Woo *et al.*, 1984; Chapman *et al.*, 1998; Gielkens *et al.*, 1998).

A recent study showed that energy intake 5½ h after breakfast was inversely related to plasma insulin before lunch in lean, but not obese subjects (Speechly and Buffenstein, 2000). Plasma insulin was >15 μU/ml in all obese but <15 μU/ml in all lean subjects. This suggested that insulin suppresses appetite in lean subjects, but that this control is lost in obesity due to resistance to the appetite controlling effects of insulin. However, we found that 50 g glucose preloads suppressed food intake to a greater extent in normal subjects with high fasting insulin (≥40 pmol/l) than in those with low fasting insulin (<40 pmol/l) despite the fact that the hyperinsulinaemic subjects had a higher body mass index (Samra *et al.*, 2004). A 75 g oral glucose load taken on another occasion elicited a twofold greater insulin response, higher GLP-1 and CCK and lower ghrelin responses in the hyperinsulinaemic than control subjects, all of which are consistent with reduced food intake (Samra *et al.*, 2004). Thus, these results are consistent with the concept that, in adults, insulin resistance is secondary to obesity and that the resulting high plasma insulin acts to help limit further weight gain.

### 7.3.2 Effect of low-carbohydrate and low-GI diets on body weight

If high insulin is important in the pathogenesis of obesity, then use of a diet which elicits a low plasma insulin response should result in weight loss. Postprandial insulin responses can be reduced either by reducing carbohydrate intake or by reducing diet GI. Indeed, one of the most popular applications of the GI is for body weight management. Scientific interest in this area has been fuelled by a number of best selling diet books which make use of the GI concept, such as the Zone, Sugar Buster's and the Montignac diet. Unfortunately, these books promote an erroneous and over-simplistic view of the GI which has caused confusion not only amongst the public, but also amongst well-known nutritional scientists about the meaning of the term 'glycaemic index'. This issue is discussed in more detail in Chapter 9, but is mentioned here because it is a prominent feature of the debate about the role of GI in weight management.

One of the most common misconceptions is that low GI means a diet which elicits a low blood glucose response. For example, a well-known group from the University of Laval in Canada published a paper entitled: 'Effect of a low-glycaemic index–low-fat–high protein diet on the atherogenic metabolic risk profile of abdominally obese men' in which a diet modelled on the Montignac diet (31% energy as protein, 32% fat, 37% carbohydrate) was fed to abdominally obese subjects for 6 days compared to an American Heart Association diet (15% protein, 30% fat, 55% carbohydrate) (Dumesnil *et al.*, 2001). The low-GI–low-fat–high-protein diet induced a spontaneous reduction in energy intake, and large falls in serum triglycerides and fasting and postprandial insulin and in increase in LDL particle diameter. These effects were attributed both to the replacement of lipids by protein rather than carbohydrate and the use of dietary carbohydrates with a low GI.

The problem with attributing the results to GI is that the GI of the experimental diets was not known. It is, therefore, very difficult for me to see how an effect can be attributed to a dietary difference which has not been assessed and about which the authors actually know nothing. This seems like a severe criticism, but it was actually stated in the table giving sample menus that the GI value of every food fed was either '*Undetermined* but probably <51' or 'Low GI, *no data available* but GI probably <30' (my emphasis). In fact, the authors were completely wrong to claim their test diet was low GI. The foods claimed to be 'low GI' (i.e. no data available but GI probably <30) were cheese, vegetables and salads, foods which are low in carbohydrate but not low GI. This perpetuates the misunderstanding that low-carbohydrate foods are low GI. In addition, it was indicated that GI values of whole-wheat bread and unsweetened jam were undetermined but probably <51. In fact, whole-wheat bread does not have a low GI (the GI of Canadian whole-wheat breads is about 70 – Wolever *et al.*, 1994a). Although the GI of unsweetened jam has not been determined, in my opinion it is likely to be about 65, since the carbohydrates in unsweetened jam consist of the sugars in the fruits from which it is made. When I calculated the GI of the two sample diets given by Dumesnil *et al.* (2001), I found that they were both virtually identical. When I pointed this out (Wolever, 2002), the authors acknowledged that they lacked directly measured GI values but felt this was merely a problem similar to that of using food tables to report the nutrient content of experimental diets. To them: 'The definition of the GI concept is not our most important concern; we care more for the epidemic proportion reached by obesity and by the need to provide patients with simple and efficient nutritional guidance'. And then they went on to affirm that in fact, ' ... the GI of our experimental diet was lower than that of our control diet' (Tremblay *et al.*, 2002).

We must disagree most emphatically with these statements! Definitions are critically important. We cannot provide useful advice unless the thing about which we provide advice is clearly defined and understood. Far from promoting simple nutritional guidance, the improper use of terms creates misunderstanding and confusion and therefore does great harm. By affirming that the GI of their experimental diet was lower than that of their control diet, Tremblay *et al.* (2002) mean that the experimental diet elicited a lower blood glucose response – a fact with which I agree. However, this was due to the fact that the diet contained less carbohydrate, not that it had a lower GI. The distinction between the terms '*glycaemic response*' and '*glycaemic index*' is important (Chapter 2, this volume, Section 2.1.1); not only do the mathematical and statistical properties of acute glycaemic responses differ from those of the GI (Wolever, 1992), the long-term effects of reducing postprandial blood glucose by reducing carbohydrate intake may differ from those of reducing GI (Wolever and Mehling, 2002, 2003).

Having ranted on about how important it is to distinguish between GI and amount of carbohydrate, it is possible that both manoeuvres, i.e. reducing carbohydrate intake and reducing diet GI (while maintaining carbohydrate intake), may reduce body weight! However, I find studies in this area notoriously difficult to interpret for two reasons. The mechanism for the weight loss is usually unclear; e.g. it is very difficult to know whether differences in weight are due to differences in energy intake because, as discussed in Chapter 6, it is impossible to measure energy intake accurately. In addition, differences in weight loss which can be seen in short-term studies tend to be lost in the long-term because of the natural tendency of people to regain the weight they have lost.

#### 7.3.2.1 Cross-sectional and prospective studies

Evidence from early epidemiological studies about the role of dietary fat tend to show a positive association between fat intake and body weight (Lissner and Heitmann, 1995). Since fat and carbohydrate intakes are inversely related, this suggests that a high carbohydrate intake is associated with a lower body weight. Recent studies support the association between high carbohydrate intake and reduced weight gain in individuals with (Toeller *et al.*, 2001) and without (Ludwig *et al.*, 1999a,b) diabetes. However, the source of the carbohydrate may be a stronger predictor of weight gain than the total carbohydrate intake.

Early studies suggested that high intake of sugars is associated with low fat intake (Rugg-Gunn *et al.*, 1991; Baghurst *et al.*, 1992) and low body mass index (Hill and Prentice, 1995). However, recent studies have found a significant association with high intake of refined sugars and obesity (Ludwig *et al.*, 2001). This has been confirmed in a clinical trial which showed that 21 overweight men and women randomized to consume drinks and foods sweetened with sucrose for 10 weeks gained significantly more body weight (+1.6 ±0.4 vs −1.0 ± 0.4 kg, $P < 0.001$) and body fat (+1.3 ± 0.5 vs −0.3 ± 0.4 kg, $P < 0.01$) than 20 subjects consuming similar drinks and foods sweetened with non-caloric sweeteners (Raben *et al.*, 2002). The weight gain was associated with, and presumably due to, a significant increase in energy intake. Subjects on sucrose increased energy intake by 418 kcal/day at 5 weeks and 492 kcal/day at 10 weeks relative to those on artificial sweeteners. This amounts to consumption of an extra 31,850 kcal over 10 weeks which would, theoretically, amount to 4.1 kg of fat; about 1.6 times the amount of body weight actually gained (Raben *et al.*, 2002).

Consistent with the association between a high intake of sugars and weight gain are findings that high intakes of dietary fibre are associated with reduced weight gain (Ludwig *et al.*, 1999a,b; Toeller *et al.*, 2001; Liu *et al.*, 2003b). In addition, weight gain in middle-aged women was inversely associated with increased intake of high-fibre, whole-grain foods, but positively related to increased intake of refined-grain foods (Liu *et al.*, 2003a,b). In studies in which it has been examined, a high-GI diet was associated with increased weight gain (Toeller *et al.*, 2001; Ma *et al.*, 2005). Thus, it may not be so much the amount of carbohydrate in the diet, but the type which is important in determining body weight gain.

#### 7.3.2.2 Effects of low-carbohydrate weight-reducing diets on body weight

Low-carbohydrate diets have been popular as a strategy for weight loss, and there is no question that they are effective. The interesting questions are: How do they work and are they any more effective than other kinds of diets? Here I am only going to discuss the results of a limited number of recent studies which illustrate the difficulty in answering these apparently simple questions.

Samaha *et al.* (2003) randomized 132 severely obese subjects to a carbohydrate-restricted diet or a conventional, calorie- and fat-restricted diet for 6 months, and followed for 1 year (Stern *et al.*, 2004). Foster *et al.* (2003) randomized 63 obese subjects to the same low-carbohydrate or conventional diets for a year. Both studies found that the low-carbohydrate diet induced significantly more weight loss than the conventional diet at 6 months (Samaha *et al.*, 2003, −5.8 vs −1.9 kg, $P = 0.002$; Foster *et al.*, 2003, −7.0% vs −3.2% of body weight, $P = 0.02$). However, by 12 months, the difference in body weight was no longer statistically significant (Stern *et al.*, 2004, −5.1 vs −3.1 kg, $P = 0.20$; Foster *et al.*, 2003, −4.4% vs −2.5%, $P = 0.26$). Dansinger *et al.* (2005) randomized 120 overweight or obese adults to the Akins, Ornish, Weight Watchers or

Zone diets for 1 year. They found a reduction in the rate of weight loss between 6 and 12 months for all diets, and, the weight loss on the low-carbohydrate diets (Atkins and Zone) was no different than that on the high-carbohydrate diets (Weight Watchers and Ornish). Figure 7.1 shows the pooled results of these three studies on body weight. Both low-carbohydrate and conventional diets produced significant weight loss; the low-carbohydrate diets resulted in significantly greater weight loss over the first 6 months, but by 12 months, there was a smaller difference in weight loss between low- and high-carbohydrate diets which was not statistically significant.

A major problem with all these studies is that 30–40% of the subjects dropped out, and thus, it is difficult to be confident about the outcomes, especially after 1 year. Foster *et al.* (2003) do not report any assessment of nutrient intakes. Samaha *et al.* (2003) and Stern *et al.* (2004) assessed nutrient intakes by 24 h. They were able to show that the subjects on the low-carbohydrate diet reported consuming significantly less carbohydrate at 6 months (37% vs 51% of energy, $P < 0.001$) and 12 months (120 vs 230 g, $P = 0.011$), and significantly more fat (41% vs 33%) and protein (22% vs 16%) than the subjects on the conventional diet at 6 months, but not 12 months. At 6 months, subjects on the low-carbohydrate diet reported eating 460 kcal less than at baseline compared to 271 kcal less than baseline for those on the conventional diet. This difference in mean energy intake, 189 kcal, amounts to a deficit of 30,800 kcal over the 6-month period on the low-carbohydrate compared to the conventional diet. Since loss of 1 kg of adipose tissue theoretically requires an energy deficit of 7700 kcal, a cumulative deficit of 30,800 kcal would result in a loss of 4.0 kg of adipose tissue, which almost exactly accounts for the 3.9 kg greater amount of weight lost on the low-carbohydrate compared to the conventional diet at 6 months! However, by 12 months (Stern *et al.*, 2004), there was a twofold greater difference in reported energy intake but half the difference in weight loss than at 6 months; subjects on the low-carbohydrate diet reported eating a mean of 413 kcal/day less than those on the conventional diet, but the difference in weight was only 2.0 kg, and neither of these differences was statistically significant. Dansinger *et al.* (2005) assessed energy and nutrient intakes using 3-day food records. Subjects on all four diets reported consuming significantly less energy than at baseline, but differences between diets were not statistically significant. Thus, reported energy intakes have to be considered, if not unreliable, at least imprecise, particularly when a difference in mean intake of over 400 kcal/day between two groups of over 40 subjects (enough to, theoretically, result in a 5 kg weight loss in 3 months) cannot be detected with statistical significance!

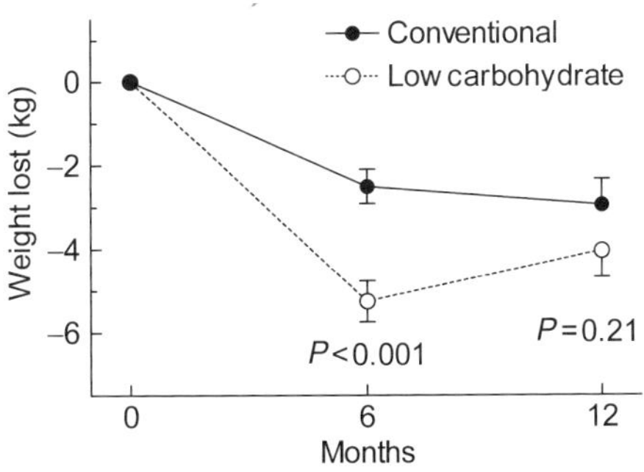


**Fig. 7.1.** Pooled results of three randomized, controlled trials (Foster *et al.*, 2003; Stern *et al.*, 2004; Dansinger *et al.*, 2005) comparing weight loss on a conventional low-fat diet with that on a ketogenic, low-carbohydrate diet. The number of subjects at each point is between 128 and 135. Points represent means ± SEM.

Dansinger *et al.* (2005) reported significant differences in carbohydrate intake, with subjects on the Atkins and Zone diets consuming less carbohydrate between 6 and 12 months (173–198 g/day) than those on Weight Watchers and Ornish diets (202–237 g/day). However, there were no differences in weight reduction for the four different diets; weight loss tended to be associated with dietary adherence rather than diet type. In addition, Dansinger *et al.* (2005) found a trend ($P = 0.08$) for fewer subjects on the more extreme diets (52% for Atkins and 50% for Ornish) to complete the study compared to those on the moderate diets (65% for Zone and 65% for Weight Watchers). By contrast, Yancy *et al.* (2004) found that significantly more subjects on a low-carbohydrate diet, 45 of 59 (76%), completed a 6-month study than those on a conventional low-fat diet, 34 of 60 (57%, $P = 0.02$).

Thus, these studies show that low-carbohydrate diets are effective for weight loss. However, because of the difficulty in measuring energy intake precisely, it is not possible to know whether the weight loss was due to a reduction in energy intake, or to some other mechanism. The theory behind low-carbohydrate diets is that reducing carbohydrate intake reduces plasma insulin and, thus inhibits the storage of fat and promotes its oxidation. However, one would expect this metabolic scenario to occur if energy intake was reduced below energy expenditure, regardless of the composition of the diet. Thus, in order to know if there is any special effect on body fat of altering the composition of the diet, it will be necessary to be able to measure and/or control energy intake precisely, a task which is impossible!

#### 7.3.2.3 *Effects of high-carbohydrate* ad libitum *diets on body weight*

There is good evidence that the inclusion of high-carbohydrate foods in the diet results in spontaneously less energy intake compared to a diet of high-fat, low-carbohydrate foods (Stubbs *et al.*, 1995). However, this is probably due to the fact that starchy high-carbohydrate foods have lower energy density than high-fat foods (Prentice, 1998). It was subsequently demonstrated that spontaneous consumption of energy from high-carbohydrate foods can be increased by increasing their energy density, and subjects consume just as much energy from a high-carbohydrate food as from a high-fat food of the same energy density (Stubbs *et al.*, 1996).

The CARMEN study was designed to see whether manipulation of the carbohydrate to fat ratio of the diet influenced body weight (Saris *et al.*, 2000). This was a multicentre trial in which 236 overweight subjects were randomized to a control diet, a low-fat high complex carbohydrate diet or a low-fat high simple carbohydrate diet for 6 months. Subjects obtained foods from the research centres resulting in fairly good ability to control and measure food intake. There was no advice for weight reduction – the only intervention was the nature of the foods consumed. The control diet group consumed ~35% energy as fat and 45% carbohydrate (~21% energy from simple carbohydrates); the low-fat high complex carbohydrate group consumed ~28% fat and 51% carbohydrate (~19% energy from simple carbohydrates) and the low-fat high simple carbohydrate group consumed ~25% fat and 55% carbohydrate (~29% energy from simple carbohydrates). Subjects lost weight on both high-carbohydrate diets but gained weight on the control diet; the change in weight on both the simple carbohydrate (−0.9 kg) and the complex carbohydrate diets (−1.8 kg) differed significantly from that on the control diet (+0.8 kg). The changes in body weight were associated with significantly more body fat loss on both high-carbohydrate diets (−1.3 and −1.8 kg for the simple and complex carbohydrate diets, respectively) than the control diet (+0.6 kg) (Saris *et al.*, 2000). Similar to the studies mentioned in the previous section, differences in reported energy intake were not correlated with and do not account for the changes in weight on the different diets. Although the reason for the greater weight loss on the high-carbohydrate diets is not clear, this study does not support the concept that a high-carbohydrate diet *per se* promotes the deposition of body fat.

#### 7.3.2.4 *Effects of low-GI weight-reducing diets on body weight*

Several studies have examined the role of low-GI diets on body weight (Fig. 7.2). We studied six subjects with diabetes who were placed on energy-restricted low-GI or high-GI diets for 6 weeks in a cross-over design (Wolever *et al.*, 1992d). There was no difference in the amount of weight lost on the low- and high-GI diets; perhaps this is not surprising, since the main aim of the study was to achieve similar weight loss on both diets to see if there were any differences in outcomes of the low- vs high-GI diets on blood glucose and lipids.

The study which supports most the hypothesis that a low-GI diet improves weight loss is that of Slabber *et al.* (1994) who gave obese females high-GI or low-GI energy-restricted diets in a 12-week parallel arm study ($n = 30$), followed by a 12-week cross-over study ($n = 16$). In the parallel study, more weight tended to be lost on low GI than high GI, 9.3 vs 7.4 kg, but the difference was not significant ($P = 0.14$); however, in the cross-over study significantly more weight was lost on low GI, 7.4 kg, than high GI, 4.5 kg ($P = 0.04$). In both studies, fasting insulin and the urinary insulin:c-peptide ratio was reduced to a significantly greater extent on the low-GI than the high-GI diet.

Bouché *et al.* (2002) studied 11 overweight men who took low- and high-GI diets for 5 weeks in a randomized, cross-over study. Although body weight at the end of the low-GI period,

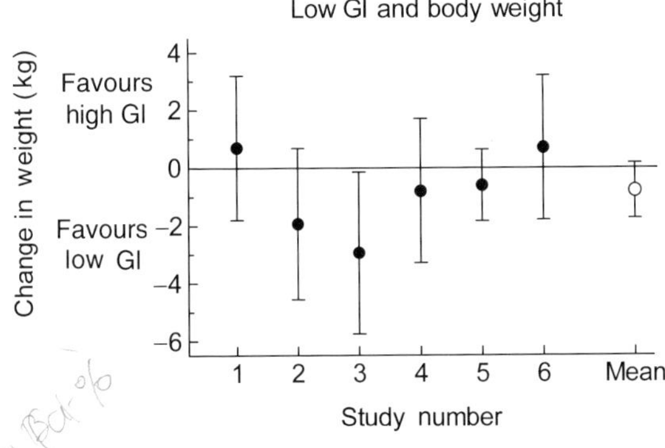


**Fig. 7.2.** Results of studies comparing weight loss on low- vs high-GI diets. Values are means and 95% confidence intervals (estimated for studies 1, 4 and 6). Study numbers: 1, Wolever *et al.* (1992d); 2 and 3, Slabber *et al.* (1994); 4, Bouché *et al.* (2002); 5, Sloth *et al.* (2004); 6, Frost *et al.* (2004).

85.7 ± 2.9 kg, did not differ significantly from that at the end of the high-GI period, 86.5 ± 2.7 kg, body fat mass, measured by dual-energy X-ray absorptiometry, was significantly lower after the low-GI than the high-GI diet (18.8 ± 1.6 vs 19.5 ± 1.6 kg, $P < 0.05$).

Ebbeling *et al.* (2003) randomized 14 obese adolescents aged 13–21 years to receive either conventional, low-fat dietary advice or dietary advice aimed at reducing dietary GL for 6 months with a 6-month follow-up. BMI and fat mass tended to increase on the conventional diet, whereas they tended to decrease on the low-GL (glycaemic load) diet. By 6 months, the difference in BMI between subjects on the low- and high-GL diets was 1 kg/m$^2$ which increased to 2 kg/m$^2$ after 1 year ($P < 0.05$). Likewise, the 3 kg reduction in body fat at 6 months ($P = 0.04$) had increased to over 4 kg by the end of 12 months. The change in body fat was significantly related to the change in diet GL, which in turn, was accomplished by both a modest reduction in carbohydrate intake (from 58% to 52% of energy) and a reduction in diet GI (from 58 to 53). Although the results of this preliminary study are impressive, I have not included it in the analysis shown on Fig. 7.1 because it involved both a reduction in carbohydrate intake and a reduction in diet GI.

Sloth *et al.* (2004) randomized 45 overweight women to receive high- or low-GI foods to replace their usual high-carbohydrate foods for 10 weeks. The GI values of the test foods were calculated from *in vitro* methods, which do not always yield accurate information (Brand-Miller and Holt, 2004). Body weight fell significantly on both diets, but the fall on low GI, −1.9 ± 0.5 kg, did not differ significantly from that on high GI, −1.3 ± 0.3 kg ($P = 0.31$).

Frost *et al.* (2004) randomized 55 subjects with CHD to healthy eating advice or a low-GI diet for 12 weeks. A difference in diet GI was achieved, with no change in carbohydrate intake. The subjects tended to be overweight, with a mean BMI of 26.9 kg/m$^2$ in the low-GI group and 28.7 kg/m$^2$ in the healthy eating group. Although both groups tended to lose weight, the healthy eating group tended to lose more weight, although this was not statistically significant.

Overall (Fig. 7.2), there appears to be no significant difference in body weight lost on low-GI vs high-GI diets, with a pooled weight change −0.78 kg (ns). For believers in the hypothesis that a low-GI diet causes weight loss, it is possible to point out flaws in the design of virtually all of these studies. However, there are other explanations for the lack of effect. In addition, even if it were true that a low-GI diet has no effect on body weight, it may still have important effects on body composition. For example, there may be a change in body fat which is not reflected in a change in body weight (Bouché *et al.*, 2002), and accounted for by an increase in the weight of lean tissue such as the intestinal tract (see below). In addition, it is possible that the true effect of a low-GI diet is so small that it is unable to be detected with the current studies. Nevertheless, small differences in body weight might have a very important impact on health. For example, between the ages of 25 and 50 years, European men generally gain, on average, about 1 pound (0.45 kg) in body weight per year. In these populations, a high amount of weight gained between the ages of 25 and 50 is associated with adverse health outcomes and poor quality of life in older age (Rosengren *et al.*, 1999; Yarnell *et al.*, 2000; Strandberg *et al.*, 2003). However, a weight gain of 1 pound per year represents only 0.1 kg over 10 weeks, which is the average length of the studies of the effect of a low-GI diet on body weight. Such an effect would be impossible to detect without thousands of subjects.

#### *7.3.2.5 Mechanisms*

There are two major mechanisms by which a low-GI diet is considered to promote weight loss: reduced appetite and food intake due to differences in plasma glucose and insulin concentrations, and reduced fat storage and increased fat oxidation secondary to reduced plasma insulin responses. I am not convinced by either of these explanations. There is some evidence that consumption of low-GI foods reduces food intake at subsequent meals, but it is not clear to me that this is due to differences in glucose and insulin responses. Also, it seems to me that the amount of body fat is regulated primarily by energy balance and I am not convinced that differences in insulin can change the amount of body fat provided that energy balance is maintained. Indeed, a recent study in which obese women were fed two meals (breakfast and lunch) of the same energy and nutrient composition, but consisting of high- or low-GI carbohydrates were associated with significant differences in plasma glucose and insulin responses, but no effect on energy expenditure or the balance of carbohydrate and fat oxidation (Díaz *et al.*, 2005).

Insulin could alter energy balance either by affecting energy intake or the efficiency of energy utilization or could alter the distribution of body fat, but these issues are not typically addressed. Another mechanism which I believe is very important is that the carbohydrate in starchy low-GI foods is less completely absorbed than that in high-GI foods, leading to a reduced efficiency of energy absorption. This might only account for 10–20 kcal/day, but over a year that adds up to 3500–7000 kcal, or 1–2 pounds of fat per year, which is about the average amount of weight that adults appear to gain in Western societies.

### 7.3.3 Low GI and appetite regulation in adults

The many external and internal factors which influence food intake are not well understood, but they include beliefs and traditions about food; time of day; factors in the environment such as the number of people eating together, the light and sounds in the room and the amount and types of food available; food sight, smell and taste; and the many neurological and physiological signals arising from the volume and chemical composition of the food consumed (Anderson, 1996). Not only physiological responses, but also the responses of individuals to environmental and psychosocial determinants of food intake appear to be influenced by genetic factors (de Castro, 2004). To help understand the factors involved, experimental paradigms have been developed to measure appetite. Normally, after eating a meal, hunger is reduced, the feeling of fullness increases and eating is inhibited, a phenomenon called post-ingestive satiety. If post-ingestive satiety did not develop normally after eating, excess energy intake may result, leading to obesity. One way of measuring post-ingestive satiety is by having subjects consumed a defined amount of food or nutrient (the preload) followed a short time later by a meal at which the subject can eat as much as desired. Appetite regulation would be perfect if the energy consumed in the preload was compensated for by an equivalent reduction in energy intake at the subsequent meal. Normal subjects compensate almost perfectly for 25–75 g sucrose consumed in a preload 1 h before an *ad libitum* meal (Woodend and Anderson, 2001). There is some evidence that the appetite of obese subjects is not suppressed as much as that of lean subjects after consumption of fat preloads (Rolls and Hammer, 1995; Speechly and Buffenstein, 2000), but that carbohydrate suppresses appetite equally in lean and obese subjects (Rolls and Hammer, 1995). However, in these studies carbohydrate and fat preloads were given to subjects mixed into yogurt. The effects of pure nutrients given alone may differ from those when the nutrients are consumed in a mixed meal. For example, when given in yogurt, fat and carbohydrate are equally satiating (Rolls and Hammer, 1995), but pure safflower oil is less satiating than sucrose (Woodend and Anderson, 2001).

Among the many factors involved in the control of post-ingestive satiety include signals derived from nerves (e.g. stretch receptors in the stomach and intestine), signals derived directly from the nutrients in foods (e.g. blood levels of glucose, amino acids and fatty acids) and signals derived from hormones of the pancreas (e.g. insulin) and gastrointestinal tract (e.g. glucagon-like polypeptide-1 (GLP-1)). Ludwig (2000) cites 16 articles to support the suggestion that low-GI foods increase satiety and reduce food intake due to differences in their blood glucose and hormonal responses. However, the results of these and other studies are not consistent (as will be discussed below), and it is very difficult to control all the factors involved, and thus isolate the effects of glucose and insulin *per se*. Among the 16 studies cited by Ludwig (2000), the 'low-GI' foods were either higher in dietary fibre, consisted of a different monosaccharide (fructose vs glucose), contained more protein, or were otherwise not matched with the high-GI foods. The following is not a comprehensive review of the literature in this field; I merely wish to illustrate the complexity of appetite regulation, and show that it is difficult to ascribe changes in appetite or food intake to differences in blood glucose and insulin *per se*.

#### *7.3.3.1 Meal volume and appetite regulation*

Filling the stomach or GI tract creates a feeling of fullness and satiety. However, when the effect of volume is studied carefully, it is found to be subtle and inconsistent. For example, instilling 300 ml of air into a test meal preload reduced food intake at a subsequent *ad libitum* meal (Rolls *et al.*, 2000), but drinking a glass of 350 ml water with a dish of chicken fricassee had no such effect (Rolls *et al.*, 1999). However, mixing exactly the same 350 ml water with exactly the same chicken fricassee before eating to create chicken soup reduced food intake at a subsequent meal compared to drinking the water with the food or eating the food alone (Rolls *et al.*, 1999)! Some of the studies cited by Ludwig (2000) to support the idea that reducing postprandial glucose results in increased satiety and/or reduced food intake compared the effects of fruits (Haber *et al.*, 1977) or vegetables (Gustafsson *et al.*, 1995a,b) processed in different ways which likely affected the distribution of nutrients in the water content of the meal, and also may have influenced the amount of chewing required, which in turn, would affect the amount of saliva and other gastrointestinal secretions produced, and hence, the volume of the meal.

Four of the studies cited by Ludwig (2000) compared test meals with or without viscous forms of dietary fibre (Krokiewski, 1984; Benini *et al.*, 1995; Lavin and Read, 1995; Rigaud *et al.*, 1998). The high-fibre test meals elicited lower glucose and insulin responses than the control test meals, but it seems unlikely that this was the cause of differences in satiety and food intake. Dietary fibre is known to affect the volume and/or gastric emptying rate of a meal (Benini *et al.*, 1995; Lavin and Read, 1995; Rigaud *et al.*, 1998), which in turn, may directly influence appetite and food intake. We have recently shown in healthy males, using test meals matched for volume, weight and nutrient content, that 40 g cereal fibre reduced food intake at 1 h by the same amount as 40 g glucose, despite no difference in blood glucose response between the high- and low-fibre test cereals (Freeland and Wolever, 2002).

#### *7.3.3.2 Fructose vs glucose*

In three of the studies cited by Ludwig (2000), the satiating effects of fructose were compared with those of glucose (Spitzer and Rodin, 1987; Rodin *et al.*, 1988; Rodin, 1991). Fructose is classified as a low-GI food and fructose consumption was consistently associated with greater satiety and less food intake than glucose. However, this does not necessarily mean that the increased satiety was due to the low and sustained glycaemic response. The pattern of postprandial glucose response elicited by fructose is rather different from that elicited by a starchy food with a low GI. After 50 g fructose, there was only a small rise in plasma glucose, but plasma glucose fell below the baseline and was identical to the plasma glucose increment 2 h after consuming 50 g glucose (Lee and Wolever, 1998). On the other hand, plasma glucose 2 h after barley remained above the baseline (Wolever and Bolognesi, 1996c). Thus, a slow sustained rise in blood glucose concentration after fructose is not seen, and cannot explain the increase in satiety. It is possible that the lack of a dynamic fall in blood glucose (see below, Section 7.3.3.3) after fructose was related to the enhanced satiety. However, it is also possible that the satiating effect of fructose is due to a special effect of fructose metabolism in the liver, compared to glucose, or to the fact that fructose is poorly absorbed by most individuals (Riby *et al.*, 1993) leading to increased colonic fermentation which could distend the large intestine and reduce appetite and food intake.

#### *7.3.3.3 Plasma glucose and insulin concentrations and appetite regulation in adults*

One of the earliest theories about how appetite is controlled, the glucostatic hypothesis, postulates that appetite increases when the blood glucose concentration falls (Meyer, 1955); this hypothesis continues to stimulate interest and gain experimental support (Campfield *et al.*, 1985, 1996). For example, recently, Melanson *et al.* (1999a,b) showed that transient and dynamic falls in blood glucose predict spontaneous meal initiation in time-blinded humans. A transient fall in glucose is defined as a fall in blood glucose of at least 5% (SD $\geq$ 2 mg/dl) below a stable baseline level (a period of at least 5 min of stable (SD $<$ 1 mg/dl) blood glucose) with the fall lasting for at least 5 min. A dynamic fall in glucose is defined as a rapid (0.023–0.070 mmol/l/min for 42–67 min) decline originating from a peak induced by nutrient ingestion. If transient or dynamic falls in glucose did trigger meal ingestion, then the pattern of a low and sustained rise of blood glucose elicited by low-GI foods might enhance satiety. This is a very attractive hypothesis. However, associations do not prove causality. Changes in blood glucose may be involved in appetite regulation postprandially, but there are also many other factors involved. In addition, the results of studies examining the effects of low-GI starchy foods on satiety and food intake are not consistent (Table 7.1) either in their overall effects or in terms of the timing of the effects in relation to the start of food intake.

Leathwood and Pollet (1988) showed that a meal made with bean flakes elicited a slow and sustained rise in blood glucose compared to one made with instant potato. The bean meal contained more protein and less carbohydrate than the potato meal, making it difficult to ascribe differences in hunger solely due to differences in blood glucose concentration (Anderson and Li, 1987). There were no differences in appetite for 2 h after the two test meals. There was a small but significant reduction in hunger at 3 and 4 h after the bean meal, but only a slight difference in stomach fullness and no effect on satiety. The largest effect was seen with 'gourmandise', i.e. the desire to eat something tasty, which was substantially less at 3 and 4 h after the bean meal than the potato meal.

Holt and Brand-Miller (1994, 1995) and Holt *et al.*, (1992, 1996) have done several studies comparing satiety responses after test meals with different glycaemic responses. In one study (Holt and Brand Miller, 1994), the effects of the particle size of wheat was studied. Glucose and insulin responses elicited by fine flour were significantly greater than those elicited by cracked wheat or whole grains. Although the insulin responses were negatively associated with the area under the satiety curve (satiety AUC) for 2 h, the differences

**Table 7.1.** Effects of low-GI foods on satiety and/or food intake.

| Intervention | Effect on glucose* | Effect on appetite* | Confounding factors | Reference |
|---|---|---|---|---|
| Bean vs potato | ↓ | Hunger ↓<br>Satiety → | Higher protein | Leathwood and Pollet (1988) |
| Wheat particle size | ↓ | Satiety → | None | Holt and Brand Miller (1994) |
| Quick-cook rice | ↑ | Satiety → | None | Holt and Brand Miller (1995) |
| High-amylose rice | ↓ | Satiety → | None | Holt and Brand Miller (1995) |
| 7 foods | ↓ GI ∝ ↑ satiety | | Fat, protein, fibre | Holt *et al.* (1992) |
| 38 foods | GI and satiety not related<br>↑ Insulin ∝ ↓ food intake | | Fat, protein, fibre | Holt *et al.* (1996) |
| Low amylose | ↓ | Satiety ↑ | None | van Amelsvoort and Weststrate (1992) |
| Glucose vs starch | ↑ | Satiety ↑ | None | Anderson *et al.* (2002) |

*↑ = significant increase; ↓ = significant decrease; → = no significant difference; ∝ = significant correlation.

in satiety AUC between the different test meals was not significant. Similarly, ordinary rice and high-amylose rice, respectively were found to elicit substantially (~50%) lower glucose and insulin responses than quick-cooking rice and low-amylose rice, but there was no significant difference in satiety AUC (Holt and Brand Miller, 1995). In a different study, the plasma glucose, insulin and CCK responses of seven different foods were negatively correlated with satiety AUC (i.e. low GI related to increased satiety) (Holt *et al.*, 1992), but in a much larger series of foods ($n$ = 38) the opposite was seen with low insulin responses being significantly associated with high food intake (Holt *et al.*, 1996).

We tested pure carbohydrates with different glycaemic responses (glucose, amylose, amylopectin) and found that the rapidly absorbed, high-GI foods produced the greatest satiety and lowest food intake (Anderson *et al.*, 2002). However, it must be pointed out that we measured food intake 1 h after the carbohydrate preload, and this does not necessarily disprove the hypothesis that a low-GI meal has a more sustained effect on satiety than a high-GI meal.

### 7.3.4 Low-GI foods and appetite regulation in children

Although the mechanism by which the effect is achieved is debatable, there are some recent studies which seem to provide quite good evidence that low-GI foods do in fact influence appetite regulation and short-term food intake.

Ludwig *et al.* (1999a,b) studied obese teenage boys on three separate occasions on which they were admitted to clinical research unit for 24 h starting at 6 pm. They were given a standard dinner, went to bed and the following morning consumed isocaloric high, medium or low 'GI' breakfast meals (GI is in inverted commas because I feel the term is not used correctly in the paper). Blood samples were taken for 5 h after which the same breakfast meal was served for lunch and then the subjects were allowed to ask for an *ad libitum* food platter if they became hungry. The high- and medium-GI breakfast meals consisted of oatmeal, sugar and milk, and were matched for nutrient content (64% energy from carbohydrate, 16% protein and 20% fat). The 160 g milk in the high-GI meal was treated with lactase '… to increase the GI of the milk sugar'. This is a misnomer because treating milk with lactase would increase the amount of carbohydrate absorbed rather than its GI, but any difference would likely be insignificant to the overall effect in these meals because milk only contributed about 13% of the meal carbohydrate. In the medium-GI meal, 63.9 g steel-cut oats and 16 g fructose were used instead of 60.9 g instant oats and 19 g dextrose. The GI value of the meals was not calculated by Ludwig *et al.* (1999a,b) and, in fact, the GI value of the steel-cut oats used is not known. On Table 7.2, I have calculated glycaemic load (GL) and GI values

**Table 7.2.** Carbohydrate content, glycaemic index (GI) and glycaemic load (GL) of test meals fed by Ludwig *et al.* (1999a,b).

| | | Carbohydrate (g) | | Glycaemic load | |
|---|---|---|---|---|---|
| Food | GI | High GI | Medium GI | High GI | Medium GI |
| Instant oats (60.9 g) | 66 | 34.0 | | 22.4 | |
| Steel-cut oats (63.9 g) (GI value not known) | 58 or 50 or 42 | | 35.7 | | 20.7 or 17.9 or 15.0 |
| Milk (160 g) | 32 | 7.7 | 7.7 | 2.5 | 2.5 |
| Cream (15 g) | 31 | 0.6 | 0.6 | 0.2 | 0.2 |
| Dextrose (19 g) | 100 | 17.1 | | 17.1 | |
| Fructose (16 g) | 20 | | 16.0 | | 3.2 |
| Total | | 59.4 | 60.0 | 42.2 | 26.6 or 23.8 or 20.9 |
| Glycaemic index | | | | 71.0 | 45.0 or 39.7 or 34.2 |

GI value of steel-cut oats is not known; calculations are shown for three different GI values taken from Foster-Powell *et al.* (2002) representing the average for oatmeal (58) the lowest value for thick flake oats (50) and the lowest value reported for oatmeal (42).

of the high-GI and medium-GI test meals. The GI value for instant oats is not given in the GI tables (Foster-Powell *et al.*, 2002), but I have used the highest value for quick cook oats (66). Swedish data suggest that the GI of thick oat flakes ranges from 50 to 55. The mean value for porridge oats is 58 with a range from 42 to 69. Thus, I have used three different GI values for steel-cut oats (58, 50 and 42). Ludwig *et al.* (1999a,b) tend to attribute their results to the presence of the steel-cut oats in the medium-GI meal. However, Table 7.2 shows that the majority of the reduction in GI and GL was achieved by the exchange of fructose for glucose which accounts for a GL difference of 17.1 − 3.2 = 13.9, which in turn, accounts for 65% to 90% of the difference in GL and GI between the two meals (depending on the GI value used for steel-cut oats). The low 'GI' meal was actually reduced in carbohydrate (40% energy from carbohydrate, 30% protein and 30% fat); according to my calculations, it contained 32 g carbohydrate and had a GI of 45 (similar or higher than that of the medium-GI meal) and GL of 14.5. Thus, the low 'GI' meal would, perhaps, more properly be termed low GL. Figure 7.3 plots the areas under the glucose response curves elicited by the three test meals as reported by Ludwig *et al.* (1999a,b) plotted against my calculated GL values. This shows that the glycaemic response was virtually proportional to the meal GL and that the GI and GL of the medium-GI meal is not sensitive to the exact GI value chosen for steel-cut oats.

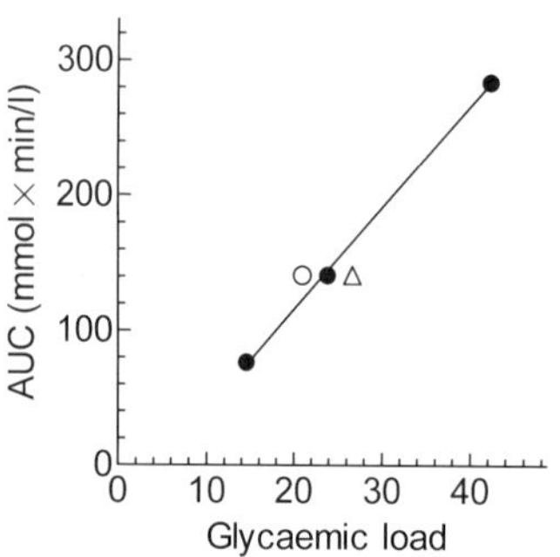


**Fig. 7.3.** Relationship between estimated glycaemic load (GL) of breakfast test meals (Table 7.2) and observed glycaemic responses (Ludwig *et al.*, 1999a,b). Line represents the linear regression. The open circle and triangle represent range of estimates of GL for the steel-cut oats test meal based on a range of GI values for steel-cut oats (see Table 7.2).

The main finding of the study was that cumulative food intake after the test lunches was reduced significantly from 5.8 mJ after high GI to 3.8 mJ after medium GI and 3.2 mJ after the low 'GI' meal. The authors consider that the observed differences in voluntary energy to intake after the low 'GI' meal can be '...primarily attributed to differences in the GI itself because similar differences...were observed...after the high-GI instant oatmeal vs the medium-GI steel-cut oatmeal. For these two oatmeal preparations, macronutrient compositions were identical and alterations in GI were obtained through differences in food structures and sugar type'. However, this is unclear because of the imprecise way that the term 'GI' is used. Based on the two test meals containing oats, I agree that this study provides evidence that a meal containing starchy foods with a lower GI may reduce food intake due to a sustained release of carbohydrate, although the major reason for the difference in GI between the high- and medium-GI meals was the switch from glucose to fructose which is associated with a difference in metabolism rather than rate of absorption. With respect to the effect of the low 'GI' meal, I am not sure if the authors really believed that their low 'GI' meal had a lower GI than that of the other meals or they actually are referring to the fact that it elicited a low glycaemic response. I find it harder than the authors to attribute the reduction in food intake after their low 'GI' meal primarily to the difference in GI or glycaemic response when several factors in the meal changed, including the amounts of protein, fat and carbohydrate as well as the nature of the carbohydrate, and the fact that the responses of plasma glucagon and satiety differed between the low and the medium 'GI' meals.

More evidence that low-GI foods reduce food intake in children comes from a study by Warren *et al.* (2003) who studied 37, 9–12 year old boys and girls in a school breakfast club. Each child received a low-GI breakfast, a low-GI breakfast plus sucrose or a high-GI breakfast in a randomized block design. The order of the blocks was randomized, and each block consisted of one of the types of breakfast served 3 days in a row. The low-GI breakfast was a choice of All Bran®, muesli, oatmeal or soya linseed bread. The low-GI plus sucrose breakfast was the same except with 5 g sucrose added per 200 kcal. The high-GI breakfast was a choice of maize flakes, Coco-Pops®, puffed rice or white bread. Each breakfast included juice, milk with cereals, or margarine with or without jelly on the bread. Intake of energy at the subsequent lunch was measured by unobtrusive observation. Lunch was a buffet-style meal which was served in the school hall where the rest of the children were eating. Intake of energy at lunch was significantly less after the low-GI and the low-GI plus sucrose breakfast than the high-GI breakfast by 145 kcal (19%) and 119 kcal (16%), respectively (Fig. 7.4). Since the energy content of the low- and high-GI breakfasts was the same, total energy intake over breakfast and lunch was reduced by the same amount as that for lunch. Although the low-GI plus sucrose contained 10% more energy than the other breakfast meals, the total energy intake of low-GI plus sucrose breakfast plus lunch was still 85 kcal less than that for the high-GI breakfast. The authors do not report the total intakes of energy at breakfast and lunch, nor whether the differences were statistically significant, but they do indicate that the study had sufficient power to detect a difference in energy intake at lunch of 54 kcal. It should be pointed out that the low-GI foods used in this study contained more dietary fibre than the high-GI foods, and this could explain the differences in food intake, rather than a difference in glycaemic response *per se*.

In summary, both the studies by Ludwig *et al.* (1999a,b) and Warren *et al.* (2003) were well designed and carefully done and show quite convincingly that altering the source and/or GI of carbohydrate at breakfast influences subsequent food intake at lunch. However, unfortunately they do not indicate the mechanism for the effect.

### 7.3.5 GI and reduced fat storage

#### *7.3.5.1 Studies in animals*

A number of investigators have used RS as a model to study the effects of a low-GI diet on body weight and fat metabolism in rats. Kabir *et al.* (1998b) fed male Sprague-Dawley rats a diet containing 575 g/kg of carbohydrate at either waxy maize starch or mung bean starch. They had previously determined that the α-amylase digestibility of and glycaemic response elicited by the maize starch was significantly greater than those of mung bean starch (Kabir *et al.*, 1998a). After 3 weeks, neither body weight nor epididymal fat pad weight differed significantly; however, fatty acid synthetase activity and gene expression were significantly higher on the maize starch than the mung bean starch diet (Kabir *et al.*, 1998b). Over a longer period of time, feeding RS to rats for 7 or 18 weeks did not influence total body weight, but resulted in a significant decrease in epididymal fat pad weight (Pawlak *et al.*, 2001) and total body fat content with a concomitant increase in lean body mass (Pawlak *et al.*, 2004).

The alteration of body composition with a higher proportion of body fat on a high-GI diet was suggested by all these authors to be due to the

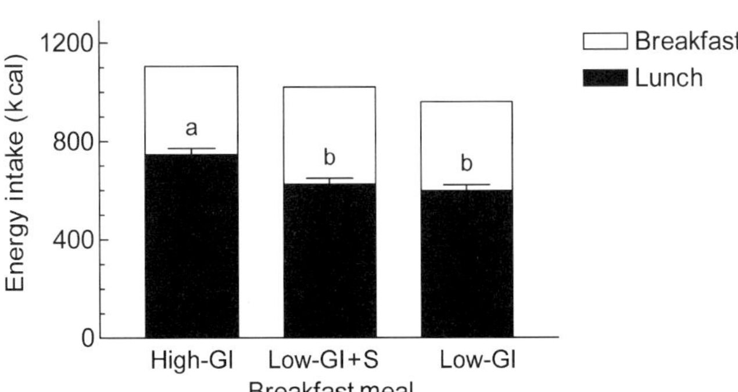


**Fig. 7.4.** Energy intakes of 37 children aged 9–12 years (means ± SEM) from low-GI, low-GI plus sucrose (low-GI + S) and high-GI breakfast meals and subsequent *ad libitum* lunches (redrawn from Warren *et al.*, 2003). Means with different letter superscripts differ significantly ($P < 0.05$).

increased insulin responses elicited by high-GI starch leading to increased lipogenesis from glucose in adipose tissue. However, the relevance of this pathway in humans is uncertain as the lipogenic capacity of adipose tissue in humans is less than in rats (Letexier *et al.*, 2003). To me the interesting question is not so much why fat mass is reduced on the low-GI starch, but what accounts for the increase in lean body mass. If there is something about the consumption of RS that causes an increase in lean body mass then, given equivalent energy intakes, the increase in lean body mass must occur at the expense of fat mass. One factor which could explain this, at least in part, is that the consumption of RS results in an increase in the mass of the gastrointestinal tract, much in the same way as the consumption of dietary fibre. For example, an 18% pectin diet increased the weight of the rat small intestine by 50–60% (Brown *et al.*, 1979) and a 2% pectin diet increased weight of the rat colon by 15% (Koruda *et al.*, 1986). However, I have not been able to determine from the literature how much changes in the weight of the intestine and its contents on high-fibre diets contribute to total body weight of the experimental animals.

#### 7.3.5.2 *Studies in humans*

Body composition was measured in only one of the studies on the effect of a low-GI diet on body weight shown in Fig. 7.1. Bouché *et al.* (2002) found that after 5 weeks of a low- or high-GI diet, body weight was lower on the low-GI diet by 0.8 kg (ns) and body fat was lower by almost an identical amount, 0.77 kg ($P < 0.05$). Two-thirds (66%) of the change in body fat was accounted for by a significant reduction in trunk fat.

### 7.3.6 GI and efficiency of energy absorption

As has been discussed in Chapter 4, carbohydrate in common foods is not completely absorbed in the small intestine, but between about 5% and 15% escapes digestion and passes into the colon where it is fermented by colonic bacteria with the production of gases such as hydrogen, methane and carbon dioxide, water, and the SCFA, acetic, propionic and butyric acids (Cummings and MacFarlane, 1991). The SCFA are absorbed from the colon (McNeil *et al.*, 1978; Wolever *et al.*, 1991b; Vogt and Wolever, 2003) providing a mechanism whereby energy from malabsorbed carbohydrates can be salvaged. It has been estimated that from 3% to 5% of human energy requirements are provided by the SCFA products of colonic fermentation (McNeil, 1984; Royall *et al.*, 1990), but this could increase at least two- to threefold depending on the nature of the carbohydrate foods consumed (McBurney *et al.*, 1987, 1988). However, the energy available in carbohydrates is not completely salvaged via colonic fermentation. Digestible carbohydrates normally provide about 4 kcal/g. During colonic fermentation, some of the energy from the fermented carbohydrate is lost to colonic bacteria, heat, gases and faeces. It has been estimated that the energy obtained from carbohydrates which are completely fermented in the colon is about 2 kcal/g (Livesey, 1992).

As discussed in Chapter 4, the amount of carbohydrate not absorbed in the small intestine is greater for low-GI than high-GI foods. The difference in absorption does not nearly account for the difference in glycaemic response, but may increase the amount of starch entering the colon by two- to threefold. Thus, since 50% of the energy from carbohydrate entering the colon is lost to the human host, the energy in low-GI foods is less efficiently absorbed than that in high-GI foods. To explore the magnitude of this effect, let us assume that the average amount of starch entering the colon from typical high-GI starchy foods is about 3–5% and that this increases to 8–10% for a mixture of low-GI foods. A typical diet contains about 250 g carbohydrate, of which about 60%, or 150 g, is starch. Therefore, on a high-GI diet, 3–5% of the starch, or 4.5–7.5 g, is fermented in the colon, whereas on a low-GI diet, 8–10% of the starch, or 12–15 g is fermented in the colon; a difference of starch availability on a low- vs high-GI diet of 7.5 g. If this 7.5 g starch was absorbed in the small intestine, as it would be on the high-GI diet, it would provide 30 kcal to the host; however, if fermented in the colon, as it would be on the low-GI diet, it provides only 15 kcal. If this scenario was true, the low-GI diet would be associated with 15 kcal less energy absorbed (assuming that energy intake is otherwise unchanged).

## 7.4 GI and Pregnancy

During pregnancy, hormones produced by the placenta oppose the action of insulin which may result in the development of gestational diabetes, a condition defined as glucose intolerance with onset or first recognition during pregnancy (Canadian Diabetes Association Clinical Practice Guidelines Expert Committee, 2003). High blood glucose concentrations during pregnancy are associated with increased birth weight and increased maternal and fetal complications even in women with normal glucose tolerance (Sermer *et al.*, 1995). Therefore, all pregnant women undergo screening for gestational diabetes (Naylor *et al.*, 1997). Treatment of gestational diabetes reduces birth weight and the complications of pregnancy (Naylor *et al.*, 1996). Because of the adverse effects of high blood glucose on pregnancy outcomes and the efficacy of reducing blood glucose concentrations, some investigators have examined the effect of a low-GI diet in pregnancy.

Scholl *et al.* (2004) examined the prospective relationship between diet GI and pregnancy outcomes in over 1000 women. Dietary GI during the course of pregnancy was positively associated with maternal glycosylated haemoglobin and plasma glucose. The average birth weight of infants for women in the lowest quintile of diet GI (<50.4) was about 116 g less than that of women in the 2nd–5th quintiles of diet GI ($P < 0.05$) after adjusting for age, parity, ethnicity, smoking, BMI, prior history of low-birth weight infant and duration of gestation. In addition, the risk of a low-birth weight infant for women in the lowest quintile of diet GI, 13.7%, was 75% higher than that of women in the 2nd–5th quintiles of diet GI ($P < 0.05$) after adjusting for confounding variables. A low-diet GI tended to reduce the risk of large-for-gestational age births, but the difference was not significant (Fig. 7.5). The results of this epidemiological study are supported by a clinical trial in which women randomized to receive a low-GI diet after 8 weeks of gestation gained significantly less weight during pregnancy (10.4 vs 18.6 kg), and gave birth to infants who were lighter (3.33 vs 4.17 kg), shorter (50.5 vs 53.1 cm) and had a smaller ponderal index (2.47 vs 2.74) (Clapp, 2002).

If a low-GI diet is associated with reduced maternal weight gain and reduced birth weight, is this beneficial? Generally, it would be considered that any treatment which increases the risk of fetal malnutrition and small babies is undesirable. A large body of literature suggests that low birth weight is associated with increased risk for heart disease, diabetes, hypertension and high serum cholesterol (Barker, 1996; Carlsson *et al.*, 1999; Leeson *et al.*, 2001; Phenekos, 2001). Against this, however, one needs to consider that the adverse effects of excess maternal weight gain, which include increased risk of adverse pregnancy outcomes and the tendency to promote obesity in the mother after delivery (Scholl *et al.*, 1995). It has been pointed out that the relationship between maternal weight gain and fetal birth weight is not clear, and concern has been expressed that women are being advised to gain too much weight during pregnancy (Feig and Naylor, 1998). Modifying diet GI might be one way to influence maternal weight gain and, hence, address this question experimentally.

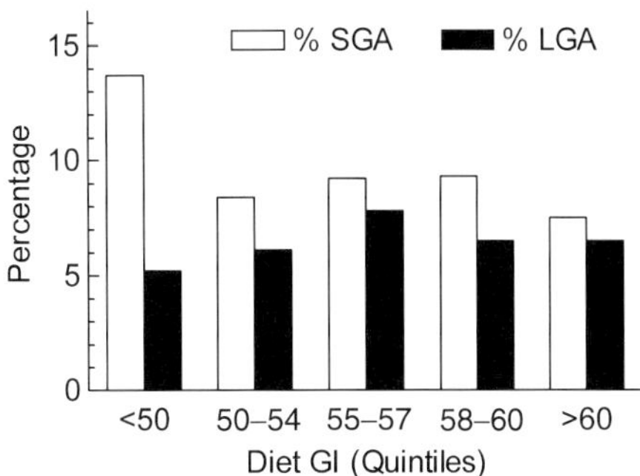


**Fig. 7.5.** Percentage of small-for-gestational age (SGA) and large-for-gestational age (LGA) births by quintile of maternal diet GI during pregnancy. Each quintile contained 216–217 women. The effect of diet GI on SGA was statistically significant, but that for LGA was not. Data from Scholl *et al.* (2004).

## 7.5 GI and Miscellaneous Conditions

### 7.5.1 GI and gastrointestinal tract function

A proportion of dietary starch enters the colon where it is fermented and influences colonic function. The consequences of this for disease mechanisms are discussed in more detail in the next chapter. However, here it is appropriate to consider the potential effects of diet GI on faecal bulk. Constipation is the commonest gastrointestinal complaint in North America, and the drugs available for treatment include the undigestible disaccharide lactulose (Canadian Pharmacists Association, 2003). Undigestible carbohydrates stimulate the growth of bacteria in the colon, and bacteria make up a large proportion of the faecal mass (Stephen and Cummings, 1980). Thus, increased intake of RS increases faecal bulk (Hylla *et al.*, 1998). It has been reported that supplementing the diet with maize starch increases faecal bulk (Shetty and Kurpad, 1986) although not all high-starch diets are necessarily associated with increased faecal bulk (Muir *et al.*, 1998). Thus, it is possible that a low-GI diet which is generally associated with increased carbohydrate fermentation (Jenkins *et al.*, 1987a,d), may increase faecal bulk and be associated with less constipation. However, no studies have examined the effect of diet GI on constipation. In North American women, a low prevalence of constipation is associated with increased physical activity and high fibre intake (Dukas *et al.*, 2003). In Asian and Japanese subjects, a low prevalence of constipation is associated with increased intake of rice (Wong *et al.*, 1999; Nakaji *et al.*, 2002).

### 7.5.2 GI and dental caries

Dental caries, or tooth decay, requires the presence of bacteria in the dental plaque, and is caused when the acid produced by these bacteria dissolve the enamel coating of the tooth leading to erosion of tooth surfaces and exposure of the underlying tissues. Dental caries is a multifactorial process involving factors such as the nature of the bacteria in the dental plaque, the properties of saliva and diet (Kandelman, 1997). Dietary carbohydrates, and particularly sugars, provide substrates from which plaque bacteria produce acid. The ability of dietary carbohydrates to be cariogenic depends on several factors: the amount and frequency of exposure of tooth surfaces to sugars and starches, the bioavailability of the starches, the nature of the microbial flora of dental plaque, the pH-lowering capacity of the plaque and the flow-rate of saliva (Lingstrom *et al.*, 2000a). Thus, it is of interest that the ability of different kinds of bread to elicit a drop in plaque pH was related to their GI, i.e. the higher the GI, the more pronounced the drop in pH (Lingstrom *et al.*, 2000b). Presumably, this may be related to the fact that higher GI starches are more readily digested by salivary amylase into sugars, stick to the tooth surfaces more or are more bioavailable to the plaque bacteria resulting in a more rapid rate of acid production.

## 7.6 Conclusions

Evidence is reviewed in this chapter that altering the GI of dietary carbohydrates directly or indirectly influences many physiological processes which are relevant to health and performance, including physical activity, cognitive function, appetite regulation, energy balance, body composition, maternal and fetal weight gain during pregnancy, gastrointestinal function and tooth decay.

## Notes

### GI and athletic performance

Recent studies further support the concept that the GI is relevant to carbohydrate metabolism during exercise and recovery, with high GI carbohydrates increasing glucose, insulin and muscle glycogen more than low GI (Stevenson *et al.*, 2005a,b; Wee *et al.*, 2005). However, although a low GI dinner improved carbohydrate tolerance the following morning, it had no effect on subsequent exercise, compared to a high GI dinner (Stevenson *et al.*, 2005c).

### GI and weight loss

Two recent studies suggest that low GI diets do not enhance weight loss beyond what is seen with energy restriction alone (Raatz *et al.*, 2005; Thompson *et al.*, 2005).

# 8

# Glycaemic Index and Disease

A large body of evidence suggests that low-GI foods may be beneficial for the prevention or treatment of a number of chronic diseases including diabetes, cardiovascular disease (CHD and stroke) and cancer. This chapter will explain briefly what is known about the pathogenesis of these disorders and review the evidence from human studies regarding the role of the GI in prevention and treatment. After discussing these points, I will then review the physiological and molecular mechanisms by which low-GI foods may influence the pathogenic processes. The mechanisms will be discussed independently of the diseases, because diabetes, cardiovascular disease and cancer are believed to have many aetiological factors in common.

## 8.1 Diabetes

Diabetes mellitus is a condition characterized by hyperglycaemia due to defective insulin secretion, defective insulin action, or both, and of a sufficient degree to be associated with an increased incidence of long-term microvascular complications in retina, nerve and kidney (Canadian Diabetes Association Clinical Practice Guidelines Expert Committee, 2003; Expert Committee on the Diagnosis and Classification of Diabetes Mellitus, 2003). The diagnosis of diabetes can be made if any one of the following three criteria is met and confirmed on at least two occasions: fasting plasma glucose (FPG) ≥7.0 mmol/l; casual (random) plasma glucose (PG) ≥11.1 mmol/l in the presence of symptoms of diabetes (such as polyuria, thirst or unexplained weight loss); plasma glucose 2 h (2 h PG) after 75 g OGTT ≥11.1 mmol/l. There are three main types of diabetes: type 1 diabetes, type 2 diabetes (which accounts for about 90% of all cases of diabetes) and gestational diabetes. In addition, a wide variety of 'other specific types' of diabetes exist, which consist mainly of specific genetic defects, other diseases or drug use.

Other related conditions include prediabetes and the metabolic syndrome. Prediabetes has been used as a convenient term for impaired fasting glucose (IFG) and impaired glucose tolerance (IGT), both of which are conditions characterized by high blood glucose levels that are below the threshold for diabetes but are still associated with clinical consequences. Isolated IFG is defined as FPG between 6.1 and 6.9 mmol/l inclusive either alone, or if an OGTT was done, with 2 h PG <7.8 mmol/l. Isolated IGT is defined as FPG <6.1 and 2 h PG between 7.8 and 11.0 mmol/l inclusive. IFG and IGT are present if FPG is 6.1–6.9 mmol/l and 2 h PG is 7.8–11.0 mmol/l. Prediabetes is associated with increased risk of developing cardiovascular disease and diabetes mellitus (Coutinho *et al.*, 1999). The metabolic syndrome is a common condition characterized by a distinctive combination of abnormalities which include abdominal obesity, hypertension, dyslipidaemia, insulin resistance and dysglycaemia. Individuals with the metabolic syndrome are at increased risk of developing cardiovascular disease and diabetes. However, there is a lack of consensus regarding the definition of the metabolic syndrome. The WHO proposed a definition that includes identification of the presence of insulin resistance (World Health Organization, 1999)

(Table 3.1), whereas the US Expert Panel on Detection, Evaluation and Treatment of High Blood Cholesterol in Adults (2001, Adult Treatment Panel III (ATP III)) provided a definition which does not require measurement of insulin resistance (Table 3.1).

When the GI was originally proposed, the major application considered was in the management of diabetes. Thus, a relatively large number of studies have been done to examine the effect of altering diet GI on glycaemic control in subjects with diabetes. Although there is good evidence that the GI may be useful in the management of diabetes, a potentially even more important application for the GI is in the prevention of type 2 diabetes or the treatment of the metabolic syndrome.

### 8.1.1 Dietary carbohydrates and prevention of type 1 diabetes

The most common form of type 1 diabetes is believed to be due to immune-mediated destruction of the insulin-producing β-cells of the pancreas, a process thought to be incited by environmental factors in genetically predisposed persons. Randomized trials testing whether administration of insulin or various drugs to people at risk of getting type 1 diabetes have been completed but no effective prevention strategy has yet been identified (Lampeter *et al.*, 1998; Christie *et al.*, 2002; Diabetes Prevention Trial Type 1 Diabetes Study Group, 2002). Nutritional factors which may be implicated include the type of milk fed during infancy, with some evidence from epidemiologic and case–control studies that breast feeding reduces the risk of developing type 1 diabetes (Schrezenmeir and Jagla, 2000). A randomized clinical trial is currently underway to test this hypothesis (Trial to Reduce IDDM in the Genetically at Risk, 2004). Interestingly, there is also evidence that breast feeding reduces risk for obesity (Armstrong *et al.*, 2003) and type 2 diabetes (Pettitt *et al.*, 1997). It is not clear whether the protective effect, if any, of breast feeding for type 1 diabetes is due to the avoidance of harmful factors in cow's milk or to the receipt of protective factors in breast milk (Kolb and Pozzilli, 1999). Recent concepts about how undigested carbohydrates influence systemic immune function (Section 8.4.4.3) suggest that the GI might have a role to play in preventing type 1 diabetes related to the proportion of carbohydrate which escapes digestion in the small intestine. This concept is compatible with the protective effects of breast milk, since breast milk is rich in various undigested carbohydrates (Brand-Miller *et al.*, 1998; Sumiyoshi *et al.*, 2003). Clearly much more research will be necessary to prove this highly speculative suggestion.

### 8.1.2 Dietary carbohydrates and prevention of type 2 diabetes

#### *8.1.2.1 Pathogenesis of type 2 diabetes*

Type 2 diabetes is associated with an inability of insulin to increase the uptake of glucose by muscle (insulin resistance), increased hepatic glucose output (sometimes known as hepatic insulin resistance) and reduced insulin secretion by pancreatic β-cells (DeFronzo, 1988). The natural history of type 2 diabetes appears to follow a course in which normal individuals destined to develop type 2 diabetes necessarily pass through a stage of IGT (Weyer *et al.*, 1999). The challenge has been to understand why the deterioration in glucose tolerance occurs. The two-step model proposed by Saad *et al.* (1991) suggested that insulin resistance is the primary defect leading to the development of diabetes and that this is followed by β-cell failure brought on by a combination of factors including genetic susceptibility, age, declining β-cell mass, glucose toxicity and β-cell exhaustion. This was the dominant model for a number of years, at least in North America, but it has been questioned recently because of evidence suggesting that β-cell dysfunction exists in the prediabetic state. The current model for the development of type 2 diabetes is that insulin resistance and β-cell dysfunction co-exist in the prediabetic state and exacerbate each other through multiple feedback mechanisms (Prentki and Corkey, 1996; Ferrannini, 1998; Gerich, 1998; Cavaghan *et al.*, 2000; Katin, 2003).

Current thinking about the pathogenesis of type 2 diabetes is more in line with Bergman (1989) who suggested that neither insulin resistance nor reduced insulin secretion alone were sufficient to cause diabetes, but that both needed to be present. Bergman's concept was that, under normal circumstances, there is a dynamic equilibrium between β-cell function and insulin sensitivity such that the normal β-cell would respond to changes in insulin sensitivity by secreting more or less insulin as required to maintain normal plasma glucose (Bergman *et al.*, 1981). Since individuals differ in their degree of insulin resistance due to genetic and environmental factors, if Bergman's idea was correct, a scatter plot of insulin sensitivity (*x*-axis) and insulin secretion in different individuals with normal blood glucose, would show that those who were insulin resistant (i.e. low insulin sensitivity) would have high insulin secretion, and those who were insulin sensitive would have low insulin secretion. There is good evidence to support a hyperbolic relationship between insulin sensitivity and insulin secretion in normal subjects (Kahn *et al.*, 1993; Clausen *et al.*, 1996) as illustrated in simple form in Fig. 8.1A. Moreover, Bergman's concept suggested that, within individuals, insulin secretion would change in response to changes in insulin sensitivity due to environmental circumstances. This is illustrated in Fig. 8.1B; let us assume point a represents the insulin sensitivity and insulin secretion of a hypothetical young female. If she begins an exercise programme, her insulin sensitivity will increase from point a to point b; this will be accompanied by a reduction in insulin secretion. If this woman now becomes pregnant, she will become more insulin resistant, i.e. she moves from point b to point c; to compensate for the reduction in insulin sensitivity her insulin secretion will increase. Thus, as long as her β-cells can respond appropriately to the changes in insulin sensitivity, her blood glucose will remain normal. Her blood glucose would only become abnormal if her β-cells were unable to increase insulin secretion in response to a reduction in insulin sensitivity, as shown at point d in Fig. 8.1C.

Many studies measuring insulin resistance do not include measurements of insulin secretion. However, a number of studies have shown that the reciprocal changes in insulin sensitivity and insulin secretion predicted by the model shown in Fig. 8.1B actually do occur. Kahn *et al.* (1990) showed that insulin sensitivity was increased by exercise training in older subjects and that this was accompanied by a reduction in insulin secretion such that glucose tolerance did not change. Catalano *et al.* (1993, 1999) studied normal women and women with gestational diabetes prior to conception and in early and late pregnancy and showed that, in both groups, pregnancy resulted in a marked decrease in insulin sensitivity with a compensatory increase in insulin secretion. Other studies show that the induction of insulin resistance obtained by treating normal men with dexamethasone (Beard *et al.*, 1984) or nicotinic acid (Kahn *et al.*, 1989) was compensated for in both cases by an increase in insulin secretion (Fig. 8.2). The models shown in Fig. 8.1B and C have also been supported by longitudinal studies in Pima Indians. Weyer *et al.* (1999) studied oral glucose tolerance, insulin action and insulin secretion on at least three occasions over 5 years in 48 Pima Indian subjects. At the start of the study, all subjects had normal glucose tolerance. By the end of the study period, 17 of the subjects had

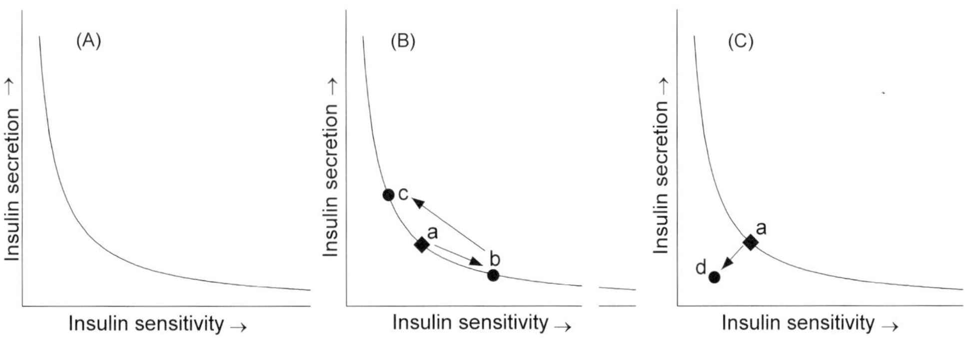


**Fig. 8.1.** A: Theoretic hyperbolic relationship between insulin sensitivity and insulin secretion in people with a normal fasting plasma glucose concentration. B: Model illustrating effect of weight loss (point a to point b) and pregnancy (point b to point c) on insulin sensitivity and insulin secretion. C: Effect of developing type 2 diabetes on insulin sensitivity and insulin secretion.

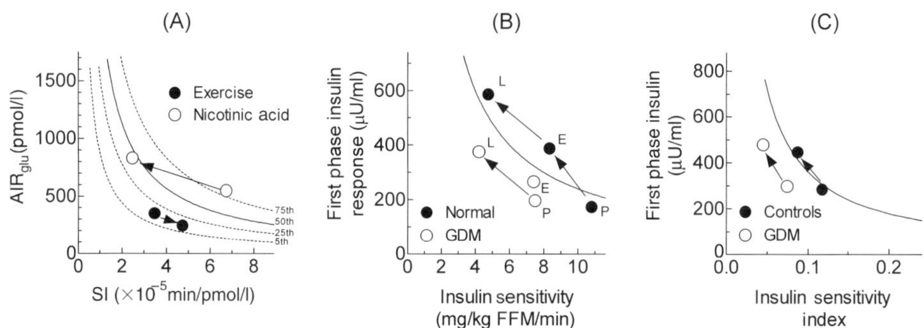


**Fig. 8.2.** Effect of various physiologic manoeuvres on insulin sensitivity and insulin secretion in human subjects: A, effect of exercise (Kahn *et al.*, 1990) and treatment with nicotinic acid (Kahn *et al.*, 1989); B, effect of pregnancy (Catalano *et al.*, 1993); C, effect of pregnancy (Catalano *et al.*, 1999). In all cases, changes in insulin sensitivity are compensated for by reciprocal changes in insulin secretion.

developed diabetes (progressors) while 31 maintained normal glucose tolerance (non-progressors). At baseline, when all subjects had normal glucose tolerance, the progressors were heavier (93.7 vs 87.9 kg) and had more body fat (38% vs 29% of body weight) than non-progressors. Over the time period of the study both groups gained weight, but the progressors gained significantly more than the non-progressors (13.2 vs 6.2 kg, $P < 0.01$). However, the % body fat gain did not differ significantly in the two groups. Although both groups tended to become more insulin resistant with time (progressors, $P < 0.0001$; non-progressors, $P = 0.06$), non-progressors compensated for the increase in insulin resistance with a significant increase in insulin secretion, whereas there was a significant decrease in insulin secretion in the progressors (Fig. 8.3). This study suggests that the difference between subjects who progress to diabetes and those who do not is not because of increased insulin resistance, but because of a failure in insulin secretion, or more precisely, a failure of the ability of the β-cell to compensate for insulin resistance by increasing insulin secretion.

### *8.1.2.2 Diet GI and risk for type 2 diabetes*

Five prospective studies have examined the effect of diet GI on the risk of type 2 diabetes (Salmerón *et al.*, 1997a,b; Stevens *et al.*, 2002; Hodge *et al.*, 2004; Schulze *et al.*, 2004) (Fig. 8.4). In four of these studies, a high-GI diet was associated with statistically significantly greater risk of developing type 2 diabetes, after adjusting for confounding variables. These four studies involved a total of over 170,000 participants, and subjects in the highest quintile or quartile of diet GI had 30–60% higher risk for diabetes than subjects in the lowest quintile or quartile of diet GI. Only one study did not report a significant effect of diet GI on diabetes risk in either white or African-American participants, but the total number of subjects in this study, 12,251, was only 7% of the number in the other four studies.

The findings of these prospective studies showing increased risk for diabetes with a high-GI diet are supported by a number of studies showing that a high-GI diet is associated with increased risk of having the metabolic syndrome, insulin resistance or a high fasting serum insulin

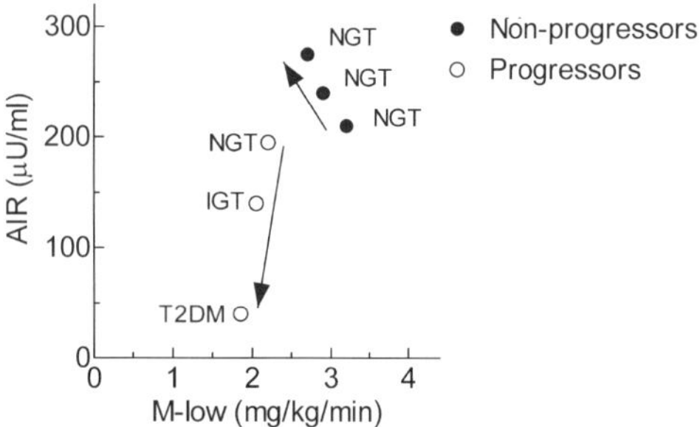


**Fig. 8.3.** Insulin sensitivity (M-low) and insulin secretion (AIR) in 38 Pima Indians studied on three occasions over 5 years. Progressors are 17 individuals who progressed from normal glucose tolerance to impaired glucose tolerance to diabetes. Non-progressors are 31 individuals whose oral glucose tolerance remained normal over the same period.

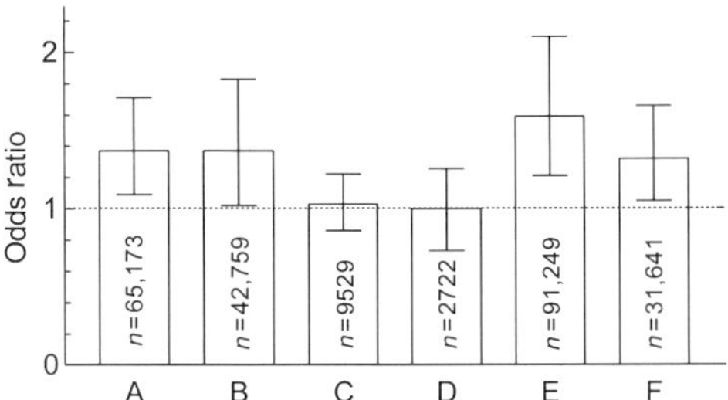


**Fig. 8.4.** Odds ratios (means ± 95% confidence intervals) for risk of developing diabetes associated with the highest quartile or quintile of diet GI, relative to the lowest quartile or quintile in six populations in five studies: A, US men (Salmerón *et al.*, 1997a); B, US women (Salmerón *et al.*, 1997b); C, US Whites (Stevens *et al.*, 2002); D, US African-American (Stevens *et al.*, 2002); E, US young/middle-aged women (Schulze *et al.*, 2004); F, Australian adults (Hodge *et al.*, 2004). The number of subjects studied is also indicated.

concentration (McKeown *et al.*, 2004; Scaglioni *et al.*, 2004).

#### 8.1.2.3 *Effect of diet GI on insulin sensitivity and insulin secretion*

It is often suggested that low-GI diets improve insulin sensitivity, but current data do not clearly support this. There have been six studies looking at the effect of a low-GI diet on insulin sensitivity; the results are difficult to compare because of the different populations studied and the different methods used to assess insulin sensitivity (Table 8.1). The best evidence that a low GI improves insulin sensitivity in subjects without diabetes is from Frost's group at the Hammersmith Hospital in London, UK. In their first study, Frost *et al.* (1996) showed that 4 weeks of a low-GI diet in individuals at risk for CHD tended to reduce the area under the plasma glucose response curve after oral glucose and significantly reduced the insulin response area. Although this is, presumably, a beneficial effect, it is difficult to know why it occurred; it could represent improved insulin sensitivity, but it could also be due to improved insulin secretion, or to a reduced rate of glucose absorption due to altered gut morphology. For example, Swinburn *et al.* (1991b) found that consuming a high-carbohydrate diet for 2 weeks reduced the areas under the plasma glucose and insulin response curves following oral glucose, but that these effects were not associated with any change in insulin sensitivity (measured using the FSIGTT and minimal model), but rather with increased glucose effectiveness and insulin secretion. A reduced rate of glucose absorption could be secondary to altered morphology of the

**Table 8.1.** Effect of low-GI diet on insulin sensitivity and β-cell function.

| | | High-GI diet | | Low-GI diet | | | | | |
|---|---|---|---|---|---|---|---|---|---|
| Subjects[a] | Design[b] | CHO (% en) | GI | CHO (% en) | GI | Method[c] | Insulin sensitivity (% diff)[d] | Insulin secretion (% diff)[d] | Reference |
| 30 CVD | 4 week, P | 45 | 65 | 45 | 54 | ISGU | +76* | – | a |
| 28 PM ♀ | 3 week, P | 50 | 62 | 51 | 49 | SITT | +44* | – | b |
| 7 N ♂ | 30 days, X | 47 | 64 | 46 | 49 | EHC | −9* | – | c |
| 34 IGT | 16 week, P | 53 | 59 | 55 | 54 | FSIGTT | +41 ns | +62*[,e] | d |
| 20 PM ♀ | 8 week, X | 51 | – | 53 | – | FSIGTT | +5 ns | +10*[,f] | e |
| 12 D ♂ | 4 week, X | 38 | 71 | 36 | 39 | EHC | +46* | – | f |

[a]CVD = cardiovascular disease; PM = postmenopausal; N = healthy normal; IGT = impaired glucose tolerance; D = type 2 diabetes.
[b]P = parallel design; X = cross-over design.
[c]ISGU = insulin-stimulated glucose uptake by adipocytes *in vitro*; SITT = short insulin tolerance test; EHC = euglycaemic hyperinsulinaemic clamp; FSIGTT = frequently sampled intravenous glucose tolerance test.
[d]$100\times(L-H)/H$, where $L$ and $H$ are the mean values after low-GI and high-GI diets, respectively.
[e]Disposition index (insulin sensitivity index times insulin AUC after intravenous glucose).
[f]Insulin AUC after intravenous glucose.
*$P < 0.05$.
References: a (Frost *et al.*, 1996); b (Frost *et al.*, 1998); c (Kiens and Richter, 1996); d (Wolever and Mehling, 2002); e (Juntunen *et al.*, 2003); f (Rizkalla *et al.*, 2004).

absorptive villi in the small intestine such as that which occurs in experimental animals fed diets containing certain types of dietary fibre (Tasman-Jones, 1993). Thus, in their next study, Frost *et al.* (1998) showed that consuming a low-GI diet for 3 weeks increased the *in vitro* insulin responsiveness of adipocytes obtained from women at risk of cardiovascular disease, and increased insulin sensitivity *in vivo*, measured using the short insulin tolerance test. However, these studies have been criticized because the method used to assess insulin sensitivity is not considered to be a 'gold-standard' method such as the euglycaemic, hyperinsulinaemic clamp.

Kiens and Richter (1996) studied a very different group of subjects, namely seven lean young men, all of whom rode bicycles for local transportation and participated in regular physical activity once or twice per week. They were given high-GI or low-GI diets for 30 days using a randomized cross-over design with euglycaemic, hyperinsulinaemic clamps performed at the end of each dietary period. Serum insulin was lower after 3 days on the low-GI diet but not after 30 days. Whole-body glucose uptake was similar for both diets at a low plasma insulin concentration (370 pmol/l), but was 9% lower (i.e. reduced insulin sensitivity) after the low-GI than the high-GI diet at the high insulin concentration (2400 pmol/l, $P < 0.05$). It is amusing to note that this study has been cited as evidence both in favour of (Brand Miller and Foster-Powell, 1999) and against (Pi-Sunyer, 2002) the use of low-GI diets! My own view is that the lack of consistency of the result for insulin sensitivity at the two levels of plasma insulin is confusing. However, the lack of difference in insulin sensitivity at the 'low' level of insulin (340 pmol/l) seems a more physiologically relevant conclusion than the reduced insulin sensitivity at a plasma insulin concentration of 2400 pmol/l because the former is more representative of the plasma insulin concentrations of healthy young men. Indeed, Kiens and Richter (1996) report maximum mean plasma insulin in their subjects during the day of about 240 pmol/l.

We did a study in subjects with IGT to see if a low-GI diet would improve insulin sensitivity (Wolever and Mehling, 2002). This study was notable in that the dietary interventions were less rigorous but were carried out for much longer (4 months) than Frost *et al.* (1996, 1998) and Kiens and Richter (1996). We measured insulin sensitivity and insulin secretion using the frequently sampled intravenous glucose tolerance test and Bergman's minimal model (method described in Chapter 3). Despite the different population, our results agreed with Kiens and Richter (1996) in that we found no effect of the low-GI diet on insulin sensitivity (Wolever and Mehling, 2002) and no reduction in mean serum insulin during the day on the low-GI diet compared to baseline (Wolever and Mehling, 2003). Indeed, mean plasma insulin decreased significantly in subjects on the high-GI diet, and this change was significantly different from the change on low GI; thus, the low-GI diet actually increased mean plasma insulin concentrations compared to the high-GI diet (Wolever and Mehling, 2003). This is consistent with our finding of a significantly improved disposition index (DI), a measure of β-cell responsiveness. DI increased from baseline by 50% ($P = 0.02$) on the high-carbohydrate, low-GI diet, with trends toward reductions on both the high-carbohydrate, high-GI diet and low-carbohydrate, high monounsaturated fat (MUFA) diets (Fig. 8.5). After adjusting for differences in baseline, the change in DI on low GI was significantly greater than those on both the other diets (Fig. 8.5, inset) (Wolever and Mehling, 2002). I believe the increase in DI on the low-GI diet is, biologically, a very significant finding, because a reduction in DI is precisely the pathogenic mechanism proposed for the development of diabetes (Figs 8.1 and 8.3).

Juntunen *et al.* (2003) did a study similar to ours (Wolever and Mehling, 2002) in which 20 healthy postmenopausal women consumed either rye or wheat bread for 8 weeks using a randomized, cross-over design. The group had previously shown that the rye bread used elicited significantly lower glucose and insulin responses than the wheat bread (Juntunen *et al.*, 2002). The test breads made up approximately 25% of total energy intake during the study. Insulin sensitivity was assessed using the frequently sampled intravenous glucose tolerance test and Bergman's minimal model. The results of Juntunen *et al.* (2003) were also similar to ours (Wolever and Mehling, 2002) in that the effects of the low-GI bread (rye bread) did not differ from those of the high-GI bread (wheat) with respect to body weight, fasting glucose, fasting insulin or insulin sensitivity index. However, the acute insulin response to

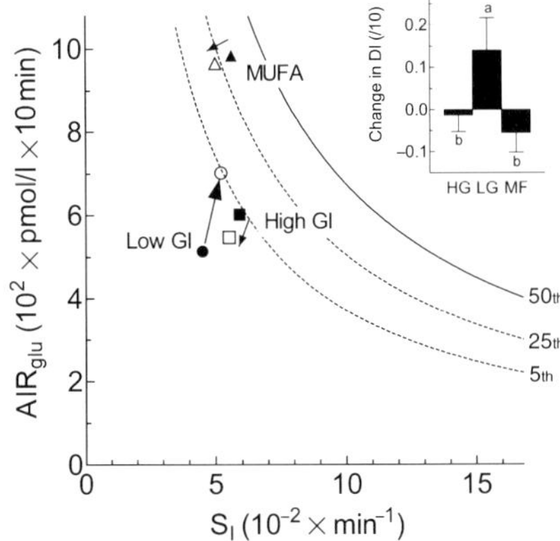


**Fig. 8.5.** Changes in insulin secretion ($AIR_{glu}$) relative to changes in insulin sensitivity ($S_I$) in subjects with impaired glucose tolerance randomized to receive, for 4 months, either a high-carbohydrate, high-GI diet (HG, $n = 11$), a high-carbohydrate, low-GI diet (LG, $n = 13$) or a low-carbohydrate, high monounsaturated fat diet (MF, $n = 11$) The curved lines represent the prediction line (50th percentile) and the 25th and 5th percentiles of the regression of $AIR_{glu}$ and $S_I$ derived from 15 control subjects. Inset: comparison of changes in disposition index ($DI = AIR_{glu} \times S_I$) in the three groups after adjustment for baseline values. Means with different letter superscripts differ significantly ($P < 0.05$) (Wolever and Mehling, 2003).

intravenous glucose increased significantly more during the rye bread period than during the wheat bread period (9.9% vs 2.8%, $P = 0.047$).

Rizkalla *et al.* (2004) found that whole-body glucose disposal, as measured by the euglycaemic, hyperinsulinaemic clamp, was significantly higher in subjects with type 2 diabetes after 4 weeks on a low-GI diet than after 4 weeks on a high-GI diet ($7 \pm 1.3$ vs $4.8 \pm 0.9$ mg/kg/min, $P < 0.001$). The difference in results between this study and those in non-diabetic subjects could be due to a difference in glucose toxicity. Although it is expected that a low-GI diet would elicit the same percentage reduction in incremental glycaemic response in normal and diabetic subjects, because subjects with diabetes have much higher glucose concentrations than normal, the reduction in absolute blood glucose concentration elicited by a low-GI diet is larger in diabetic than normal subjects. Thus, there could be a larger reduction in glucose toxicity in diabetic than normal subjects. Rizkalla *et al.* (2004) found that average blood glucose during an 8-h metabolic profile in their subjects with diabetes was reduced by about 1.3 mmol/l, relative to the change on the high-GI diet, whereas Wolever and Mehling (2003) found a difference of only about 0.3 mmol/l in subjects with IGT, and Kiens and Richter (1996) found no difference in normal subjects.

Even if it cannot be shown that a low-GI diet improves insulin sensitivity, this does not mean that a low-GI diet has no role to play in preventing diabetes. As discussed in Section 8.1.2.1, changes in insulin sensitivity, if accompanied by compensatory changes in insulin secretion, may have no impact on diabetes risk. β-Cell responsiveness (DI – the product of insulin sensitivity and insulin secretion) appears to be the key factor which needs to be increased to prevent type 2 diabetes (Finegood and Topp, 2001).

### 8.1.3 Effect of diet GI on glycaemic control in diabetes

#### *8.1.3.1 Cross-sectional studies*

Diet GI was positively associated with overall glycaemic control in three different cross-sectional studies in individuals with diabetes.

We studied the correlation between habitual diet assessed by two 3-day food records and glycaemic control in 354 patients with type 2 diabetes from seven centres in Canada (Wolever *et al.*, 1995b). In the 75 subjects treated with diet alone glycated haemoglobin (A1c) was inversely related to carbohydrate intake as a % of energy ($r = -0.302$, $P = 0.01$) and positively related to diet GI ($r = 0.321$, $P < 0.01$). There was no significant correlation between A1c and diet GI in the 87 subjects on insulin, but A1c was negatively related to carbohydrate as a % of energy ($r = -0.303$, $P < 0.01$) and dietary fibre intakes ($r = -0.345$). There was no relationship between carbohydrate or GI and A1c in the 82 subjects on metformin or the 98 subjects treated with sulphonylurea.

We also studied 272 subjects with type 1 diabetes from seven centres in Canada treated with a mixture of regular and NPH insulins before breakfast and supper and who adjusted their doses of insulin using a standardized algorithm based on the results of home blood glucose monitoring 2–4 times daily, and the amount of dietary carbohydrate in the dietary prescription provided by a registered dietitian (Wolever *et al.*, 1990). Neither nutrient intake, diet GI nor insulin dose was related to A1c. However, day-to-day variation in carbohydrate ($P = 0.0097$) and starch ($P = 0.0016$) intakes and diet GI ($P = 0.033$) were positively related to A1c, and the associations remained significant when adjusted for age, sex, duration of diabetes and BMI. Since, in this study, the insulin dose was adjusted based on the *prescribed* amount of carbohydrate in the diet (which in turn, was based on the habitual intake), the results show that consistency in the GI and the amount of dietary carbohydrate from day to day (and hence closer adherence to the prescribed diet) are associated with improved glycaemic control in type 1 diabetes.

The largest cross-sectional study to examine the relationship between diet and glycaemic control in people with diabetes was the EURODIAB study which involved 2810 subjects with type 1 diabetes from 31 European centres. In all 2810 subjects, diet GI was positively related to A1c ($P = 0.0001$) (Buyken *et al.*, 2001). The difference in median GI between the highest and lowest quartiles (64 vs 54) was associated with an 11% reduction in A1c in southern European centres and a 6% reduction in A1c in northern, western and eastern European centres.

#### *8.1.3.2 Clinical trials*

At least 17 clinical trials have been published comparing the effect of high-carbohydrate, low-GI diets with those of high-carbohydrate, high-GI diets in the treatment of diabetes. These studies suggest that low-GI diets have a modest but statistically significant effect in improving glycaemic control in subjects with type 1 or type 2 diabetes. The results of 14 of these have been summarized in a meta-analysis by Brand-Miller *et al.* (2003b). These studies included 356 subjects and utilized either randomized cross-over or randomized parallel designs of 12 days to 12 months duration (mean 10 weeks). Low-GI diets significantly reduced A1c in the nine studies in which it was measured by an absolute amount of 0.43% (95% CI 0.72–0.13). When data for A1c and fructosamine were pooled, low-GI diets reduced glycated proteins by an average of 7.4% of the baseline value (95% CI 8.8–6.0).

Since the publication of this meta-analysis, three other studies have appeared, the results of which are consistent with those of the previous studies. Heilbronn *et al.* (2002) placed 45 overweight (mean BMI, 33.8 kg/m$^2$) subjects with type 2 diabetes on energy-restricted diets for 12 weeks. All subjects consumed a run-in diet containing 50% energy as carbohydrate for the first 4 weeks, during which time average weight loss was 3.6 kg. Subjects were then randomized to an energy restricted, high-carbohydrate, high-GI diet (carbohydrate intake, 61% energy; GI, 75) or an energy-restricted high-carbohydrate, low-GI diet (carbohydrate intake, 59% energy; GI, 43) for the next 8 weeks. During the 8-week experimental phase, weight loss was equivalent on the high- and low-GI diets (4.8 vs 4.4 kg, respectively). The reduction in glycated haemoglobin on the low-GI diet, 6.65–6.04%, was twice that on the high-GI diet, 6.32–6.08%, but the difference was not statistically significant ($P = 0.17$).

Jimenez-Cruz *et al.* (2003) studied 14 obese or overweight subjects with type 2 diabetes using a randomized cross-over design who followed high-carbohydrate (64% energy), high-GI (56) diets or high-carbohydrate (60% energy), low-GI (44) diets for 6 weeks each. There was no significant change in blood lipids, but HbA1c fell significantly more on the low-GI diet (8.5–8.1%) than on the high-GI diet (8.6–8.6%) ($P < 0.008$).

Rizkalla *et al.* (2004) placed 12 men with type 2 diabetes on high-GI and low-GI diets for 4 weeks each using a randomized cross-over design. HbA1c was reduced from 7.57% after the high-GI diet to 7.17% after the low-GI diet ($P < 0.01$). Relative to the high-GI diet, the low-GI diet also significantly reduced fasting total and low-density lipoprotein (LDL) cholesterol, apoB, FFAs and plasminogen activator inhibitor-1 (PAI-1) activity.

## 8.2 Cardiovascular Disease

Cardiovascular disease includes many conditions, but the present discussion will be about angina, myocardial infarction, peripheral vascular disease and stroke all of which are caused by the narrowing of arteries by atherosclerotic plaques or their occlusion by vascular thrombosis.

### 8.2.1 Pathogenesis of cardiovascular disease

Three factors, known as Virchow's triad, are involved in the development of vascular thrombosis: changes in the blood vessel wall (atherosclerosis), changes in blood flow (vasomotor tone and endothelial function) and changes in the constituents in the blood (lipids, clotting factors and cytokines). All of these factors may be able to be modified by diet, including changes in the GI of dietary carbohydrate.

#### *8.2.1.1 Atherosclerotic plaques*

Atherosclerosis plaques are lesions containing a necrotic lipid core within the intima of the artery and separated from the lumen by the fibrous cap, an endothelial layer with variable amounts of fibrocellular tissue. In smaller arteries, such as coronary or cerebral arteries, plaques are often eccentric in cross section and can fill much of the artery lumen. Once a plaque has reduced the area of the lumen by more than about 45%, the natural ability of the artery to dilate and remodel is lost, and lumen stenosis develops which reduces blood flow (Dickson and Gotlieb, 2003). Vascular thrombosis occurs when an unstable or vulnerable plaque ruptures leading to activation of platelets and the formation of a blood clot which occludes the lumen of the artery.

The early stages of the development of atherosclerotic plaques involve the accumulation of cholesterol within the intima due to a disruption in the balance between cholesterol influx and efflux in the plaque. As the condition progresses, atherosclerosis becomes a chronic inflammatory process with unstable atherosclerotic lesions being characterized by the presence of inflammatory cells (macrophages and T lymphocytes), proliferation of smooth muscle cells and extracellular matrix and neovascularization. These changes may be initiated by the uptake and accumulation of cholesterol by macrophages within the plaque, which, over time, leads to the formation of foam cells which ultimately die and form the necrotic lipid core. The cholesterol-filled macrophages release a number of factors which accelerate the growth and development of the atherosclerotic plaque, including growth factors that promote neovascularization, cytokines that stimulate smooth muscle cell proliferation and attract lymphocytes, and metalloproteinases that can weaken the plaque cap leading to rupture (Vaughan *et al.*, 1996).

#### *8.2.1.2 Endothelial function*

The endothelium is the layer of cells lining the lumen of the artery and it is involved in the regulation of vasomotor tone, thrombosis, fibrinolysis and platelet activity. The endothelium produces nitric oxide, which normally causes vasodilation and reduced arterial stiffness, and endothelin-1, which has the opposite effects. Increased arterial stiffness increases cardiovascular risk, particularly in older subjects (Wilkinson and McEniery, 2004). Endothelial function is disrupted in atheromatous arteries, such that stimuli which would normally dilate a healthy artery cause atheromatous arteries to constrict. Lowering blood cholesterol with statins (HMG-CoA reductase inhibitors) improves myocardial perfusion in patients with coronary artery disease within periods of just a few weeks. Since this is too short an interval for anatomic regression to occur, the improved blood flow is presumed to be due to improved endothelial vasomotor function (Vaughan *et al.*, 1996).

The effect of altering dietary GI on endothelial function has not been studied. However, it is known that high-fat meals acutely impair endothelial function. Vogel *et al.* (1997) studied normal subjects after a high-fat meal (an Egg McMuffin®, Sausage McMuffin® and two hash brown patties; 50 g fat, 14 g saturated fat) and an isocaloric low-fat meal (Frosted Flakes®, skimmed milk and orange juice; 0 g fat) on two occasions. Flow-mediated brachial artery vasoactivity did not change for 6 h after the low-fat meal, but decreased significantly between 2 and 4 h after the high-fat meal. The changes in vasoactivity were negatively correlated with changes in postprandial triglycerides, i.e. large reductions in endothelial function were associated with large increases in postprandial triglycerides. Treatment of subjects with coronary artery disease with folic acid for 4 months (Title *et al.*, 2000) and treatment of hypercholesterolaemic subjects with ω-3 fatty acids for 4 months (Goodfellow *et al.*, 2000) improved endothelial function.

#### 8.2.1.3 Changes in constituents of blood – blood lipids

The main lipid constituent of the atherosclerotic plaque is cholesterol. LDL cholesterol is the major cholesterol-carrying lipoprotein in the circulation, and, hence the main route by which cholesterol reaches atherosclerotic plaques. Cholesterol accumulates in plaques when its rate of influx exceeds its rate of efflux. Factors which increase the influx of cholesterol into the plaque include a high concentration of LDL in the blood, altered structure of LDL particles, such as oxidation (Witztum, 1994) or glycation (Lyons, 1992; Cai *et al.*, 2004) or the presence of small, dense LDL (Austin, 2000). Factors which reduce the rate of efflux of cholesterol from the artery wall include increased uptake into macrophages (retention of the cholesterol within the lesion) and reduced reverse cholesterol transport which could be due to a defect in the ATP-binding cassette transporter 1 (ABCA1) which transports cholesterol out of cells or to a defect in the composition or metabolism of HDL cholesterol which accepts cholesterol from cells and transports it in the blood to the liver for excretion (Ng, 2004). Recent clinical trials showing that LDL-lowering therapy reduces risk for CHD (Durrington, 2003) provide very strong evidence that LDL cholesterol is a major cause of CHD.

A low concentration of HDL in the blood is associated with high risk for CHD, possibly by virtue of reduced reverse cholesterol transport. Typically, low HDL is associated with high serum triglycerides, and manoeuvres which reduce serum triglycerides tend to increase HDL (e.g. Garg, 1998; Sørensen *et al.*, 1998; Rubins *et al.*, 1999). This is because of the interaction between VLDL and HDL particles in the circulation (Ng, 2004). Cholesterol is transported out of cells by ABCA1, accepted by nascent HDL particles and esterified by the enzyme lecithin–cholesterol acyltransferase (LCAT). Esterification of the cholesterol is critical to allow the HDL particle to continue to accept cholesterol from peripheral cells. The HDL particle obtains the fatty acids necessary to esterify cholesterol from VLDL particles via the action of cholesteryl-ester transfer protein (CETP) which transfers triglyceride from VLDL to HDL in exchange for transfer of cholesteryl ester from HDL to VLDL. In this way, cholesterol from peripheral cells is transferred to VLDL, which is metabolized to LDL and eventually taken up by the liver where the cholesterol can be converted into bile acids and excreted in the stool. However, the transfer of triglyceride and cholesteryl ester between VLDL and HDL, as mediated by CETP, is an equilibrium reaction. If the concentration of triglyceride in blood is high, then excess amounts of triglyceride are transferred to HDL which becomes abnormally enriched with triglyceride. Triglyceride-enriched HDL is more rapidly cleared from the circulation than normal HDL (Lamarche *et al.*, 1999), explaining why serum triglyceride concentrations are often inversely associated with serum HDL cholesterol concentrations.

High serum triglycerides are also associated with the presence of small, dense LDL particles which are more atherogenic than large, buoyant LDL particles (Austin, 2000). This phenomenon may be partly related to overproduction of apoB by the liver yielding more VLDL particles, and partly due to increased activity of hepatic lipase which can remove triglyceride from LDL particles, thus decreasing their size. It has been suggested that one of the most common causes of high blood triglycerides is impaired trapping of FFAs by adipocytes during the hydrolysis of chylomicrons by LPL (Sniderman *et al.*, 1998) resulting in an increased blood FFA concentration which stimulates VLDL and apoB production. Other factors which may increase blood FFA concentrations, such as a high saturated fat diet and visceral adiposity, also increase hepatic lipase activity (Deeb *et al.*, 2003).

#### 8.2.1.4 Changes in constituents of blood – non-lipid components

A number of non-lipid components have been associated with increased risk for CHD, including high blood glucose concentrations, even within the non-diabetic range (Coutinho *et al.*, 1999), high blood homocysteine concentrations (Hankey and Eikelboom, 1999) and high levels of inflammatory markers such as c-reactive protein (CRP). High levels of CRP may confer as much risk for CHD as the presence of the metabolic syndrome (Sattar *et al.*, 2003) or high LDL cholesterol (Ridker *et al.*, 2005). Platelet activity and factors regulating thrombosis and fibrinolysis, such as PAI-1 (Vaughan *et al.*, 1996), are also important modulators of cardiovascular disease risk.

### 8.2.2 Effect of GI on risk for cardiovascular disease

Three prospective and one case–control studies have examined the effect of dietary GI on risk of developing cardiovascular disease (Fig. 8.6). In the largest study for CHD (Liu *et al.*, 2000), high-GI diet was associated with about 30% increased risk for CHD. The other two studies showed no significant effect, but, with only 1/50th the number of subjects as in the study by Liu *et al.* (2000) had much less power to detect an effect. A high diet GI tended to be associated with an increased rate of progression of coronary atherosclerosis in postmenopausal women, but the effect was not significant ($P = 0.11$, Mozaffarian *et al.*, 2005). Diet GI had no effect on the risk for stroke in women (Oh *et al.*, 2005).

### 8.2.3 Effect of GI on cardiovascular disease risk factors

#### 8.2.3.1 *Epidemiological studies*

A number of prospective and cross-sectional studies have found consistently that high diet GI is associated with high serum triglycerides and/or low serum HDL cholesterol. In the Nurse's Health Study, the highest quintile of diet GI was associated with 18% higher serum triglycerides than the lowest quintile of diet GI (Liu *et al.*, 2001). Frost *et al.* (1999) studied 1420 British adults and showed that diet GI was significantly and negatively associated with serum HDL cholesterol in both men and women. Mehalski *et al.* (2003) studied over 9000 patients with existing CHD recruited to participate in a trial of the effect of pravastatin on CHD outcomes. HDL cholesterol measured during the baseline period, before being randomized to active or placebo treatment, was significantly and inversely related to diet GI. HDL cholesterol was also found to be inversely correlated with diet GI in a group of 11–25-year-old males and females ($P = 0.048$) (Slyper *et al.*, 2005).

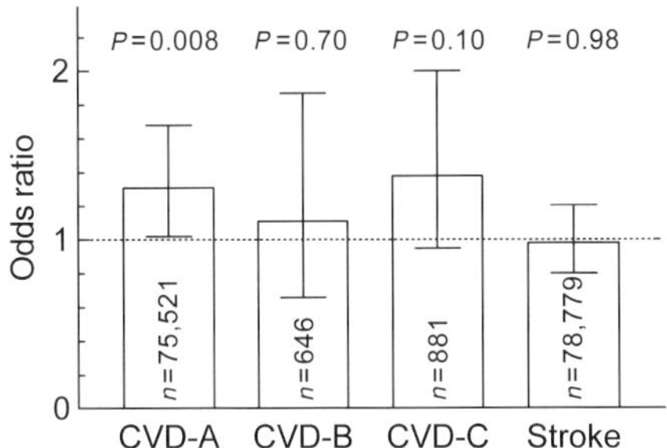


**Fig. 8.6.** Odds ratios (means ± 95% confidence intervals) for risk of developing cardiovascular disease associated with the highest tertile or quintile of diet GI, relative to the lowest tertile or quintile in four studies: CVD-A, US women (Liu *et al.*, 2000); CVD-B, Dutch elderly men (van Dam *et al.*, 2000); CVD-C, Italian men and women, case–control study in 433 cases and 448 controls (Tavani *et al.*, 2003); Stroke, US women (Oh *et al.*, 2005).

One prospective study (Liu *et al.*, 2002) showed that plasma CRP levels in 244 women in the Women's Health Study were directly related to dietary GI, going from 1.8 mg/l in the lowest quintile of diet GI to 2.8 mg/l in the highest ($P < 0.01$). Diet GI had no significant association with plasma adiponectin concentrations in 532 male participants in the Health Professionals Follow-up Study (Pischon *et al.*, 2005). There have been no epidemiological studies looking at the relationship between diet GI and factors influencing blood clotting.

#### 8.2.3.2 *Clinical trials*

Two meta-analyses have been conducted summarizing the effects of 16 (Opperman *et al.*, 2004) or 15 (Kelly *et al.*, 2004) clinical trials on major risk factors for cardiovascular disease (Table 8.2). Both analyses showed a significant effect of a low-GI diet in reducing total cholesterol and glycated haemoglobin, but no significant effects on LDL or HDL cholesterol, triglycerides, body weight or FPG or insulin. Kelly *et al.* (2004) concluded that there is weak evidence that low-GI diets reduce CHD risk, but acknowledged that many of the trials used were short-term studies of poor quality conducted on small sample sizes. Thus, there is a need for well-designed adequately powered studies to assess the effects of low-GI diets on risk for CHD.

Recently, Ebbeling *et al.* (2005) published the results of a pilot study designed to assess the effect of a low-GL diet on cardiovascular disease risk factors in obese young adults. Subjects aged 18–35 with a BMI > 27 kg/m$^2$ were randomized to receive a conventional weight reducing diet or

**Table 8.2.** Results from two meta-analyses of the effect of low-GI diets on cardiovascular risk factors.

| | Kelly *et al.* (2004) | | Opperman *et al.* (2004) | |
|---|---|---|---|---|
| Risk factor | Effect size[a] | *P* | Effect size[a] | 95% CI (*P*) |
| Total cholesterol (mmol/l) | −0.17 | 0.03 | −0.33 | <0.0001 |
| LDL cholesterol (mmol/l) | −0.07 | 0.5 | −0.15 | 0.06 |
| HDL cholesterol (mmol/l) | 0.04 | 0.4 | −0.04 | 0.20 |
| Triglycerides (mmol/l) | −0.02 | 0.7 | 0.04 | 0.57 |
| Glycated haemoglobin (%) | −0.45 | 0.02 | −0.27 | 0.01 |
| Body weight (kg) | 0.14 | 0.7 | – | – |
| Fasting glucose (mmol/l) | 0.18 | 0.13 | – | – |
| Fasting insulin (pmol/l) | 9.0 | 0.3 | – | – |

[a]A negative value indicates that the mean on low GI was less than that on high GI.

an experimental diet with a low GL for 1 year with 12 subjects on the conventional diet and 11 on the experimental diet completing the trial. On the conventional diet subjects reduced energy intake with an increase in % energy from carbohydrate and reduction in % energy as fat (Table 8.3). On the experimental diet subjects reduced energy intake with a moderate reduction in GI and % energy from carbohydrate, and moderate increases in % energy from fat and protein (Table 8.3). Weight loss was comparable in both diet groups. Although changes in total, LDL and HDL cholesterol did not differ between groups, fasting triglycerides and PAI-1 concentrations fell significantly more in subjects on the experimental than the conventional diet (Fig. 8.7). While it is not possible to ascribe these beneficial effects to a change in any single dietary component, a reduced diet GI was an important component of the intervention.

Two clinical trials showed that a low-GI diet substantially reduced concentrations of serum PAI-1 in subjects with diabetes (Järvi *et al.*, 1999; Rizkalla *et al.*, 2004). There have been no clinical trials looking at the effect of a low-GI diet on inflammatory markers.

## 8.3 Cancer

It has been known since at least 1919 that patients with cancer have abnormal glucose tolerance (Rohdenburg *et al.*, 1919; Glicksman and Rawson, 1956; Marks and Bishop, 1957; Weisenfeld *et al.*, 1962) due to decreased insulin sensitivity (Bishop and Marks, 1959; Copeland, G.P., Leinster, S.J., Davis, J.C. and Hipkin, L.J. (1987) Insulin resistance in patients with colorectal cancer. *British Journal of Surgery* 74, 1031-1035. Although this could be a result of the disease process, recent concepts suggest that insulin resistance contributes to the cause of carcinogenesis.

Diet has been implicated in origin of many cancers, particularly those of the colon, breast and prostate. We (Bruce *et al.*, 2000) recently noted that, with respect to colon cancer it is generally held that a sedentary lifestyle and a diet high in

**Table 8.3.** Composition of conventional and low glycaemic load diets consumed by young adults for 1 year.[a]

| Variable | Experimental diet ($n = 11$) | | Conventional diet | | Group × time |
|---|---|---|---|---|---|
| ($n = 12$) | Baseline | 12 months | Baseline | 12 months | interaction (*P*) |
| Energy (kcal) | 1860 | 1494 | 1802 | 1472 | 0.76 |
| Glycaemic index | 56.2 | 46.3 | 56.6 | 52.9 | 0.004 |
| Carbohydrate (% en) | 52.7 | 45.5 | 54.8 | 58.3 | <0.001 |
| Total fat (% en) | 32.6 | 35.4 | 30.0 | 24.3 | 0.006 |
| Saturated fat (% en) | 11.3 | 10.6 | 10.7 | 7.6 | 0.18 |
| Protein (% en) | 15.7 | 20.5 | 16.1 | 18.1 | 0.07 |

[a]Data from Ebbeling *et al.* (2005).

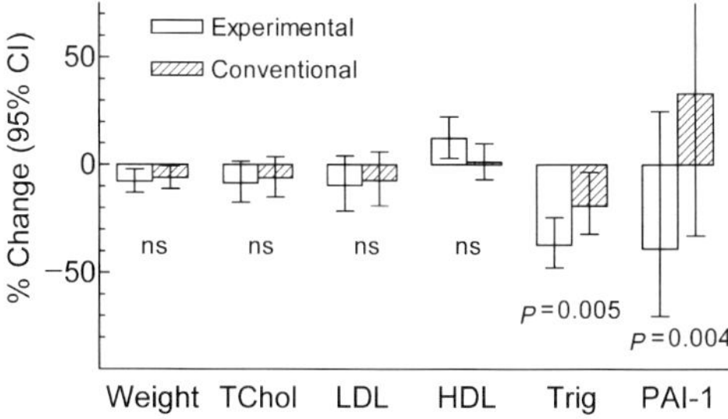


**Fig. 8.7.** Changes (% of baseline value with 95% confidence intervals) in body weight and fasting serum total (TChol), low-density lipoprotein (LDL) and high-density lipoprotein (HDL) cholesterol, triglycerides (Trig) and plasminogen activator inhibitor 1 (PAI-1) concentrations in young adults randomized to receive conventional or experimental (low glycaemic load) diets for 1 year. The composition of the diets is shown in Table 8.3. Data from Ebbeling *et al.* (2005).

meat and fat and low in grain, fruit, vegetables and dietary fibre are factors that increase risk. Traditionally these factors have been thought to act by luminal mechanisms, i.e. by directly interacting with colon cells. Fat and meat are thought to increase risk by means of increased levels of toxic bile acids and increased exposure to carcinogenic heterocyclic amines formed when meat is cooked. The protective effects of grain, fruit and vegetables have been attributed to their content of antioxidants or inhibitory compounds such as allyl sulphides. The protective effects of fibre have been attributed increased faecal bulk diluting the concentrations of toxic compounds in the faecal stream, and to the beneficial effects of the SCFA products of fibre fermentation. However, McKeown-Essen (1994) and Giovannucci (1995) noted that the risk factors for colon cancer were similar to those for insulin resistance. We (Bruce *et al.*, 2000) proposed a link between insulin resistance and cancer based on the systemic effects of insulin resistance which may affect risk for cancer in many parts of the body. Evidence suggests that diets high in energy, saturated fat and high-GI carbohydrates and low in fibre and *n*-3 fatty acids can lead to insulin resistance which is associated with hyperinsulinaemia, hyperglycaemia and hypertriglyceridaemia. These factors may promote cancer because high levels of insulin, triglycerides and FFAs could lead to increased growth of colon cancer precursor lesions.

Since then, a good number of case–control and prospective studies have emerged looking at the effect of a high diet GI on the risk of developing cancer in various different cites (Fig. 8.8). Most of the studies (7 of 11) show that a high-GI diet is associated with a statistically significant increase in risk of developing cancer in colon and rectum, the upper aero-digestive tract (mouth, pharynx, larynx and oesophagus), breast, prostate, ovary and endometrium (Augustin *et al.*, 2001, 2003a,b, 2004a,c; Franceschi *et al.*, 2001; Silvera *et al.*, 2005). Diet GI had no effect on risk of gastric cancer (Augustin *et al.*, 2004b) or pancreatic cancer (Michaud *et al.*, 2002). Of the two studies on colorectal cancer, one showed no statistically significant effect of diet GI (Higginbotham *et al.*, 2004), although the relative risk, 1.7 ($P = 0.12$), was the same as in the other study in which the effect was statistically significant ($P < 0.001$, Franceschi *et al.*, 2001). One study on breast cancer showed a

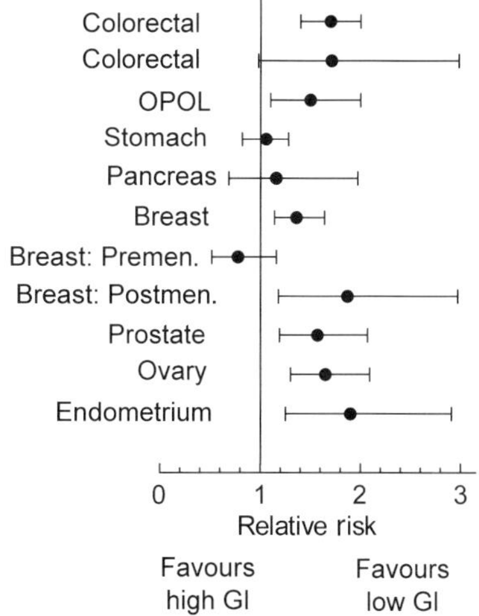


**Fig. 8.8.** Relative risk of developing various types of cancer for subjects with a diet GI in the highest quintile vs those in the lowest quintile of diet GI. References for studies, top to bottom: Colorectal, Franceschi *et al.* (2001)*; Higginbotham *et al.* (2004)**; OPOL (oral, pharyngeal, oesophagus and larynx), Augustin *et al.* (2004a)*; Stomach, Augustin *et al.* (2004a)*; Pancreas, Michaud *et al.* (2002)**; Breast (men. = menopausal), Augustin *et al.* (2001)*, Silvera *et al.* (2005a)**; Prostate, Augustin *et al.* (2004b)*; Ovary, Augustin *et al.* (2003a)*; Endometrium, Augustin *et al.* (2003b)*. * = case–control studies; ** = prospective studies.

statistically significant ($P = 0.01$) interaction between diet GI and menopausal status such that a high diet GI increased risk only in postmenopausal women (Silvera *et al.*, 2005a).

## 8.4 Mechanisms of Action of Low-GI Foods

The major diseases discussed in this chapter, diabetes, cardiovascular disease and cancer, share common aetiological factors. The following will briefly review some of the physiological mechanisms by which changing the GI of dietary carbohydrate may influence the risk of developing chronic diseases or may be useful in the treatment of these and other conditions.

### 8.4.1 Reduced glucose toxicity

Glucose toxicity refers to damage caused to tissues by high concentrations of glucose *per se* which may contribute, at least in part, to the pathogenesis of insulin resistance, β-cell failure, diabetes complications, endothelial dysfunction and atherosclerosis. Several mechanisms have been proposed by which glucose toxicity occurs, including increased glucose flux through the polyol and glucosamine pathways, increased non-enzymatic glycation products and glycosylation of certain proteins, activation of diacylglycerol and protein kinase C, reduced production of nitric oxide and increased oxidative and carbonyl stress (Ceriello, 1998; Baynes and Thorpe, 1999; Gerich, 2003). It has been proposed that some of these effects are caused not only by a high concentration of blood glucose but also by a high magnitude of glucose fluctuations (Heine *et al.*, 2004). For example, more apoptosis was seen in umbilical vein cells exposed to intermittent high glucose concentrations than in cells exposed to a constant high glucose concentration (Risso *et al.*, 2001). In addition, reducing the postprandial rises in blood glucose by treating subjects with type 1 diabetes with pramlintide (a synthetic analogue of human amylin) reduced measures of postprandial oxidative stress (Ceriello *et al.*, 2005).

Additional evidence that reducing postprandial glucose fluctuations has clinical relevance for diabetes and CHD in humans comes from studies showing that postprandial spikes in glucose may be more closely correlated with atherosclerosis than fasting glucose or HbA1c (Temelkova-Kurtschiev *et al.*, 2000; DECODE Study Group, 2001). We showed that acarbose, a drug which reduces postprandial glucose excursions by reducing the rate of glucose absorption, reduced postpandial glucose and insulin concentrations, increased insulin sensitivity in subjects with IGT (Chiasson *et al.*, 1996), reduced the rate of conversion of IGT to diabetes (Chiasson *et al.*, 2002) and reduced the incidence of hypertension and cardiovascular events in subjects with IGT (Chiasson *et al.*, 2003; Zeymer *et al.*, 2004).

### 8.4.2 Reduced plasma insulin concentration

The role of high plasma insulin, *per se*, in the pathogenesis of cardiovascular disease, diabetes and obesity is controversial and is discussed in more detail in Chapters 3 and 7.

### 8.4.3 Acute effects on gut hormone secretion

The gastrointestinal tract is the source of a large number of hormones. Some of these, such as ghrelin (Wren *et al.*, 2001), peptide YY (PYY) (Batterham *et al.*, 2003a), pancreatic polypeptide (Batterham *et al.*, 2003b), oxyntomodulin (Cohen *et al.*, 2003) and cholecystokinin (CCK) (Reidelberger, 1994) are mostly known for their effects in regulating gut function and appetite. However, GIP (Nauck *et al.*, 2004) and GLP-1 (Drucker, 1998) are known to have important effects on insulin sensitivity and secretion and may be implicated in the pathogenesis of diabetes. Since most of the gut hormones are secreted in response to the presence of nutrients in the gastrointestinal tract, it is logical to suppose that factors which influence the digestion and absorption of foods may influence the secretion of gut hormones acutely. Indeed, there is evidence that slowly absorbed carbohydrates induce lower acute responses of GIP and GLP-1 (Jenkins *et al.*, 1982b, 1990; Juntunen *et al.*, 2002). Altering the rate of glucose absorption does not appear to affect pancreatic polypeptide responses (Jenkins *et al.*, 1990), but the addition of viscous fibre in the form of beans (Bourdon *et al.*, 2001) or barley (Bourdon *et al.*, 1999) increased postprandial CCK responses. However, perhaps of more importance than the acute effects of low-GI foods on gut hormone secretion are potential chronic effects which may be mediated by increased colonic fermentation.

### 8.4.4 Increased colonic fermentation

Carbohydrate which escapes digestion in the small intestine enters the colon where it is fermented by colonic bacteria with the production of gases such as hydrogen and methane, and the SCFA acetate, propionate and butyrate (Cummings and MacFarlane, 1991). Carbohydrate substrates for colonic bacteria include dietary fibre, undigestible oligosaccharides and RS. About 3–5% of the starch in high-GI starchy foods such as cooked potatoes and white bread escapes digestion in the small intestine. However, since the starch in low-GI starchy foods is slowly digested, more starch from low-GI foods 'leaks' out into the colon than does starch from high-GI foods. The amount of starch in various foods escaping digestion in the small intestine and the degree to which this accounts for the reduction in glycaemic responses will be discussed in more detail in Chapter 9. The point to be made here is that low-GI starchy foods are associated with an increased amount of carbohydrate escaping digestion in the small intestine (Wolever *et al.*, 1986b; Jenkins *et al.*, 1987d) and hence an increase in colonic fermentation (Jenkins *et al.*, 1987a; Wolever *et al.*, 1992b). This, in turn, has a number of local and systemic effects which could contribute to the mechanism for the putatively beneficial effects of low-GI foods in diabetes, cardiovascular disease and cancer.

#### *8.4.4.1 Effects of fermentation on colonic luminal events*

Carbohydrates entering the colon are the major energy sources for colonic bacteria; hence, if more carbohydrate is provided to colonic bacteria, their growth is stimulated. Specific types of carbohydrates may stimulate the growth of specific types of bacteria, for example, fructo-oligosaccharides stimulate the growth of bifidobacteria (van Loo *et al.*, 1999; Bouhnik *et al.*, 2004). When colonic bacterial growth is stimulated by the provision of undigestible carbohydrate as an energy source, the bacteria use blood urea, which diffuses freely into the colonic lumen, for protein synthesis, thus trapping urea nitrogen in the faeces (Birkett *et al.*, 1996) and reducing urinary urea excretion. We have demonstrated both in subjects with and without diabetes that urinary urea excretion is reduced on a low-GI compared to a high-GI diet (Jenkins *et al.*, 1987a; Wolever *et al.*, 1992b).

The SCFA produced during colonic fermentation are weak acids, and hence, acidify the colonic luminal contents. An early hypothesis relating to the protective effect of dietary fibre on colon cancer risk was that a low colonic pH would reduce the activity of 7-dehydoxylase and hence reduce the formation of toxic metabolites of bile acids (Hill and Fernandez, 1986; Bartram *et al.*, 1991). The same argument could be advanced for low-GI foods. However, current thinking about the protective role of SCFA for colon cancer is focused on the ability of butyrate to inhibit the proliferation and promote the differentiation of tumour cells (Young and Gibson, 1995). Since starch fermentation produces more butyrate than the fermentation of other substrates (Cummings and MacFarlane, 1991), low-GI foods may particularly stimulate butyrate production in the colon. There is no evidence that this occurs in humans but we were able to show that acarbose increased serum butyrate concentrations in subjects with IGT (Wolever and Chiasson, 2000).

Another mechanism by which dietary fibre is thought to reduce risk for colon cancer is by bulking the stool and reducing transit time, hence reducing the concentration of toxic components in the lumen and the amount of time the epithelium is exposed to them (Hill and Fernandez, 1986). A similar mechanism could be proposed for low-GI foods by virtue of the increase in bacterial cell mass stimulated by increased colonic fermentation (Scheppach *et al.*, 1988a).

#### *8.4.4.2 Effect of fermentation on nutrient absorption from the colon*

Colonic fermentation provides a mechanism for salvaging energy and other nutrients which are not absorbed in the small intestine. The SCFA produced during colonic fermentation are absorbed from the colon (Vogt and Wolever, 2003) and provide energy to the host. It has been estimated that about 3–5% of energy requirements are provided by colonic SCFA on a normal low-fibre, western diet, and that this could increase to 10% or more with increased intakes of slowly digested starch and dietary fibre (McNeil, 1984; McBurney *et al.*, 1988; Royall *et al.*, 1990). The energy value of undigestible carbohydrates depends on the extent to which they are fermented and the products of fermentation. Generally speaking, completely fermentable carbohydrates provide about 2 kcal/g. For Western diets, in which about 70% of the unavailable carbohydrates are fermented, it has been estimated that every gram of unavailable carbohydrate provides about 1.7 kcal to the host as SCFA with about 0.14 kcal being lost as hydrogen and methane gases, 0.14 kcal lost as heat, and 2.1 kcal lost in the faeces, 0.86 kcal in bacterial matter and 1.24 kcal as unfermented carbohydrate (Livesey and Elia, 1995). If low-GI starchy foods are consumed, perhaps 5–10% more starch escapes digestion in the small intestine than the high-GI starchy foods they replace. Assuming 100 g/day starch intake from low-GI foods, the excess amount of starch entering the colon and providing only 2 kcal/g instead of 4 kcal/g would be about 5–10 g/day; this results in an energy 'deficit' of 10–20 kcal/day, which, as mentioned in Chapter 7, over a year adds up to the energy contained in 1 pound of fat, the rate at which weight tends to be gained by adults in Western societies (Rosengren *et al.*, 1999; Yarnell *et al.*, 2000; Strandberg *et al.*, 2003).

The absorption of SCFA from the colon not only provides energy to the host but also stimulates the absorption of minerals such as calcium from the colon (Trinidad *et al.*, 1996, 1999). Thus, feeding unabsorbed carbohydrates such as lactulose increases overall calcium absorption in postmenopausal women (Van den Heuvel *et al.*, 1999). SCFA may also stimulate the absorption of other minerals such as potassium, magnesium (Demigné and Rémésy, 1985), copper, zinc and selenium (Ducros *et al.*, 2005). Increased calcium absorption is of obvious potential relevance for the maintenance of bone mass and the prevention of osteoporosis. However, calcium, potassium and/or magnesium have also been implicated in the regulation of energy metabolism (Zemel, 2004) and blood pressure (Appel *et al.*, 1997; Logan, 2000) and in the risk for cardiovascular disease (Iso *et al.*, 1999; Al-Delaimy *et al.*, 2004; Lopez-Ridaura *et al.*, 2004). Thus, increased mineral absorption from the colon secondary to the increased colonic fermentation associated with a low-GI diet provides another possible mechanism by which low-GI foods may influence risk for obesity, diabetes and cardiovascular disease.

Another interesting effect of colonic fermentation is that it may increase folate availability to the human host. Adequate folate availability is considered necessary to help reduce risk of cardiovascular disease by promoting a normal plasma homocysteine concentration (Boushey *et al.*, 1995; Malinow *et al.*, 1998; Robinson *et al.*, 1998; Hankey and Eidelboom, 1999). Serum folate concentrations have been found to be positively related to NSP intake in females (Houghton *et al.*, 1997). Thus, it was suggested that NSP promotes the growth of colonic bacteria which can synthesize folate (Kim *et al.*, 2004), which in turn, is absorbed from the large intestine and utilized by the host to help maintain folate status. We obtained some evidence that starch malabsorption increases folate status in humans by showing that, in patients with type 2 diabetes, miglitol, an α-glucosidase inhibitor, prevented the fall in serum folate which occurred upon treatment with metformin (Wolever *et al.*, 2000).

#### *8.4.4.3 Systemic effects of colonic fermentation*

Increased colonic fermentation could affect systemic metabolism via the effects of the SCFA absorbed, or by virtue of immune responses elicited by altered interactions between colonic bacteria and colonic endothelial cells.

Butyrate is believed to be taken up and metabolized by colonic epithelial cells with only very low levels appearing in peripheral blood (Scheppach *et al.*, 1991). Nevertheless, butyrate can be detected in peripheral blood and we have shown that serum butyrate concentrations increase in subjects with IGT after treatment with acarbose (Wolever and Chiasson, 2000) and in subjects with type 2 diabetes after 6-month consumption of a high-fibre breakfast cereal (Wolever *et al.*, 2002b). Thus, low-GI foods may affect colonic butyrate production.

Propionate appears in portal blood in substantial amounts (Scheppach *et al.*, 1991), but is believed to be taken up primarily by liver, so that very little appears in peripheral blood (Scheppach *et al.*, 1988b). Thus, propionate could influence metabolism in the liver. We have shown that rectally infused propionate inhibits the incorporation of rectally infused acetate into blood lipids (Wolever *et al.*, 1995c) and that rectally infused propionate, which is a gluconeogenic substrate, raises blood glucose (Wolever *et al.*, 1991b). Specific unabsorbed carbohydrates, such as rhamnose, may increase blood propionate levels (Vogt *et al.*, 2004a,b), but increased intake of wheat bran and psyllium (Wolever *et al.*, 2002b) and malabsorbed starch (Wolever and Chiasson, 2000) do not appear to do so. Thus, low-GI foods probably do not affect colonic propionate production.

Acetate is the only SCFA to reach peripheral blood in reasonable amounts. Rectal infusion of acetate reduces plasma FFAs and raises serum cholesterol and triglyceride concentrations (Wolever *et al.*, 1991b). Acetate does not appear to have any direct effects on insulin secretion (Wolever *et al.*, 1991b) or glucose metabolism (Scheppach *et al.*, 1988c) in humans. However, the reduction in FFA provides a mechanism whereby colonic acetate could have an indirect effect on glucose metabolism. High serum FFA reduces peripheral glucose uptake, increases hepatic glucose output (Ferrannini *et al.*, 1983; Boden *et al.*, 1994) and in the long term, reduces insulin secretion (Zhou and Grill, 1994; Carpentier *et al.*, 1999). It has been suggested that consuming a meal rich in fermentable carbohydrates in the evening improves glucose tolerance the following morning (Wolever *et al.*, 1988a) via a reduction in hepatic glucose output (Thorburn *et al.*, 1993) or increase in insulin sensitivity (Robertson *et al.*, 2003) mediated by reduced FFA as a result of increased colonic fermentation. However, consumption of the unavailable sugars lactulose and rhamnose had no effect on serum FFA concentrations throughout the day (Vogt *et al.*, 2004b).

The effect of colonic fermentation on blood lipids is controversial. In our recent studies, we have found that long-term (4–6 months) consumption of low-GI foods (Wolever and Mehling, 2003) or a high fibre intake tended to increase serum triglycerides, an effect which was related to the change in serum acetate (Wolever *et al.*, 2002b). However, these results are not consistent with studies in which the diet is supplemented with unavailable oligosaccharides. Animal studies show that unavailable oligosaccharides reduce serum triglycerides (Delzenne *et al.*, 2002), whereas, the results of nine human studies reviewed recently are inconsistent (Williams and Jackson, 2002) with three findings no effects on serum cholesterol and triglycerides, three showing significant reductions in triglycerides and four showing modest reductions in cholesterol.

Colonic fermentation may also influence systemic metabolism via the effects of SCFA on the entero-insulin axis. Animal studies suggest that a high-fibre diet upregulates GLP-1 secretion, possibly via the SCFA products of the fermentation of fibre in the colon (Reimer and McBurney, 1996). It has also been shown that human subjects who have had their colons removed, but with minimal small bowel resection have lower GLP-1 and higher postprandial plasma glucose and glucagon concentrations during a 9-h metabolic profile than normal subjects (Robertson *et al.*, 1999). This could be because the colon itself secretes GLP-1, but could also be explained by a lack of SCFA in the subjects without a colon. Whether stimulating SCFA production results in increased GLP-1 secretion in humans is not known. However, studies in animals show that GLP-1 increases pancreatic β-cell mass (Perfetti *et al.*, 2000; Trumper *et al.*, 2001) and delays the onset of diabetes in db/db mice, an animal model which spontaneously develops diabetes (Wang and Brubaker, 2002). This is consistent with the finding that a low-GI diet increased β-cell function and increased postprandial insulin concentrations significantly in normal subjects (Juntunen *et al.*, 2003) and subjects with IGT (Wolever and Mehling, 2002, 2003) compared to a high-GI diet.

Finally, events in the colon that can be modulated by colonic fermentation are known to influence inflammation and immunity, which in turn, can have local and systemic effects (Schley and Field, 2002). One mechanism by which colonic fermentation may influence inflammation is by altering the bacterial species in the colon. For example, oral administration of a mixture of various strains of lactobacilli, bifidobacteria and streptococci reduced inflammation in ileal pouch–anal anastomoses in subjects with previous ulcerative colitis (Gionchetti *et al.*, 2000). This may occur because non-pathogenic strains of bacteria can reduce the synthesis of inflammatory cytokines by gut epithelial cells by blocking NF-κB activation (Xavier and Podolsky, 2000). SCFA may also have direct effects on inflammatory processes; for example, it has been shown that physiological concentrations of butyrate modulated NF-κB activity in human colonic cells (Inan *et al.*, 2000). However, whether these effects influence the pathogenesis of atherosclerosis, diabetes or cancer is not known.

## 8.5 Conclusions

There is evidence that low-GI dietary carbohydrates reduce risk for developing diabetes, cardiovascular disease and cancer and may be useful in their treatment. The quality of the evidence varies; there is moderately strong evidence from clinical trials showing that low-GI diets improve blood glucose control in diabetes, there is only weak evidence from clinical trials that low-GI diets improve traditional risk factors for cardiovascular disease, and there is only epidemiological evidence that low-GI diets reduce the risk for cancer. These conditions share multiple aetiologies, and biologically plausible mechanisms exist whereby altering the GI of dietary carbohydrates can influence many of these processes. There is some evidence that the nature of dietary carbohydrates may be relevant in the prevention or treatment of other diseases, such as osteoporosis, renal failure and liver disease, and there may be other conditions for which GI is relevant.

## Notes

### GI and risk for type 2 diabetes

Two recent papers explored the cross-sectional relationships between GI, GL and carbohydrate intake and measures of glucose metabolism; one suggested a positive association between GI and risk for diabetes (Sahyoun *et al.*, 2005), while the other suggested there was no effect (Lau *et al.*, 2005). However, conclusions of the latter study are not supported by any data showing the GI of the diets of the subjects in the study.

### GI and insulin economy

A recent study showed that use of low GI, high fibre bread for 3 weeks reduced the plasma insulin response to intravenous glucose, with no change in glucose, in women with impaired glucose tolerance (Ostman et al., 2005).

### GI and cancer

Three recent studies found no significant association between diet GI and risk of breast (Giles *et al.*, 2005; Lajous *et al.*, 2005) or pancreatic cancer (Silvera *et al.*, 2005b).

### GI and gall stone disease

Recent papers show that, compared with the lowest quintile, the highest quintile of dietary GI is associated with 18% ($P = 0.04$) increased risk of symptomatic gall stones in men (Tsai *et al.*, 2005a) and 32% ($P < 0.0001$) increased risk for cholecystectomy in women (Tsai *et al.*, 2005b).

# 9
# Glycaemic Index vs Glycaemic Load

The concept of the GL originated in 1997 in papers from Harvard University showing that high GL was associated with an increased risk of diabetes (Salmerón *et al.*, 1997a,b). Subsequently other papers appeared from this group that linked high GL with increased risk of cardiovascular disease (Liu *et al.*, 2000) or cardiovascular risk factors (Liu *et al.*, 2001, 2002) and colorectal cancer (Higginbotham *et al.*, 2004). GL was defined as food GI times the amount of carbohydrate (g) divided by 100, i.e.:

$$GL = g \times GI/100$$

The concept has been enthusiastically accepted by some (Bell and Sears, 2003) and extended to include benefits for obesity (Ebbeling *et al.*, 2003). However, before accepting the GL concept wholeheartedly, it should be evaluated critically. In this chapter, I will review the definition of GL and whether it is useful for predicting short-term glycaemic responses and longer-term outcomes such as glycaemic control, insulin sensitivity, insulin secretion, plasma FFAs and blood lipids. We will see that GL is being calculated differently by different authors. I will show that GL is not proportional to acute glycaemic responses. Most importantly, since GL is the product of GI and grams of carbohydrate, advice to reduce diet GL would only be valid if reducing diet GI had the same short- and long-term metabolic effects as reducing the amount of available carbohydrate in the diet. However, evidence suggests that this is not so.

## 9.1 Definition of GL

The GL was originally defined as the sum, for all foods in the diet, of the products of the carbohydrate content per serving of each food in the diet times the average number of servings of that food per day times its GI. The resulting GL variable was adjusted for total energy using the residuals method (Salmerón *et al.*, 1997b). On the other hand, when being applied to diets in intervention studies, the resulting GL variable is sometimes adjusted for energy using the residuals method (Wolever and Mehling, 2002) and sometimes by dividing by 1000 kcal (Ebbeling *et al.*, 2003). When applied to individual foods, the GL is defined as GI times grams of carbohydrate divided by 100 (Foster-Powell *et al.*, 2002; Bell and Sears, 2003; Brand-Miller *et al.*, 2003a). If, for a single meal, GL is GI times grams of carbohydrate (not adjusted for energy), then the GL for the day's diet would be the sum of the GL for each meal (not adjusted for energy). However, in epidemiological studies, the GL values for the day are adjusted for energy. Which method is correct, and does it matter?

This situation is analogous to the well-known problem of how to adjust macronutrient intakes for energy. It is clear that different methods of adjusting macronutrient intakes for energy can yield different interpretations from the same data set (Beaton *et al.*, 1997; Willett *et al.*, 1997). The same holds true for GL, and is illustrated for GL in Fig. 9.1 which shows mean values for diet GL from a study we performed in subjects with IGT

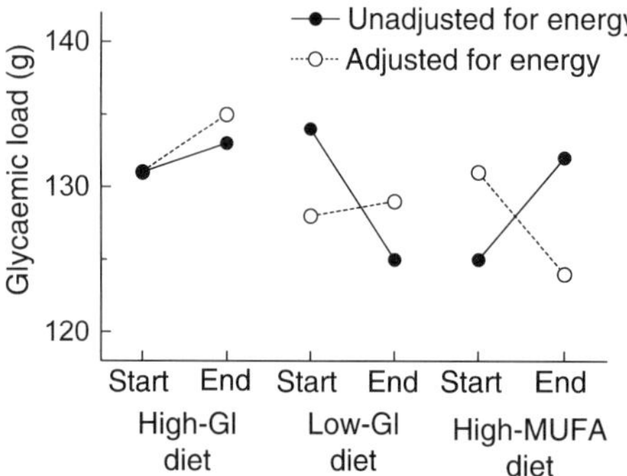


**Fig. 9.1.** Glycaemic load (GL) of diets of subjects in a clinical trial on three different diets. High GI = high-GI, high-carbohydrate; Low GI = low-GI, high-carbohydrate; High MUFA = low-carbohydrate, high monounsaturated fatty acid (MUFA). The graph shows the difference between adjusting GL values for energy or not. Adjustment was done by the method of residuals. Data from Wolever and Mehling (2002).

(Wolever and Mehling, 2002). We reported GL values adjusted for energy, because that is how GL was defined by Salmerón *et al.* (1997b). However, doing so changed the direction of change of GL on both the low-GI and low-carbohydrate, high-MUFA diets. On the low-GI diet, recorded carbohydrate intake in grams remained constant but GI fell, resulting in a reduction in unadjusted GL; however, recorded energy intake tended to fall on the low-GI diet, which, after adjustment, offset the reduction in GL. On the other hand, on the MUFA diet, recorded carbohydrate intake in grams tended to increase with no change in GI, leading to an increase in unadjusted GL; however, recorded energy intake increased significantly, which resulted in a reduction in diet GL after adjustment for energy.

Most of the evidence about GL comes from epidemiological prospective studies in which GL values are adjusted for energy. As is apparent from the example above, if GL was not adjusted for energy intake, then the results of the epidemiological studies could be completely different. Thus, if the effects expected from reducing GL suggested by the epidemiological studies are to be realized, GL as practically applied must be calculated in the same way as was done in those epidemiological studies, i.e. adjusted for energy intake. In practice, however, GL values of foods are calculated without adjusting for energy, and these values are naturally summed to give GL values for meals. If we consider individual foods, adjusting for energy leads to a curious result. The GL of one slice of bread containing 20 g carbohydrate and GI of 71 is $20 \times 71/100 = 14.2$. Therefore, the GL of two slices of bread is $40 \times 71/100 = 28.4$. But, since two slices of bread contains twice as much energy as one slice, adjusting for energy results in one slice of bread having the same GL as two slices! Clearly, this is not consistent either with current practice (Brand-Miller *et al.*, 2003a; Liu *et al.*, 2003a,b) or with the intention of the GL concept! But it leaves me wondering exactly what the GL concept means.

These considerations suggest that translation of the GL concept from epidemiological studies to real diets is not straightforward. GL as currently used in practice by multiplying a food GI times its carbohydrate content is not the same quantity as the GL defined in the epidemiological studies in which the values were adjusted for energy intake.

## 9.2 Glycaemic Load and Acute Glycaemic Responses

The purpose of the paper in which the term GL was coined (Salmerón *et al.*, 1997b) was to test '... the hypothesis that diets leading to a high insulin demand would influence the risk of NIDDM....' In the methods section of that paper, GL was defined as '... an indicator of a glucose response or insulin demand induced by the total carbohydrate intake', while in the discussion, it was suggested that GL '... may be interpreted as a measure of dietary insulin demand' (Salmerón *et al.*, 1997b). Curiously, there was no attempt to validate whether the GL was actually an indicator of blood glucose or insulin responses (the latter presumably considered to be analogous to 'insulin demand'). However, this can be done quite simply by looking at the relationship between GL and the observed blood glucose and insulin responses elicited by a range of amounts of different sources of carbohydrate. Data from two of our studies are ideal for this purpose. We measured glucose and insulin responses of normal subjects after consuming 0 to 100 g carbohydrate from barley, spaghetti, bread or instant potato (Wolever and Bolognesi, 1996a) or bread, glucose, sucrose and fructose (Lee and Wolever, 1998). When the GL of the test meals was calculated and plotted against the mean glycaemic responses, it is apparent not only that the data from both studies appear to fall along a single curve, but also that the shape of that curve is not linear (Fig. 9.2). The figure shows the results of three regression models: linear (dotted line, $r = 0.946$, $P < 0.0001$), second order polynomial of the form $y = ax + bx^2 + c$ (dashed line, $r = 0.958$) and exponential association of the form $y = a \times (1-e^{-bx})$ (solid line, $r = 0.959$). Elsewhere in this book and in the literature, we have used the exponential model to describe glycaemic dose–response data because it can be extrapolated beyond the data more reliably than the polynomial model. Unfortunately, it is not easy to compare statistically the goodness of fit of an exponential model with that of a linear model. Thus, the polynomial model is included here because the goodness of fit of the model to the data can be compared with that of a linear model. The result of that analysis showed that the polynomial model fits the data statistically significantly better than a linear model, ($F_{(1,23)} = 6.59$, $P = 0.017$). Thus, GL is not proportional to the glucose responses elicited by different types and amounts of carbohydrate foods, at least when glycaemic response is expressed as IAUC and measured over 2 h. The polynomial model is very similar to the exponential model (Fig. 9.2), but the fit of the exponential model to the data is somewhat better; thus, I believe it as the best relatively simple model to use to describe glucose dose–response data.

By contrast, the mean AUC values for plasma insulin were linearly related to GL for these test meals (Fig. 9.2), which is consistent with the notion of Salmerón *et al.* (1997b) that GL is a reflection of insulin demand. However, it is of interest that, despite the fact that the glucose responses of the two studies fit almost exactly along the same non-linear regression line, the slopes of the regression lines for insulin responses differed significantly for the starchy foods vs the sugars ($P = 0.012$). It seems unlikely and can be explained by the fact that starchy foods contain protein and fat which stimulate more insulin for a given glycaemic response because different doses of white bread were included in the sugars study (Lee and Wolever, 1998). The open circles in Fig. 9.2 represent glucose and insulin responses of different doses of glucose, sucrose, fructose and white bread but all the points, including those for bread, fit very closely along the same regression line. Thus, it seems more likely that the difference in regression slopes for the starchy foods vs the sugars reflects heterogeneity of pancreatic β-cell function in the different groups of

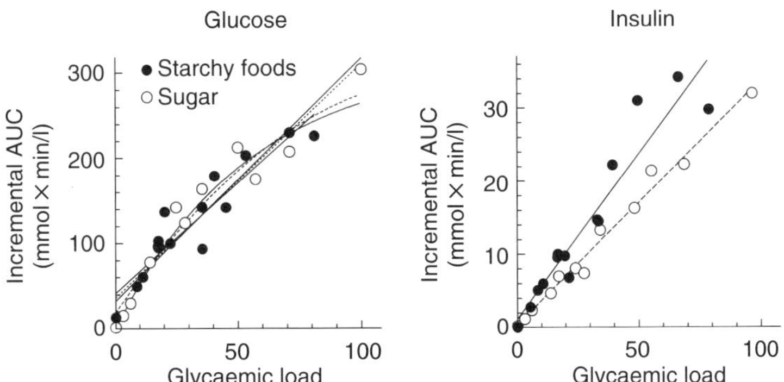


**Fig. 9.2.** Relationship between glycaemic load and plasma glucose (left) and insulin (right) responses in normal subjects. Closed circles represent different doses of starchy foods (Wolever and Bolognesi, 1996a). Open circles represent different doses of sugars and white bread (Lee and Wolever, 1998). Lines of graphs represent regression models. On the glucose graph, dotted line represents linear model; dashed line represents second-order polynomial model; solid line represents exponential model; the goodness of fit for the polynomial model is significantly better than that for the linear model ($P = 0.017$, see text for more details). On the insulin graph, solid line represents linear regression for starchy foods and dashed line represents linear regression for the sugars and white bread; the slopes of the two regression lines differ significantly ($P = 0.012$).

subjects that participated in the different studies. Thus, if the concept of 'insulin demand' is interpreted as insulin response, the notion would only hold for comparing relative insulin responses within a single individual of group of individuals; GL would not reflect insulin responses in different individuals.

The GL of a food is not proportional to the glycaemic response it elicits (Fig. 9.2); in this context, it is of interest to note that although GL is determined both by the GI and the grams of carbohydrate consumed, the relationship between GI and AUC differs from that between grams of carbohydrate and AUC. Figure 9.3 shows the mean IAUC for seven foods (fructose, sucrose, glucose, barley, spaghetti, bread and instant potato) plotted against their GI values at three levels of carbohydrate intake (Wolever and Bolognesi,1996a; Lee and Wolever, 1998). The linear correlations (solid lines) not only virtually superimpose upon the non-linear regression lines (dashed) for all three doses but also the departure from linearity is not statistically significant in any case. Thus, AUC is linearly related to GI at any level of carbohydrate intake. On the other hand, the increase in IAUC is not proportional to the amount of carbohydrate consumed, but rather increases in a curvilinear fashion (Figs 4.1, 4.2 and 9.4). Thus, increases in GL due to changes in GI would be expected to be linearly related to AUC, but changes in GL due to differences in carbohydrate intake would not.

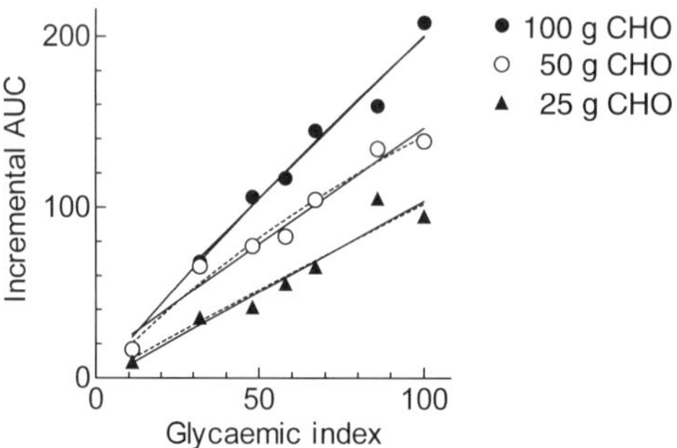


**Fig. 9.3.** Relationship between GI and glycaemic response AUC for fructose, sucrose, glucose, barley, spaghetti, bread and instant potato at each of three levels of carbohydrate intake. Solid lines are linear regressions, dotted lines are non-linear regressions (exponential model). Regressions do not depart significantly from linearity.

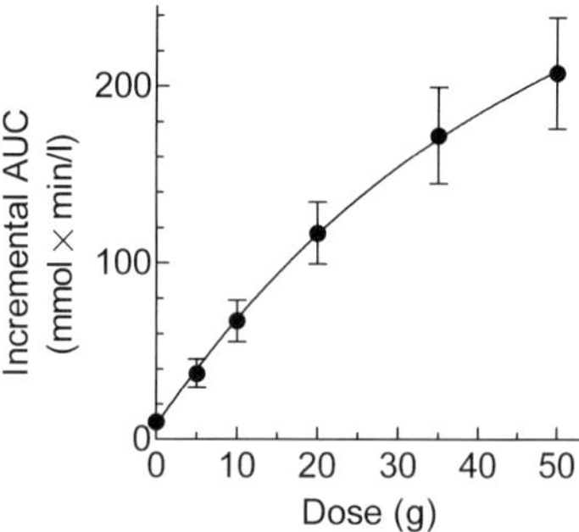


**Fig. 9.4.** Glycaemic responses elicited by 0, 5, 10, 20, 35 and 50 g available carbohydrate doses of white bread in ten normal subjects. Values are means ± SEM. Line is non-linear regression equation: AUC $= 293 \times (1-e^{-0.0230g}) + 8$, where g is the grams of carbohydrate.

### 9.2.1 Validity of the GL concept

Recently Brand-Miller *et al.* (2003a) conducted a study to test the validity of the GL concept and concluded that their data '... support the concept of dietary glycemic load as a measure of overall glycemic response and insulin demand'. This appears to be inconsistent with my conclusion that GL is not linearly related to glycaemic response. Since Brand-Miller *et al.* (2003a) measured glucose responses over 2 h and calculated AUC in the same way as we did the data are directly comparable with ours. Brand-Miller *et al.* (2003a) reported the results of two separate studies. In one, a group of ten subjects consumed ten different carbohydrate foods in amounts which delivered the same GL as contained in one slice of white bread. In the other study, two groups of subjects were fed 1–6 units of GL from nine different carbohydrate foods, where 1 unit is the GL (GI × g) in one slice of white bread (13 g carbohydrate). Thus, 6 units are equivalent to 81 g of carbohydrate from white bread.

If the GL concept is valid, then the glycaemic responses elicited by the ten foods should have been the same, since all the test meals had the same GL. However, the mean AUC values differed significantly for the different foods, varying over nearly a fourfold range from about 20 (red lentils) to about 75 mmol/l × 2 h (ice cream). If these two foods are excluded, the responses of the other eight foods do not differ significantly, nevertheless, the mean AUC values still vary over nearly a twofold range suggesting that the power of the study to detect differences was not large, possibly because such a low amount of carbohydrate was used. Therefore, I do not find this first study to be a convincing demonstration of the validity of the GL.

The second study (Brand-Miller *et al.*, 2003a) showed that the glucose AUC was related to the dose of GL fed, which varied from 1 to 6 arbitrary units. There was a strong linear trend ($P < 0.001$) and the authors indicate that the fit was not significantly improved when a quadratic (non-linear) equation was fitted. Nevertheless, the data clearly appear to fall along a curve (Fig. 9.5). However, the results of Brand-Miller *et al.* (2003a) agree with ours in showing that the plasma insulin responses are linearly related to the GL.

Before moving on, it is of interest to see how closely the data of Brand-Miller *et al.* (2003a) agree with our dose–response data. Brand-Miller *et al.* plotted the glucose response AUC on the dose level (1 through 6). One dose level was defined as having the same GL as one slice of bread which contains 13 g carbohydrate. Thus, to see if the exponential association model we derived from our data fit the data of Brand-Miller *et al.* (2003a), the $x$-axis units have to be converted to grams of carbohydrate which was done by multiplying each dose level by 13 g (Fig. 9.5). The exponential model is of the form:

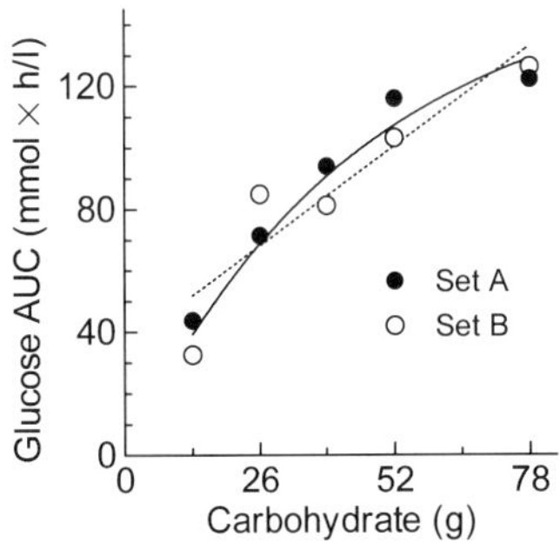


**Fig. 9.5.** Dose–response of observed glucose response on glycaemic load equivalent to one, two, three, four and six slices of white bread (each slice contains 13 g carbohydrate). Subjects consumed two sets of five foods in a balanced 5 × 5 Greco-Latin square design. Data from Brand-Miller *et al.* (2003a). Dotted line, linear regression ($r = 0.929$, $P < 0.001$). Solid line, exponential model with rate constant fixed at the same value as in Fig. 4.2 ($r = 0.968$).

$$\text{AUC} = A \times (1 - e^{-Kg})$$

where $A$ is the maximum value for AUC at an infinitely large dose and $K$ is the rate constant, which determines the curvature of the line. The value of $A$ will vary for different experiments since it is related to the glucose tolerance status of the subjects in the study. However, if the equation is universally applicable, the value for $K$ should be a constant. The estimate of $K$ from our data is 0.0222 (Fig. 4.2). The value of $K$ in Fig. 9.4 is very similar (0.023). When we fit an exponential model to the data of Brand-Miller *et al.* (2003a), with the value of $K$ fixed at 0.0222, the resulting curve fits the data very well (Fig. 9.5), with $r^2$ for the exponential model being 0.936 compared to 0.863 for the linear model.

### 9.2.2 Glycaemic glucose equivalent

Recently, Monro (2002) has introduced the concept of glycaemic glucose equivalent (GGE) which was defined as the weight of glucose having the same glycaemic impact as a given weight of food. GGE was calculated as follows:

$$\text{GGE} = \text{foodwt. (g)} \times (\%\text{CHOAVL} \times \text{GI})/10{,}000$$

where %CHOAVL = available carbohydrate per 100 g of food, a formula which reduces to:

$$\text{GGE} = \text{g} \times \text{GI}/100$$

where g = grams available carbohydrate and GI = GI of the food. Thus, I interpret GGE to be equivalent to GL. However, Monro distinguishes between GGE and GL by saying that GGE '... refers specifically to the acute glycaemic effect of a single food intake event and is designed for use in glycaemia management, whereas glycaemic load is a measure of the cumulative exposure to glycaemia as a risk factor in disease'.

#### *9.2.2.1 Published study on the validity of GGE*

Liu *et al.* (2003a) tested the validity of the GGE and concluded: 'GGE content predicted glycaemic impact of foods over a practical range of carbohydrate intakes'. They addressed the question of whether GGE predicts the glycaemic impact of foods by designing a study to test three main hypotheses: (i) different foods with the same GGE content elicit similar glycaemic responses in a group of subjects; (ii) doubling the GGE results in double the glycaemic response; and, perhaps most importantly, (iii) that GGE equals RGE. A group of 12 normal and 11 diabetic subjects were studied on ten different occasions with glycaemic responses being measured after five different foods, with each food being fed at two different GGE levels. This is a large and comprehensive study which was adequate to test the hypotheses. However, examination of the data presented by Liu *et al.* (2003a) shows that the results do not support any of the three hypotheses.

The first hypothesis was that different foods with the same GGE content would elicit the same glycaemic responses (Liu *et al.*, 2003a,b). To address this, they fed five different foods each at two levels of GGE to a group of normal subjects and a group of subjects with diabetes. There were significant differences in glycaemic response for foods with the same GGE. In subjects with diabetes at both levels of GGE the incremental areas under the plasma glucose response curves elicited by foods fed at the same GGE level varied over more than a twofold range and the differences were statistically significant. In normal subjects, statistically significant differences in glycaemic response occurred at one of the two GGE levels (Fig. 9.6). Thus, the glycaemic responses elicited by different foods fed at the same level of GGE were not similar, but differed significantly from each other in three of four cases.

The second hypothesis was that doubling the GGE intake would double the glycaemic response. The results showed that doubling GGE, by doubling the portion size of each food, significantly increased the glycaemic response.

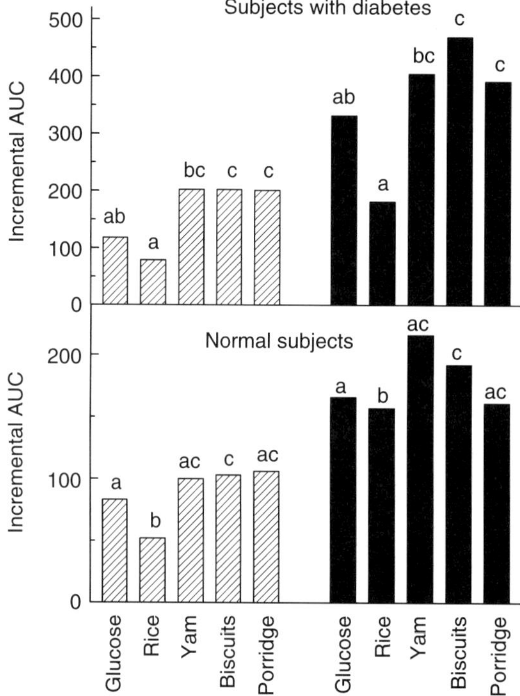


**Fig. 9.6.** Incremental areas under the glycaemic response curves elicited by amounts of five different foods containing 10 glycaemic glucose equivalents (GGE; hatched bars) and 20 GGE (filled bars) in subjects with diabetes (top) and subjects without diabetes (bottom). Theoretically, foods with the same level of GGE should elicit the same glycaemic response. Means with different letter superscripts differ significantly ($P < 0.05$) (Liu *et al.*, 2003a,b).

However, the question asked was whether the increase in glycaemic response was *proportional* to the increase in GGE. The authors approached this problem by expressing the glycaemic response of the portion of each food containing 20 or 48 GGE as a ratio of that for a portion containing ten or 24 GGE. When the GGE doubled, the glycaemic response ratios should have been equal to 2.0. Liu *et al.* (2003a) describe the results for the ratios as follows: 'In the subjects with type II diabetes, the ratio of dose 1:dose 2 approached 1:2 for most foods, although it was about 1:1.6 in the case of noodles'. This is curious since the ratios for normal subjects were not described and the ratio for noodles in subjects with diabetes is given as 1.5 in the table (not 1.6 as in the text). There is no statistical analysis of the ratios comparing either the ratios among the different foods or comparing the observed ratios with the expected ratio of 2.0. In fact, the response ratios varied from 1.5 to 2.7 in subjects with diabetes and from 1.5 to 2.2 for normal subjects. The ratios tended to become smaller as the amount of carbohydrate increased and the correlation was significant for the subjects with diabetes ($r = -0.865$, $P < 0.05$) (Fig. 9.7). The authors suggested that this may be an artefact based on the fact that the study was only 2-h long and so the glycaemic response curve did not reach baseline. However, the results of Christensen *et al.* (1972) suggest that the dose–response of AUC elicited by 25, 50, 100 and 200 g doses of glucose is curved even though, in that study, glycaemic responses were measured for 6 h, by which time blood glucose had returned to baseline after all four treatments (Fig. 4.5). An exponential dose–response curve would predict that doubling the dose of carbohydrate would increase AUC by less than twofold yielding a ratio of dose 1:dose 2 of <2. Most of the ratios observed by Liu *et al.* (2003a) were higher than would be predicted by the exponential model, and indeed, more than half were higher than 2 (Fig. 9.7).

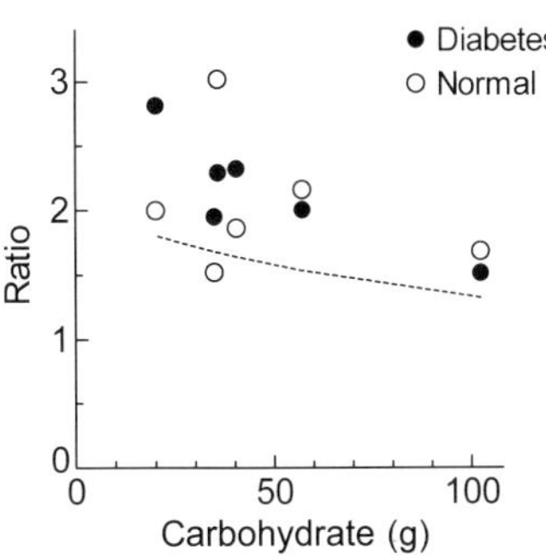


**Fig. 9.7.** Relationship between the ratio of glycaemic responses elicited by different foods fed at two doses and the amount of carbohydrate in the higher dose. For each food, the higher dose (dose 2) contained twice as much carbohydrate at the lower dose (dose 1); ratio is the AUC for dose 2 divided by the AUC for dose 1. Each food was tested in subjects with and without diabetes (Liu *et al.*, 2003a). The dotted line represents the expected ratios based on the exponential model from Fig. 4.2 used to assess the data of Brand-Miller *et al.* (2003a) in Fig. 9.5.

The third hypothesis of Liu *et al.* (2003a) was that GGE = RGE. RGE was defined as AUC divided by the glycaemic sensitivity factor (AUC/GGE), where AUC is the observed IAUC. The glycaemic sensitivity factor was taken as the average of the values of AUC/GGE for all foods tested by each individual. RGE, therefore, is intended to correct the relative glycaemic effects by the individuals' glycaemic sensitivity. According to the authors, 'Therefore, if GGE accurately predicted glycaemic response, the numbers for GGE intake and RGE should be the same'. They concluded that: 'In most cases, the correspondence between GGE intake and relative glycaemic effect was quite close ... ' (Liu *et al.*, 2003a, p. 1144, bottom of right column). This statement gives the impression that the correspondence between RGE and GGE is quite good 'in most cases'. However, I do not believe that the data support such a strong statement. In order to determine whether RGE equals GGE, I used the approach of considering how many times the GGE fell within the 95% CI of RGE (Wolever, 2004b). If it is assumed that RGE values are normally distributed, then the 95% CI represents the range within which the true value for RGE is expected to occur 95% of the time. The 95% CI of the various estimates of RGE can be calculated as:

$$\mathrm{CI} = \mathrm{mean} \pm \mathrm{SEM} \times t_{0.05(2),\, n-1}$$

where mean and SEM are given in Table 4 by Liu *et al.* (2003a), and $t_{0.05(2),\, n-1}$ equals the critical value of the *t*-distribution for two-tailed $P = 0.05$ with $n-1$ degrees of freedom. Figure 9.8 shows the mean and 95% CI of the RGE values at the 24 different levels of GGE intake. If the hypothesis that RGE = GGE is true, then GGE should fall

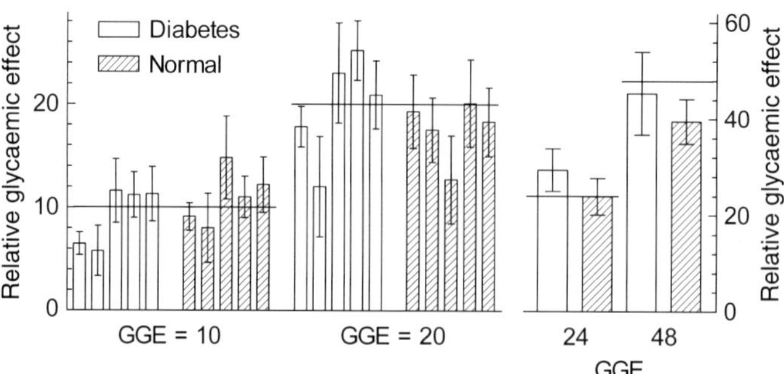


**Fig. 9.8.** Mean ± 95% confidence intervals (CI) of relative glycaemic effect (RGE) in normal and diabetic subjects of different foods consumed at different intakes of glycaemic glucose equivalent (GGE) (Liu *et al.*, 2003a). RGE = AUC/*F*, where AUC is the glycaemic response elicited by the food and *F* is the glucose sensitivity factor which is the average value of AUC/GGE for all foods tested by each individual. Solid lines indicate the levels of GGE intake for the various tests. If, according to the authors' hypothesis, RGE equals GGE, then there should be a 95% probability that GGE is within the 95% CI for RGE. Figure from Wolever (2004b).

within the 95% CI of RGE 95% of the time, i.e. 23 out of 24 times. However, it is apparent from Fig. 9.8 that GGE falls within the 95% CI of RGE for only 16 of the 24 tests (6 of 12 for subjects with diabetes and 10 of 12 for normal subjects). Thus, with this set of data, the probability that RGE = GGE is $<0.001$ by Fisher's exact test. In diabetic subjects, if RGE = GGE, then the chance of GGE being within the 95% CI of RGE at most 6 of 12 times is $P < 0.0001$, and the corresponding probability for normal subjects (10 of 12) is $P < 0.1$. This suggests the hypothesis that RGE = GGE should be rejected (at least in diabetic subjects). Therefore, Liu *et al.* (2003a) provide no good evidence that GGE accurately predicts glycaemic responses (RGE).

### 9.2.2.2 *Theoretical considerations about the validity of GGE*

Ideally, for Monro (2003), GGE would be measured directly to avoid the errors involved in measuring the carbohydrate content of a food and its GI. Thus, the GGE content of one serving of a food would be determined as follows:

$$\text{GGE} = 50 \times F/G$$

where $F$ is the glycaemic response elicited by a serving of the food and $G$ is the glycaemic response elicited by 50 g glucose.

Monro (2005) claims GGE to be valid, accurate and precise. In the preceding section, I have shown the conclusion that GGE is a valid predictor of the glycaemic impact of foods is not supported by the data. Here, I would like to address the question of accuracy. To say that a value is accurate is to say that it is equal to the true value. GGE is defined as the weight of glucose in grams that would elicit a glycaemic response equal to that elicited by the food. Surprisingly, whether this is actually so or not has not been assessed! However, I believe that GGE is not accurate and overestimates the amount of glucose which would elicit such a glycaemic response. The reason for this is illustrated in Fig. 9.9. The points show the glycaemic responses elicited by 0, 25 and 50 g glucose from a recent study of ours (Lee and Wolever, 1998); the mean AUC elicited by 50 g glucose was 213 mmol × min/l. The actual glycaemic response elicited by glucose at doses between 0 and 50 g is represented by the solid curved line whose equation is: AUC = 282 × $(1-e^{-0.028g})$.

As an example, let us calculate the amount of glucose which would elicit the same glycaemic response as a food with a GGE of 20. First, we need to calculate the AUC elicited by a food with a GGE of 20, assuming that the GGE of the food was tested in the same group of subjects who tested the glucose. Since GGE = 50 × $F/G$, where $F$ = AUC after the food and $G$ = AUC after 50 g glucose, therefore, $F = \text{GGE} \times G/50$. Since, in this group of subjects $G = 213$, thus, for a food with a GGE of 20 (Fig. 9.9, dotted line A), AUC = 20 × 213/50 = 85.2 (Fig. 9.9, dotted line B).

We have just calculated that a food with a GGE of 20 would elicit a glycaemic response AUC of 85.2 mmol × min/l in this group of subjects; now we need to calculate how much glucose would elicit the same AUC in the same group of subjects. From the dose–response curve for glucose, $\text{AUC} = 282 \times (1-e^{-0.028g})$, therefore $g = \ln(1-[\text{AUC}/282])/-0.028$. Solving for AUC = 85.2 gives a value for $g$ of 12.8 g (Fig. 9.9, dotted line C). This suggests that 12.8 g glucose would elicit the same glycaemic response as a food with a calculated GGE of 20, and thus, that the GGE overestimates the true glycaemic impact of the food by 56%. Performing a similar calculation for a range of GGE values shows that the amounts of glucose which elicit the same glycaemic response as foods with various GGE values are as follows:

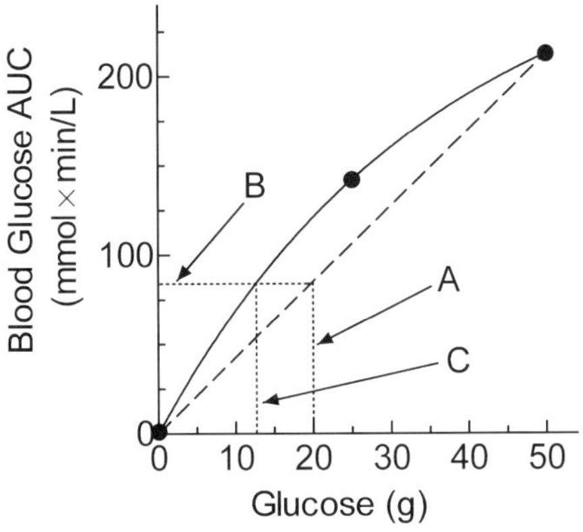


**Fig. 9.9.** Theoretical evaluation of accuracy of glycaemic glucose equivalent (GGE). GGE is the amount of glucose which would elicit the same glycaemic response as a serving of the food. Filled circles represent mean areas under the glycaemic response curves (AUC) of normal subjects after consuming 0, 25 and 50 g glucose (Lee and Wolever, 1998). GGE = 50 × *F*/*G* where *F* is the AUC elicited by a serving of a food and *G* is the AUC elicited by 50 g glucose. Therefore, dotted lines A and B show that the AUC for a food with a GGE of 20 would be about 85 mmol × min/l. Dotted line C shows that the amount of glucose which would elicit an AUC of 85 is about 13 g. Thus, GGE overestimates the true glycaemic impact of foods (see text, Section 9.2.2.2).

GGE 2 g, glucose 1.1 g (82% overestimate); GGE5 g, glucose 2.8 g (78% overestimate); GGE 10 g, glucose 5.8 g (72% overestimate); GGE 15 g, glucose 9.2 g (61% overestimate); GGE 30 g, glucose 21.6 g (39% overestimate); and GGE 40 g, glucose 33.1 g (21% overestimate). This suggests that GGE overestimates the true glycaemic impact of foods by a substantial amount (20–80%), and, therefore that GGE is not accurate.

### 9.2.3 Concluding remarks about GL and GGE

Recent data attempting to validate GL and GGE as markers of the acute glycaemic effects of foods are not convincing, despite conclusions to the contrary. Nevertheless, although GL has not yet been shown to be *quantitatively* accurate, it is a useful way of thinking about how carbohydrate foods influence *acute* postprandial glucose responses, at least *qualitatively*. For example, foods with a high GI do not impact on the blood glucose response very much if the amount of carbohydrate consumed is low, as is the case for certain vegetables. Thus, these concepts may be clinically useful in some situations, although proof of this is lacking. In addition, the validity and accuracy of GL and GGE values need to be demonstrated more convincingly and, to achieve this, methodological improvements may be required.

## 9.3 Does Low GI Equal Low Carbohydrate Beyond Acute Responses?

It has been suggested that it is beneficial for health to reduce diet GL (Bell and Sears, 2003). Diet GL can be reduced either by reducing diet GI without changing carbohydrate intake, or by reducing carbohydrate intake without reducing GI, or both. We have already seen that both these manoeuvres can reduce acute glucose and insulin responses. The question is whether reducing diet GI has the same effects on longer-term physiological effects and metabolic outcomes as reducing carbohydrate intake. Evidence from epidemiological studies, second-meal studies and dietary intervention studies (clinical trials) suggest that they do not.

### 9.3.1 Evidence from epidemiological studies

Table 9.1 summarizes the results of studies looking at the association between dietary GI, GL and carbohydrate intake of the risk of developing type 2 diabetes, cardiovascular disease and cancer. A high diet GI was associated with a significantly increased risk of diabetes in three of four studies, cardiovascular disease in one of three studies, insulin resistance syndrome in one study, and cancer in seven of ten studies. By contrast, high diet GL was associated with a significantly increased risk of diabetes in only one of four studies and cardiovascular disease in one of three studies, and was not associated with insulin resistance syndrome in one study. However, diet GL was associated with cancer risk in five of 11 studies. Increased intake of carbohydrate intake was not associated with significantly increased risk of diabetes, heart disease or insulin resistance in any of five studies in which it was assessed, but was associated with increased risk of cancer in two of four studies in which it was assessed.

Since GL = GI × carbohydrate intake, then, if high GI was associated with increased risk of disease, but carbohydrate intake has no effect, then one would expect that to be an effect of diet GL because of the effect of diet GI. In the diabetes and cardiovascular disease studies, high GI increased risk but carbohydrate intake had no effect. In addition, in none of these studies there was a significant association between GL and risk in the absence of a significant association between GI and risk. This suggests that, for these conditions, diet GI influences risk but the amount of carbohydrate in the diet does not.

**Table 9.1.** Effects of dietary glycaemic index, carbohydrate intake and glycaemic load on risk of type 2 diabetes, cardiovascular disease and cancer.

| | Relative risk[a] (*P*-value) | | | |
|---|---|---|---|---|
| Condition | Glycaemic index | Carbohydrate | Glycaemic load | Reference |
| Type 2 diabetes | 1.37 (0.03) | 0.85 (0.33) | 1.25 (0.17) | Salmerón *et al.* (1997a) |
| | 1.37 (0.005) | 1.04 (0.83) | 1.47 (0.003) | Salmerón *et al.* (1997b) |
| | 1.00 | – | 1.00 | Stevens *et al.* (2002) |
| | 1.59 (0.001) | 0.89 (0.69) | 1.33 (0.21) | Schulze *et al.* (2004) |
| Cardiovascular disease | 1.31 (0.008) | 1.23 (ns) | 1.98 (<0.001) | Liu *et al.* (2000) |
| | 1.11 (0.70) | – | | van Dam *et al.* (2000) |
| | 1.38 (0.10) | – | 1.08 (0.69) | Tavani *et al.* (2003) |
| Insulin resistance syndrome | 1.41 (0.04) | 0.92 (0.97) | 0.82 (0.74) | McKeown *et al.* (2004) |
| Cancer (site) | | | | |
| Breast | 1.4 (<0.01) | – | 1.3 (<0.01) | Augustin *et al.* (2001) |
| Breast (pre-)[b] | 0.78 (0.12) | – | 0.96 (0.44) | Silvera *et al.* (2005) |
| Breast (post-) | 1.87 (0.01) | – | 1.08 (0.68) | Silvera *et al.* (2005) |
| Colorectal | 1.7 (<0.001) | – | 1.8 (<0.001) | Franceschi *et al.* (2001) |
| Colorectal | – | 1.01 (0.66) | 1.05 (0.94) | Terry *et al.* (2003) |
| Colorectal | 1.71 (0.04) | 2.41 (0.02) | 2.85 (0.004) | Higginbotham *et al.* (2004) |
| Pancreas | 1.16 (0.53) | 1.30 (0.25) | 1.53 (0.14) | Michaud *et al.* (2002) |
| Pancreas | 1.08 (0.83) | – | 0.87 (0.43) | Johnson *et al.* (2005) |
| Ovary | 1.65 (<0.01) | 1.62 (<0.01) | 1.65 (<0.01) | Augustin *et al.* (2003a) |
| Endometrium | 1.90 (0.009) | – | 1.10 (0.78) | Augustin *et al.* (2003b) |
| OPOL[c] | 1.5 (<0.05) | – | 1.8 (<0.05) | Augustin *et al.* (2004a) |

[a]Relative risk for highest vs lowest level (usually quintiles) of intake after adjusting for all confounding variables.
[b]pre- = premenopausal; post- = postmenopausal women (significant interaction between effect of GI and menopausal status).
[c]Total of oral, pharyngeal, oesophagus and larynx.

The results of the cancer studies are somewhat different in that for two of four studies there were significant positive associations between carbohydrate intake and cancer risk. In both of these, however, there were also significant positive associations between GI and GL and cancer risk, suggesting that there may be independent contributions of GI and carbohydrate to risk. However, in the two studies with no effect of carbohydrate intake, there was also no effect of GI or GL. In the seven studies in which the effect of carbohydrate intake was not assessed, there was no case where there is a significant effect of GL in the absence of a significant effect of GI, but there were two cases where there was a significant effect of GI in the absence of an effect of GL.

Table 9.2 summarizes the associations between GI, GL and carbohydrate intake and blood lipids and other risk factors for cardiovascular disease. Diet GI was negatively related to serum HDL cholesterol in three of five studies. van Dam *et al.* (2000) found no relationship between GI and HDL, and did not examine the effects of GL or carbohydrate. Liu *et al.* (2001) found a significant association between GL and HDL in the absence of significant effects of GI and carbohydrate. Frost *et al.* (1999) found a significant relationship between GI and HDL, but did not study GL. Ford and Liu (2001) found significant effects of both GI and GL on HDL but did not report the association between carbohydrate and HDL. Slyper *et al.* (2005) found significant effects of GI, GL and carbohydrate on HDL. Thus, the effects of GI on HDL, as opposed to carbohydrate and GL, are inconsistent in these studies.

There are only two studies for triglycerides; van Dam *et al.* (2000) found no effect of GI and did not examine carbohydrate or GL. On the other hand, Liu *et al.* (2001) found that GI, carbohydrate and GL all were positively related to serum triglycerides. In one study, serum CRP was positively related to GI, carbohydrate intake and GL (Liu *et al.*, 2002). In normal men, plasma adiponectin concentrations were negatively related to carbohydrate intake and GL, but not to GI (Pischon *et al.*, 2005), but in men with diabetes both GI and GL were negatively related to plasma adiponectin (Qi *et al.*, 2005).

In healthy schoolchildren, diet GI, but not diet GL was associated with plasma insulin concentrations (Scaglioni *et al.*, 2004). In healthy adults, both GI and GL were positively associated with HOMA-derived insulin resistance index, but dietary carbohydrate had no effect (McKeown *et al.*, 2004).

Thus, it appears that the effects of GI, carbohydrate and GL on risk vary with the disease. GI appears to be more important for diabetes risk and insulin resistance than carbohydrate or GL. The results of studies on CVD are not consistent; on the one hand GI or GL were significantly

**Table 9.2.** Relationships between dietary glycaemic index, carbohydrate and glycaemic load intakes and blood lipids and other risk markers in healthy adults.

| | Direction (*P*-value)[a] | | | |
|---|---|---|---|---|
| Marker | Glycaemic index | Carbohydrate | Glycaemic load | Reference |
| HDL | −ve, <0.0001 | −ve, 0.06 | – | Frost *et al.* (1999) |
| HDL | 0.81 | – | – | van Dam *et al.* (2000) |
| HDL | −ve, <0.001 | – | −ve, <0.001 | Ford and Liu (2001) |
| HDL | −ve, 0.10 | 0.76 | −ve, 0.03 | Liu *et al.* (2001) |
| HDL | −ve, 0.043 | −ve, 0.021 | −ve, 0.009 | Slyper *et al.* (2005) |
| Triglycerides | 0.44 | – | – | van Dam *et al.* (2000) |
| Triglycerides | +ve, 0.03 | +ve, 0.005 | +ve, <0.001 | Liu *et al.* (2001) |
| LDL | 0.56 | 0.60 | – | Frost *et al.* (1999) |
| CRP | +ve, <0.01 | +ve, <0.01 | +ve, <0.01 | Liu *et al.* (2002) |
| Adiponectin | 0.21 | −ve, 0.05 | −ve, 0.02 | Pischon *et al.* (2005) |
| Adiponectin | −ve, 0.005 | 0.26 | −ve, 0.004 | Qi *et al.* (2005) |
| Insulin | +ve, 0.03 | – | 0.5 | Scaglioni *et al.* (2004) |
| HOMA-IR | +ve, <0.001 | 0.52 | +ve, 0.03 | McKeown *et al.* (2004) |

[a]Direction of association (e.g. −ve = higher intake associated with lower blood lipid).

related to increased risk in only about half of the studies, and on the other hand, the concordance between the effects of GI, carbohydrate and GL differ in different studies. For cancer risk, there appears to be more consistency in that both GI and GL are associated with increased risk in six of the seven studies where the effects of both were reported.

### 9.3.2 Evidence from second-meal studies

The second-meal effect is an experimental paradigm in which metabolic events elicited by one meal influence metabolic responses elicited by the next meal. For example, it is known that the hypothalamic response of serotonin in response to carbohydrate or protein in the rat depends on the composition of the previous meal and the interval between meals; a meal of carbohydrate increased hypothalamic serotonin secretion if taken first, but decreased serotonin secretion if taken 2 h after a protein meal. Likewise, a meal of protein decreased hypothalamic serotonin secretion if taken first, but increased it if taken 2 h after a carbohydrate meal. However, if the interval between meals is increased to 4 h, the effects of carbohydrate and protein at the second meal are not affected by the composition of the first meal (Fernstrom and Fernstrom, 1995; Rouch *et al.*, 2003). In addition, plasma glucose, insulin and fatty acid responses elicited by a second meal depend on the type and amount of fatty acids consumed in the first (Ercan *et al.*, 1994; Jackson *et al.*, 2001, 2002; Robertson *et al.*, 2002). However, I am here mostly interested in comparing the effect that changing the amount of carbohydrate vs changing the rate of absorption of carbohydrate in the first meal has on the glycaemic response elicited by the next meal.

The hypothesis that varying the amount or rate of absorption of carbohydrate could influence the response to a subsequent meal was derived from the concept of the glucose–fatty acid cycle (Randle *et al.*, 1963) in which the oxidation of fatty acids was proposed to inhibit the oxidation of carbohydrate and *vice versa*. Thus in the fasting state blood glucose, insulin levels are low and the primary fuel for the body is the FFA derived from the hydrolysis of triglyceride in adipose tissue. The oxidation of FFA inhibits the use of glucose by muscle, thus sparing the limited supply of glucose for tissues which require it, such as brain. After a carbohydrate-containing meal, blood glucose and insulin levels rise. Insulin inhibits the hydrolysis of triglyceride in adipose tissue, and hence, inhibits the release of FFA, thus reducing blood FFA concentrations. The reduction in blood FFA facilitates insulin-stimulated glucose uptake into adipose tissue and muscle. In adipose tissue, glucose is converted to glycerol and used to re-esterify FFA to triglyceride reducing FFA output into the circulation even further. In muscle, glucose replaces FFA as the primary fuel. However, when the rate of uptake of glucose from the blood exceeds the rate of absorption of carbohydrate from the intestine, blood glucose and insulin levels begin to fall. Once the insulin concentration has returned to the fasting level, the inhibition of lipolysis in adipose tissue is relieved and blood FFA increases leading to increased fat oxidation and an inhibition in the use of glucose. According to this concept, then, the role of insulin was not so much to control the utilization of glucose directly, but rather to control the output of FFA from adipose tissue which in turn, influenced the disposal of glucose.

Early studies showed that after meals of 100 g glucose or sucrose, plasma FFA levels fell to reach a nadir within 1–2 h, and rebounded to reach fasting levels by 5–6 h. However, the rebound of FFA was significantly slower after ingesting starch than glucose, due, it was suggested, to slower gastrointestinal absorption of glucose (Swan *et al.*, 1966). We hypothesized, therefore, that if glucose was supplied to the body slowly over a long period of time FFA levels would remain suppressed for longer than if the same amount of glucose was provided to the body rapidly over a short period of time. Thus, after a meal containing slowly absorbed carbohydrate, the disposal of glucose after a subsequent meal would be facilitated, compared to that after the same amount of rapidly absorbed carbohydrate. We tested this by comparing the glycaemic response elicited by oral glucose taken 4 h after the consumption of oral glucose with or without the addition of guar gum (Jenkins *et al.*, 1980b). When guar was taken at the first meal, the plasma glucose response elicited by the second meal was reduced by 50%. When 50 g glucose was sipped continuously over a 3.5-h period, plasma FFA levels 4 h later were suppressed compared to a bolus of 50 g glucose, and the rate of disposal of glucose after an intravenous glucose load was improved (Jenkins *et al.*, 1990).

We first compared the effects of slowly absorbed carbohydrate vs a reduced amount of carbohydrate by examining the second-meal effect after consuming meals containing whole wheat bread or lentils (Jenkins *et al.*, 1982b). To see whether the effect of lentils could be explained better by slow absorption or malabsorption, we mimicked slow absorption by having subjects nibble the bread meal slowly over 4 h, and we mimicked malabsorption by reducing the amount of bread by 75%. The glucose AUCs elicited by lentils, slow bread, and 25% bread were similar to each other and all significantly less than that elicited by the control bread meal (Fig. 9.10). However, the shape of the response curves differed; the rise in blood glucose was slow and sustained after lentils and slow bread compared to a marked peak and undershoot after 25% bread (Fig. 9.10). The second-meal glycaemic response tended to be reduced after lentils and slow bread compared to the control bread meal, whereas the second-meal response after 25% bread was significantly higher than after the control bread meal.

Collier *et al.* (1987) did a second-meal study showing that doubling the amount of bread consumed in the first meal tended to decrease the second-meal glycaemic response, but that adding the same amount of calories as fat (butter) tended to increase the second-meal response (Fig. 9.11). Thus, both reducing carbohydrate content and increasing the fat content tended to impair the second-meal glycaemic response.

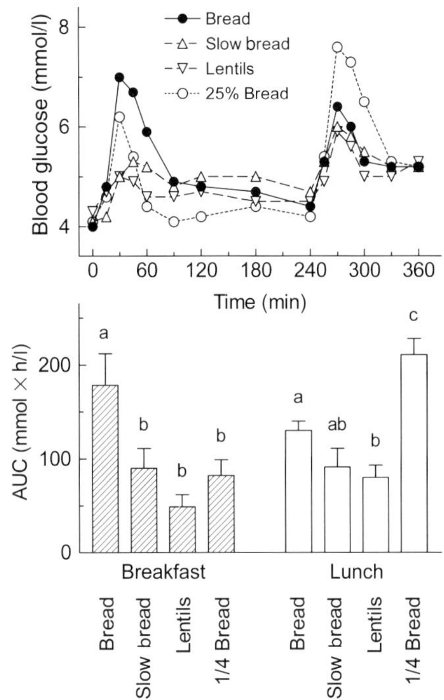


**Fig. 9.10.** Mean blood glucose responses in seven normal subjects elicited by breakfast test meals of lentils, whole wheat bread and cheese (consumed within 20 min or slowly nibbled over 4 h) and a meal containing 25% the amount of bread, followed by a standard lunch. The lentils and bread meals contained 127 g carbohydrate, 26–29 g dietary fibre, 13–18 g fat and 57 g protein; the 25% bread breakfast contained 39 g carbohydrate, 8 g fibre, 12 g fat and 38 g protein. Top, blood glucose responses; Bottom, incremental AUC after breakfast and lunch meals (means with different letter superscripts differ significantly). Data from Jenkins *et al.* (1982b).

Although the results of Jenkins *et al.* (1982b) and Collier *et al.* (1987) supported the hypothesized second-meal glycaemic effects of slowing carbohydrate absorption and reducing carbohydrate intake, the effects of these manoeuvres on postprandial FFA were not measured until 13 years later when we compared the effects of reducing meal GI and reducing carbohydrate content in a Latin square design (Wolever *et al.*, 1995a). Four isocaloric breakfast meals were designed; two contained about 84 g carbohydrate and differed in GI (72 vs 49) by exchanging a low-fibre for a high-fibre breakfast cereal. The other two meals had GI values of 66 and 50, and contained half the amount of carbohydrate, with the difference in calories made up by fat from margarine. The glucose, insulin and FFA responses are shown in Fig. 9.12. There were statistically significant interactions between the effects of carbohydrate and GI on the plasma glucose and FFA responses; low GI significantly reduced glucose responses after breakfast and lunch with high-carbohydrate meals, but not low-carbohydrate meals. The FFA rebound was significantly lower after the low-GI, high-carbohydrate breakfast compared to high-GI, high-carbohydrate; however, after the low-GI, low-carbohydrate breakfast, the FFA rebound was significantly higher than after high-GI, low-carbohydrate. The results of this study cannot be used to draw conclusions about the difference

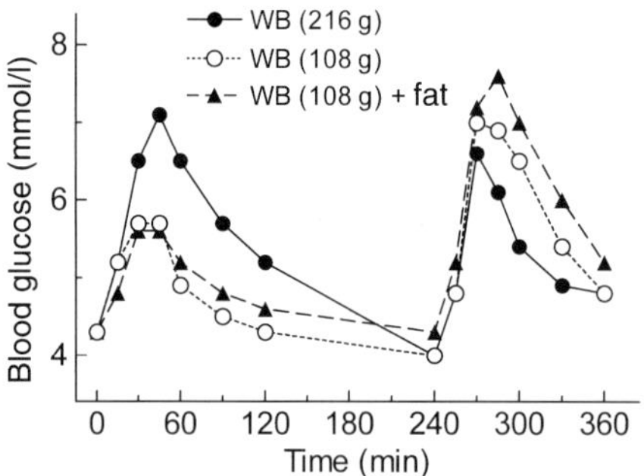


**Fig. 9.11.** Mean glycaemic responses of six normal subjects after breakfast test meals of bread and cheese (108 g bread, 52 g carbohydrate, 1 g fat and 23 g protein; 216 g bread, 101 g carbohydrate, 2 g fat and 22 g protein) or bread and cheese plus butter (52 g carbohydrate, 26 g fat, 23 g protein), followed by a standard lunch (Collier *et al.*, 1987).

between the effects of slowing carbohydrate vs reducing the amount consumed alone, since the amounts of fat in the meals differed, and Collier *et al.* (1987) showed that this influenced the second-meal response. However, the study did suggest that acute modulation of the FFA rebound by manipulating the source and amount of carbohydrate in a breakfast meal significantly influenced the mean blood glucose concentration after lunch, with FFA concentration 4 h after breakfast being significantly related to the mean plasma glucose concentration between 4 and 6 h (Fig. 9.13). In all of these cases, the use of slow-release carbohydrate improved second-meal carbohydrate tolerance, and, where measured, significantly prolonged the suppression of plasma FFA concentrations. By contrast, 4 h after meals containing a reduced amount of carbohydrate, FFA concentrations were significantly increased and second-meal carbohydrate tolerance was impaired. Thus, it appears that the second-meal effect differs depending on whether glycaemic responses are reduced by slowing carbohydrate absorption, or by reducing the amount of carbohydrate absorbed.

Other investigators have also found that delaying carbohydrate absorption at breakfast reduced the glycaemic response elicited by a subsequent standard lunch meal; methods used to delay absorption include the addition of lactic acid (Östman *et al.*, 2002), the use of spaghetti vs white bread (Liljeberg and Björck, 2000) and the addition of psyllium (Pastors *et al.*, 1991). Shaheen and Fleming (1987) compared the effect of breakfast meals consisting of kidney beans, bran cereal or white bread, and were unable to detect a significant second-meal effect, but they were also unable to demonstrate any significant difference between the glycaemic responses elicited by the breakfast test meals.

Liljeberg *et al.* (1999) conducted an elegant study examining the effect of varying the GI and the amount of RS in nine different breakfast test meals on the glycaemic response to the second meal. All the breakfast meals contained 50 g total starch, with the amount of digestible starch varying from 38.8 to 49.9 g and the GI varying from 37 to 71. The glycaemic response elicited by the second meal was significantly influenced by the GI, but was not affected by altering the amount of RS. Thus, the authors concluded that slow absorption of starch from the breakfast meal, but not the content of indigestible carbohydrates in the breakfast meal, improved glucose tolerance at the second meal (Liljeberg *et al.*, 1999). This further shows that the metabolic effects of reducing the rate of absorption differ from those of reducing the amount of carbohydrate absorbed.

### 9.3.3 Evidence from dietary intervention studies

Clinical trials clearly show that reducing diet GI has different long-term metabolic effects than reducing carbohydrate intake. However, it is difficult to generalize about the effects because there are many different ways of implementing low-GI and low-carbohydrate interventions. Based on current evidence, it is difficult to say which type of intervention is more beneficial.

Reducing dietary GI is accomplished by replacing carbohydrate foods in the diet with foods with a lower GI. Since one carbohydrate food is being exchanged for another, an experimental change from a high- to a low-GI diet can be achieved with little or no change in the overall macronutrient composition of the diet, although in some studies use of low-GI foods was associated with a higher intake of dietary fibre and small increases in carbohydrate and protein intakes and a reduction in fat (Frost *et al.*, 1994; Wolever and Mehling, 2002).

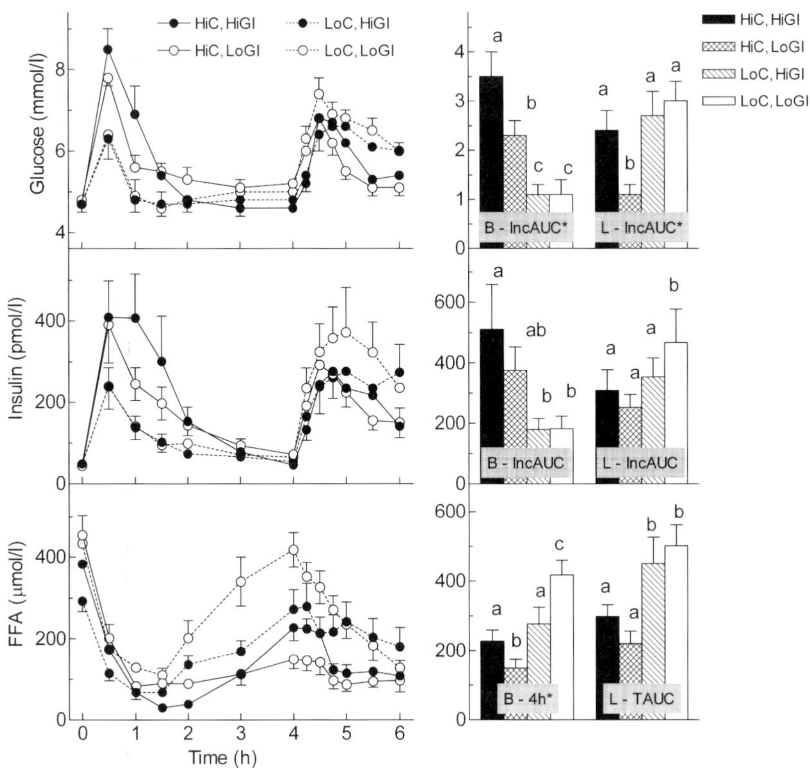


**Fig. 9.12.** Responses of plasma glucose, insulin and free-fatty acids (FFAs) of eight normal subjects after four different breakfasts followed by a standard lunch. The isocaloric breakfast meals followed a 2 × 2 factorial design and contained 84 g (HiC) or 41 g (LoC) carbohydrate with a high (HiGI) or low (LoGI) glycaemic index. Bar graphs show glucose and insulin incremental areas under the curve (IncAUC) after breakfast (B) or lunch (L) and, for FFA, the mean concentration at 4 h, and the total area under the curve after lunch. * Indicates statistically significant interaction between amount of carbohydrate and GI ($P < 0.05$). Data from Wolever *et al.* (1995a).

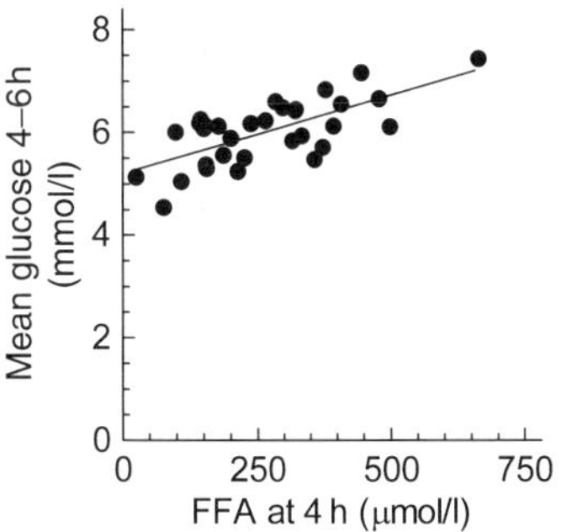


**Fig. 9.13.** Relationship between plasma FFA concentration 4 h after breakfast and mean plasma glucose after lunch (4–6 h) ($r = 0.691$, $P < 0.0001$). Data from Wolever *et al.* (1995a).

By contrast, reducing carbohydrate intake can be achieved in many different ways, and the overall effect probably depends on with what the carbohydrate is replaced. It is possible to replace the carbohydrate with nothing, in which case weight will be lost. Indeed, when considering weight loss diets, the metabolic effects may depend more on the amount of weight lost than the composition of the weight-reducing diet (Dansinger *et al.*, 2005). However, if the diet is to be weight-maintaining, one has to replace the carbohydrate calories with something else, which could be mixed fat sources (Swinburn *et al.*, 1991b; Ireland *et al.*, 1992), MUFA (Garg, 1998) or protein (Seino *et al.*, 1983; Skov *et al.*, 1999). In addition, one can replace available carbohydrates with unavailable ones such as RS (Jenkins *et al.*, 1999). These different dietary manoeuvres likely have different long-term metabolic effects, but for most of them too few data are available to make a reliable comparison between the effects of reducing dietary carbohydrate with those of reducing diet GI. However, a number of studies have looked at the effects of reducing carbohydrate intake and replacing it with MUFA.

Figure 9.14 compares the metabolic effects of low-carbohydrate/high-MUFA diets with those of low-GI diets in different studies, based on several meta-analyses (Garg, 1998; Wolever, 2003; Kelly *et al.*, 2004). These data suggest that both MUFA and low-GI diets reduce serum total cholesterol. However, MUFA significantly increased HDL and reduced triglycerides, whereas low GI had no effect on these measures. On the other hand, low GI significantly reduced mean blood glucose (measured as glycated proteins) whereas MUFA had no effect.

We performed two studies which directly compared the effects of reducing dietary carbohydrate (CHO) (replaced by MUFA) or reducing dietary GI. Tsihlias *et al.* (2000) used a breakfast

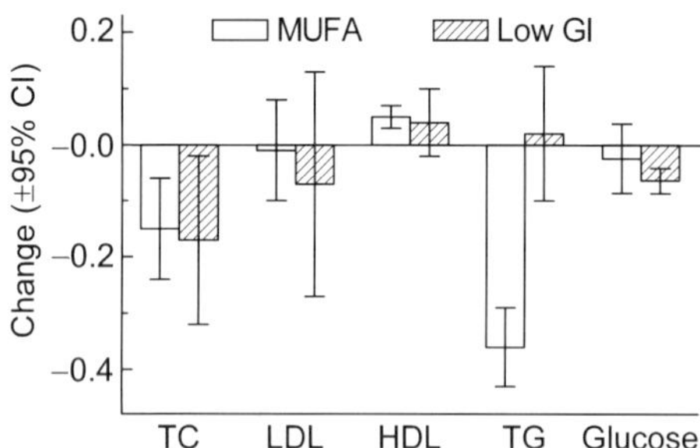


**Fig. 9.14.** Comparison of long-term metabolic effects of reducing dietary carbohydrate intake and replacing the energy with monounsaturated fatty acid (MUFA) or reducing dietary GI, keeping total carbohydrate intake constant. Based on results of several meta-analyses, changes (mmol/l) in TC (total cholesterol), LDL (low-density lipoprotein cholesterol), HDL (high-density lipoprotein cholesterol) and TG (triglycerides) for MUFA based on 10 studies reviewed by Garg (1998), and for low GI based on 15 studies reviewed by Kelly *et al.* (2004). Changes in glucose (glycated proteins %/100) based on review of 7 studies of MUFA and 14 studies of low GI reviewed by Wolever (2003).

cereal high in psyllium and wheat bran to reduce diet GI in subjects with type 2 diabetes. Wolever and Mehling (2002, 2003) used low-GI starchy foods to reduce diet GI in subjects with IGT. Both studies used olive oil and canola oil margarines to increase MUFA intake. Both studies showed that reducing dietary carbohydrate had different long-term metabolic effects than reducing diet GI. In both studies, low-carbohydrate and low-GI diets affected mean postprandial glucose to almost exactly the same extent (in the diabetes study, postprandial glucose increased from baseline on both treatments, but the increase tended to be less than on the high-carbohydrate/high-GI control diet). However, in both studies, compared to the low-carbohydrate diet, low-GI tended to increase postprandial insulin and triglycerides and decrease postprandial FFA and each of these effects was significant in at least one of the studies (Fig. 9.15). In the subjects with diabetes, 6 months on a high-fibre, low-GI diet had significantly different effects than 6 months on a low-carbohydrate, high-MUFA diet, respectively, on fasting HDL cholesterol ($-0.05 \pm 0.02$ vs $+0.08 \pm 0.03$ mmol/l, $P = 0.002$) (Tsihlias *et al.*, 2000), fasting HDL triglyceride ($+0.03 \pm 0.01$ vs $0.00 \pm 0.01$ mmol/l, $P = 0.045$), fasting triglycerides ($+0.32 \pm 0.11$ vs $-0.22 \pm 0.17$ mmol/l, $P = 0.007$), LDL cholesterol ($-0.02 \pm 0.08$ vs $0.43 \pm 0.14$ mmol/l, $P = 0.01$) and LDL particle size ($-0.45 \pm 0.12$ vs $-0.31 \pm 0.13$ nm, $P = 0.032$) (Wolever *et al.*, 2003b). In subjects with IGT, 4 months on a high-carbohydrate, low-GI diet had significantly different effects than 4 months on a low-carbohydrate, high-MUFA diet, respectively, on diastolic blood pressure ($-3.6 \pm 1.1$ vs $+4.7 \pm 2.5$ mmHg, $P < 0.05$) and β-cell function measured as DI (DI = SI × $AIR_{glu}$, where SI is insulin sensitivity index and $AIR_{glu}$ is the area under the insulin response curve for 10 min after intravenous glucose) ($+0.17 \pm 0.07$ vs $-0.09 \pm 0.08$, $P = 0.019$) (Wolever and Mehling, 2002). Consistent with the diabetes study, there were non-significant trends for reduced HDL cholesterol and higher serum triglycerides on the low-GI diet compared to the MUFA diet.

Thus, evidence from epidemiological studies and short- and long-term metabolic studies all show that the metabolic effects of reducing diet GI differ in some ways from those of reducing carbohydrate intake.

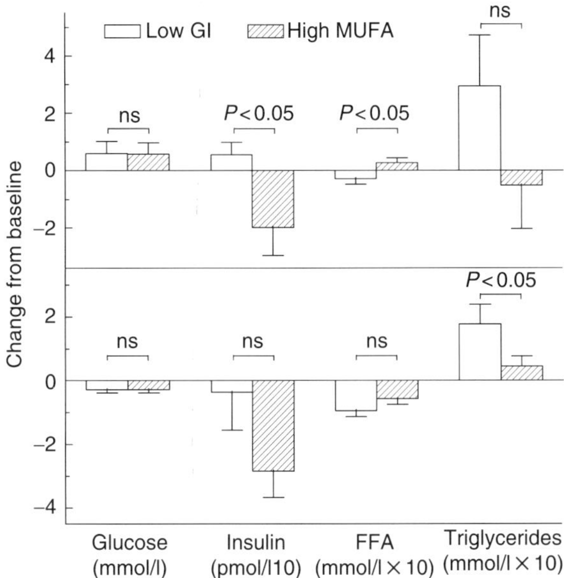


**Fig. 9.15.** Comparison of effects of reducing dietary GI with those of reducing carbohydrate intake and replacing with monounsaturated fatty acid (MUFA) in subjects with type 2 diabetes (top) (Tsihlias *et al.*, 2000) and subjects with impaired glucose tolerance (bottom) (Wolever and Mehling, 2003) on mean concentrations of plasma glucose, insulin, free-fatty acids (FFAs) and triglycerides during an 8-h metabolic profile. Values represent the difference between concentrations while consuming low-GI or MUFA meals at the end of the study and the concentrations while consuming high-carbohydrate, high-GI meals at baseline.

## 9.4 Clinical Utility of GI vs GL and GGE

GI is a qualitative measure of the blood glucose raising potential of the available carbohydrate in foods which is independent of the amount of carbohydrate consumed. It has been suggested that the GI is difficult to understand, especially for consumers, because GI is independent of the amount of carbohydrate consumed, and thus, is not a measure of the glycaemic response elicited by a food (Monro, 2003). Recently, Monro (2005) has gone so far as to conclude that the GI is not valid, accurate or even safe! Therefore, it has been suggested that the concept should be altered to indicate the glycaemic response elicited by 50 g of food, i.e. the GGE (Monro, 2003). GGE, like GL, is intended to be a quantitative measure of the glycaemic impact of a specific amount of food.

The general tenet upon which the GL and GGE are based is that reducing the glycaemic impact of foods is beneficial. However, there are many different ways to reduce glycaemic responses, which, as shown above, do not have the same short- or long-term metabolic effects. Thus, reducing the glycaemic response *per se* is not necessarily beneficial; whether it is beneficial or not depends on the mechanism by which the reduction in blood glucose occurs. Thus, GGE or GL are not specific enough to be useful tools for providing nutritional advice with the aim of promoting long-term health. There are many different ways to reduce GGE and GL which may or may not have beneficial effects depending on the method chosen to reduce GL. On the other hand, lowering diet GI, but keeping the overall macronutrient composition of the diet fairly constant by exchanging the types of starchy carbohydrate foods, is a specific nutritional manoeuvre which has been shown to have a number of beneficial effects. Retaining the concept of GI according to its original definition is, therefore, a useful measure of the 'quality' of dietary available carbohydrates independent of their amount.

One implication of this is that the definition of the term 'GI' should be retained and continue to refer to the glycaemic effects of the available carbohydrate in foods. This means that unavailable carbohydrates should be excluded from the available carbohydrate load used to determine GI. Thus, partly digestible or indigestible carbohydrates which elicit a low glycaemic response cannot necessarily be said to have a low GI; rather, they could be considered to have a low GL or low GGE. Completely undigestible carbohydrates cannot be said to have a GI value at all because they do not contain any available carbohydrate; however, they too can be considered to have a low GL (or GGE). This is not to say that it is inappropriate or harmful to reduce glycaemic responses by exchanging available for unavailable carbohydrates. Indeed, such manoeuvres may be useful. However, there are few data about the long-term physiological effects of replacing available carbohydrates with unavailable or partly available carbohydrates, and such data would be very welcome to help guide dietary recommendations in this area. What I am saying, however, is that we cannot ascribe the same long-term health benefits to, for example, sugar alcohols based on clinical trials of low-GI diets because low-GI foods and sugar alcohols do not reduce blood glucose by the same mechanisms. Low-GI diets and sugar alcohols share the common physiologic mechanism of increased colonic fermentation, but we do not know the importance of this mechanism in determining the overall metabolic effects of low-GI diets. In addition, the types and amounts of substrates fermented on a low-GI diet differ from those after consuming sugar alcohols, and we do not know the implications of that.

It is clear that GL and GGE are more useful than GI alone for determining the acute glycaemic response elicited by a food, and such information might be useful in certain situations such as calculating the amount of insulin in a person with type 1 diabetes prior to a meal. However, there are a number of problems with this. First, GL and GGE may greatly overestimate the glycaemic impact of foods (see Section 9.2.2.2) which, if true, could be dangerous because it would result in an overestimate of the amount of insulin injected and, thus, increase the risk of hypoglycaemia. Another problem is that GL and GGE are influenced by the amounts of fat and protein in foods, and, as has been reviewed in Chapter 5, there is good evidence that these nutrients do not have the same effects in people with diabetes as in normal subjects, or even in people with type 1 diabetes compared to those with type 2 diabetes. This is also a problem when determining the GI of foods, such as food bars, which contain considerable amounts of protein and fat, and this issue has not been resolved. However, for high-carbohydrate starchy foods we know that GI values are the same in normal and diabetic subjects (Chapter 2, this volume).

Another problem with the clinical utility of GL and GGE for adjusting insulin doses in people with diabetes is that it may not be enough to know the GI and the amount of carbohydrate to calculate the appropriate amount of insulin to elicit a normal glycaemic response. This is because GI, GL and GGE are all based on AUC, and this does not indicate the shape of the glycaemic response curve. People with type 1 diabetes not only need to avoid hyperglycaemia but also hypoglycaemia. To see how GI and the proportion of carbohydrate absorbed as glucose (Pg) affected glycaemic responses in subjects with type 1 diabetes treated with the rapid acting insulin analogue insulin lispro, we compared glycaemic responses elicited by 50 g available carbohydrate portions of four starchy foods (instant potato, bread, spaghetti and barley) and pineapple juice in eight subjects (Mohammed and Wolever, 2004). The mean incremental area under the glucose response curve was highly related to the published GI values of the foods ($r = 0.98$, $P < 0.01$), but the shape of the glycaemic response curves differed for the juice (Pg = 0.5) compared to the starchy foods (Pg = 1.0). Blood glucose increased significantly more rapidly after pineapple juice than the starchy foods, but also fell most rapidly, leading to a significantly higher occurrence of hypoglycaemia after pineapple juice (seven of eight trials, 88%), than the other four foods (10 of 32 trials, 31%, $P = 0.0016$). This suggests that knowing GL is not enough to optimize insulin adjustment in type 1 diabetes, and that further information about the nature of the carbohydrate absorbed may be necessary.

## 9.5 Conclusions

Reducing diet GI is a specific dietary manoeuvre involving exchange of high-carbohydrate foods with little change in the overall macronutrient content of the diet. On the other hand, reducing diet GL or reducing GGE, are not specific. Since GL and GGE are calculated as the product of GI times grams of carbohydrate consumed, they can be altered either by changing GI or by changing the amount of carbohydrate consumed, or both. If carbohydrate intake is reduced, it can be replaced by other nutrients such as protein, saturated fat, MUFA or unavailable carbohydrates, or by nothing. The effects on metabolism and health of reducing carbohydrate intake depend on what, if anything, is consumed in its stead. Thus, the health effects of advice to reduce diet GL cannot be predicted, and should not be equated with the effects of reducing diet GI. Indeed, epidemiological studies and short- and long-term clinical trials all show that the effects of altering diet GI are not the same as those of altering the amount of carbohydrate. Further research is required to determine not only if GL and GGE to predict acute glycaemic responses but also whether specific methods of reducing diet GL, other than by reducing GI, are beneficial.

# References


Abdallah, L., Chabert, M. and Louis-Sylvestre, J. (1997) Cephalic phase responses to sweet taste. *American Journal of Clinical Nutrition* 65, 737–743.

Akgün, S. and Ertel, N.H. (1980) A comparison of carbohydrate metabolism after sucrose, sorbitol and fructose meals in normal and diabetic subjects. *Diabetes Care* 3, 582–585.

Akinmokun, A., Selby, P.L., Ramaiya, K. and Alberti, K.G. (1992) The short insulin tolerance test for determination of insulin sensitivity: a comparison with the euglycaemic clamp. *Diabetic Medicine* 9, 432–437.

Al-Delaimy, W.K., Rimm, E.B., Willett, W.C., Stampfer, M.J. and Hu, F.B. (2004) Magnesium intake and risk of coronary heart disease among men. *Journal of the American College of Nutrition* 23, 63–70.

Allen, F.M. (1920) Experimental studies on diabetes. Series I. Production and control of diabetes in the dog. 2. Effects of carbohydrate diets. *Journal of Experimental Medicine* 31, 381–402.

Alles, M.S., Hautvast, J.G., Nagengast, F.M., Hartemink, R., Van Laere, K.M. and Jansen, J.B. (1996) Fate of fructo-oligosaccharides in the human intestine. *British Journal of Nutrition* 76, 211–221.

American Diabetes Association (1994) Nutrition recommendations and principles for people with diabetes mellitus (Position Statement). *Diabetes Care* 7, 519–522.

American Diabetes Association (2002) Evidence-based nutrition principles and recommendations for the treatment and prevention of diabetes and related complications. *Diabetes Care* 25 (Suppl. 1), S50–S60.

Anderson, G.H. (1996) Regulation of food intake. In: Shils, M.E., Olson, J.A. and Shike, M. (eds) *Modern Nutrition in Health and Disease*, 8th edn. Lea & Febiger, Philadelphia, Pennsylvania, pp. 524–536.

Anderson, G.H. and Li, E.T.S. (1987) Protein and amino acids in the regulation of quantitative and qualitative aspects of food intake. *International Journal of Obesity* 11 (Suppl. 3), 97–108.

Anderson, I.H., Levine, A.S. and Levitt, M.D. (1981) Incomplete absorption of the carbohydrate in all-purpose wheat flour. *New England Journal of Medicine* 304, 1339–1346.

Anderson, G.H., Catherine, N.L.A., Woodend, D.M. and Wolever, T.M.S. (2002) Inverse association between the effect of carbohydrates on blood glucose and subsequent short-term food intake in young men. *American Journal of Clinical Nutrition* 76, 1023–1030.

Andersson, H. (1992) The ileostomy model for the study of carbohydrate digestion and carbohydrate effects on sterol excretion in man. *European Journal of Clinical Nutrition* 46 (Suppl. 2), S69–S76.

Andersson, H.B., Ellegård, L.H. and Bosaeus, I.G. (1999) Nondigestibility characteristics of inulin and oligofructose in humans. *Journal of Nutrition* 129, 1428S–1430S.

Anonymous (1995) UK prospective diabetes study 16. Overview of 6 years' therapy of type II diabetes: a progressive disease. UK Prospective Diabetes Study Group. *Diabetes* 44, 1249–1258.

Anonymous (1998a) Intensive blood-glucose control with sulphonylureas or insulin compared with conventional treatment and risk of complications in patients with type 2 diabetes (UKPDS 33). UK Prospective Diabetes Study (IKPDS) Group. *Lancet* 352, 837–853.

Anonymous (1998b) Effect of intensive blood-glucose control with metformin on complications in overweight patients with type 2 diabetes (UKPDS 34). UK Prospective Diabetes Study Group. *Lancet* 352, 854–865.

Appel, L.J., Moore, T.J., Obarzanek, E., Vollmer, W.M., Svetkey, L.P., Sacks, F.M., Bray, G.A., Vogt, T.M., Cutler, J.A., Windhauser, M.M., Lin, P.-H., Karanja, N. and the DASH Collaborative Group (1997) A clinical trial of the effects of dietary patterns on blood pressure. *New England Journal of Medicine* 336, 1117–1124.

Armario, A., Marti, O., Molina, T., de Pablo, J. and Valeds, M. (1996) Acute stress markers in humans: response of plasma glucose, cortisol and prolactin to two examinations differing in the anxiety they provoke. *Psychoneuroendocrinology* 21, 17–24.

Armstrong, L.E. (2002) Caffeine, body fluid–electrolyte balance, and exercise performance. *International Journal of Sport Nutrition and Exercise Metabolism* 12, 189–206.

Armstrong, J., Rielly, J.J. and the Child Health Information Team (2003) Breastfeeding and lowering the risk of childhood obesity. *Lancet* 359, 2003–2004.

Ascaso, J.F., Pardo, S., Real, J.T., Lorente, R.I., Priego, A. and Carmena, R. (2003) Diagnosing insulin resistance by simple quantitative methods in subjects with normal glucose metabolism. *Diabetes Care* 26, 3320–3325.

Asp, N.-G.L. (1995) Classification and methodology of food carbohydrates as related to nutritional effects. *American Journal of Clinical Nutrition* 61(Suppl.), 930S–937S.

Astrup, A. (1998) The American Paradox: the role of energy-dense fat-reduced food in the increasing prevalence of obesity. *Current Opinion in Clinical Nutrition and Metabolic Care* 1, 573–577.

Augustin, L.S., Dal Maso, L., La Vecchia, C., Parpinel, M., Negri, E., Vaccarella, S., Kendall, C.W., Jenkins, D.J. and Franceschi, S. (2001) Dietary glycemic index and glycemic load, and breast cancer risk: a case–control study. *Annals of Oncology* 12, 1533–1538.

Augustin, L.S.A., Polesel, J., Bosetti, C., Kendall, C.W., La Vecchia, C., Parpinel, M., Conti, E., Montella, M., Franceschi, S., Jenkins, D.J.A. and Dal Maso, L. (2003a) Dietary glycemic index, glycemic load and ovarian cancer risk: a case–control study in Italy. *Annals of Oncology* 14, 78–84.

Augustin, L.S.A., Gallus, S., Bosetti, C., Levi, F., Negri, E., Franceschi, S., Dal Maso, L., Jenkins, D.J.A., Kendall, C.W. and La Vecchia, C. (2003b) Glycemic index and glycemic load in endometrial cancer. *International Journal of Cancer* 105, 404–407.

Augustin, L.S.A., Gallus, S., Franceschi, S., Negri, E., Jenkins, D.J.A., Kendall, C.W., Dal Maso, L., Talamini, R. and La Vecchia, C. (2003c) Glycemic index and load and risk of upper aero-digestive tract neoplasms (Italy). *Cancer Causes and Control* 14, 657–662.

Augustin, L.S.A., Gallus, S., Negri, E. and La Vecchia, C. (2004a) Glycemic index, glycemic load and risk of gastric cancer. *Annals of Oncology* 15, 581–584.

Augustin, L.S.A., Galeone, C., Dal Maso, L., Pelucchi, C., Ramzzotti, V., Jenkins, D.J.A., Montella, M., Talamini, R., Negri, E., Franceschi, S. and La Vechia, C. (2004b) Glycemic index, glycemic load and risk of prostate cancer. *International Journal of Cancer* 112, 446–450.

Austin, M.A. (2000) Triglyceride, small, dense low-density lipoprotein, and the atherogenic lipoprotein phenotype. *Current Atherosclerosis Reports* 2, 200–207.

Baghurst, K.I., Baghurst, P.A. and Record, S.A. (1992) Demographic and nutritional profiles of people consuming varying levels of added sugars. *Nutrition Research* 12, 1455–1465.

Balkau, B., Charles, M.A., Drivsholm, T., Borch-Johnsen, K., Wareham, N., Yudkin, J.S., Morris, R., Zavaroni, I., van Dam, R., Feskins, E., Gabriel, R., Diet, M., Nilsson, P., Hedblad, B. and European Group for the Study of Insulin Resistance (EGIR) (2002) Frequency of the WHO metabolic syndrome in European cohorts, and an alternative definition of an insulin resistance syndrome. *Diabetes Metabolism* 28, 364–376.

Bantle, J.P., Laine, D.C., Castle, G.W., Thomas, W., Hoogwerf, B.J. and Goetz, F.C. (1983) Postprandial glucose and insulin responses to meals containing different carbohydrates in normal and diabetic subjects. *New England Journal of Medicine* 309, 7–12.

Barker, D.J.P. (1996) Growth *in utero* and coronary heart disease. *Nutrition Reviews* 54, S1–S7.

Barrett-Connor, E. (1991) Nutrition epidemiology: how do we know what they ate? *American Journal of Clinical Nutrition* 54, 182S–187S.

Bartram, H.-P., Scheppach, W., Heid, C., Fabian, C. and Kasper, H. (1991) Effect of starch malabsorption on fecal bile acids and neutral sterols in humans: possible implications for colonic carcinogenesis. *Cancer Research* 51, 4238–4242.

Basu, A., Alzaid, A., Dinneen, S., Caumo, A., Cobelli, C. and Rizza, R.A. (1996) Effects of a change in the pattern of insulin delivery on carbohydrate tolerance in diabetic and nondiabetic humans in the presence of differing degrees of insulin resistance. *Journal of Clinical Investigation* 97, 2351–2361.

Batterham, R.L., Cohen, M.A., Ellis, S.M., Le Roux, C.W., Withers, D.J., Frost, G.S., Ghatei, M.A. and Bloom, S.R. (2003a) Inhibition of food intake in obese subjects by peptide YY3-36. *New England Journal of Medicine* 349, 941–948.

Batterham, R.L., Le Roux, C.W., Cohen, M.A., Park, A.J., Ellis, S.M., Patterson, M., Frost, G.S., Ghatei, M.A. and Bloom, S.R. (2003b) Pancreatic polypeptide reduces appetite and food intake in humans. *Journal of Clinical Endocrinology and Metabolism* 88, 3989–3992.

Baynes, J.W. and Thorpe, S.R. (1999) Role of oxidative stress in diabetic complications: a new perspective on an old paradigm. *Diabetes* 48, 1–9.

Beard, J.C., Halter, J.B., Best, J.D., Pfeifer, M.A. and Porte, D. Jr (1984) Dexamethasone-induced insulin resistance enhances B cell responsiveness to glucose levels in normal men. *American Journal of Physiology* 247, E592–E596.

Beaton, G.H. (1994) Approaches to analysis of dietary data: relationship between planned analyses and choice of methodology. *American Journal of Clinical Nutrition* 59 (Suppl. 1), 253S–261S.

Beaton, G.H., Burema, J. and Ritenbaugh, C. (1997) Errors in the interpretation of dietary assessments. *American Journal of Clinical Nutrition* 65, 1100S–1107S.

Beaugerie, L., Flourié, B., Marteau, P., Pellier, P., Franchisseur, C. and Rambaud, J.-C. (1990) Digestion and absorption in the human intestine of three sugar alcohols. *Gastroenterology* 99, 717–723.

Beebe, C. (1999) Diets with a low glycemic index: not ready for practice yet! *Nutrition Today* 34, 82–86.

Behall, K.M., Scholfield, D.J. and Canary, J. (1988) Effect of starch structure on glucose and insulin responses in adults. *American Journal of Clinical Nutrition* 47, 428–432.

Behme, M.T. and Dupre, J. (1989) All bran vs corn flakes: plasma glucose and insulin responses in young females. *American Journal of Clinical Nutrition* 50, 1240–1243.

Bell, S.J. and Sears, B. (2003) Low-glycemic-load diets: impact on obesity and chronic diseases. *Critical Reviews in Food Science and Nutrition* 43, 357–377.

Benini, L., Castellani, G., Brighenti, F., Heaton, K.W., Brentegani, M.T., Casiraghi, M.C., Sembenini, C., Pellegrini, N., Fioretta, A., Minniti, G., Porrini, M., Testolin, G. and Vantini, I. (1995) Gastric emptying of a solid meal is accelerated by the removal of dietary fibre naturally present in food. *Gut* 36, 825–830.

Benton, D. and Nabb, S. (2003) Carbohydrate, memory, and mood. *Nutrition Reviews* 61, S61–S67.

Benton, D. and Parker, P.Y. (1998) Breakfast, blood glucose and cognition. *American Journal of Clinical Nutrition* 67 (Suppl.), 772S–778S.

Benton, D., Ruffin, M.-P., Lassel, T., Nabb, S., Messaoudi, M., Vinoy, S., Desor, D. and Lang, V. (2003) The delivery rate of dietary carbohydrates affects cognitive performance in both rats and humans. *Psychopharmacology* (Berl) 166 (1), 86–90.

Bergman, R.N. (1989) Lilly Lecture 1989: toward physiological understanding of glucose tolerance: minimal model approach. *Diabetes* 38, 1512–1527.

Bergman, R.N., Phillips, L.S. and Cobelli, C. (1981) Physiologic evaluation of factors controlling glucose tolerance in man: measurement of insulin sensitivity and beta-cell glucose sensitivity from the response to intravenous glucose. *Journal of Clinical Investigation* 68, 1456–1467.

Bergman, R.N., Finegood, D.T. and Ader, M. (1985) Assessment of insulin sensitivity *in vivo*. *Endocrine Reviews* 6, 45–86.

Bergman, R.N., Prager, R., Volund, A. and Olefsky, J.M. (1987) Equivalence of the insulin sensitivity index in man derived by the minimal model method and the euglycemic glucose clamp. *Journal of Clinical Investigation* 79, 790–800.

Bergstrom, J., Hermansen, L., Hultman, E. and Saltin, B. (1967) Diet, muscle glycogen and physical performance. *Acta Physiologica Scandinavica* 71, 140–150.

Berkus, M.D., Stern, M.P., Mitchell, B.D., Newton, E.R. and Langer, O. (1990) Does fasting interval affect the glucose challenge test? *American Journal of Obstetrics and Gynecology* 163, 1812–1817.

Bernard, C. (1848) Nouvelle fonction du foie. *Compte rendu Acadamie du Sciences*, Paris 27, 249, 253, 514.

Bernard, C. (1855) *Leçons de physiologie expérimentale appliqué a la medicine, faite au Collége de France.* J.B. Baillière, Paris.

Berne, C., Fagius, J., Pollare, Y. and Hemjadhl, P. (1992) The sympathetic response to euglycemic hyperinsulinemia. *Diabetologia* 35, 873–879.

Bertelsen, J., Christiansen, C., Thomsen, C., Poulsen, P.L., Vestergaard, S., Steinov, A., Rasmussen, L.H., Rasmussen, O. and Hermansen K. (1993) Effect of meal frequency on blood glucose, insulin and free fatty acids in NIDDM subjects. *Diabetes Care* 16, 4–7.

Biliaderis, C.G. (1991) The structure and interactions of starch with food constituents. *Canadian Journal of Physiology and Pharmacology* 69, 60–78.

Bingham, S.A., Day, N.E., Luben, R., Ferrari, P., Slimani, N., Norat, T., Clavel-Chapelon, F., Kesse, E., Nieters, A., Boeing, H., Tjønneland, A., Overvad, K., Martinez, C., Dorronsoro, M., Gonzalez, C.A., Key, T.J., Trichopoulou, A., Naska, A., Vineis, P., Tumino, R., Krogh, V., Bueno-de-Mesquita, H.B., Peeters, P.H., Berglund, G., Hallmans, G., Lund, E., Skeie, G., Kaaks, R. and Riboli, E. (2003) Dietary fibre in food and protection against colorectal cancer in the European Prospective Investigation into Cancer and Nutrition (EPIC): an observational study. *Lancet* 361, 1496–1501.

Birkett, A., Muir, J., Phillips, J., Jones, G. and O'Dea, K. (1996) Resistant starch lowers fecal concentrations of ammonia and phenols in humans. *American Journal of Clinical Nutrition* 63, 766–772.

Bishop, J.S. and Marks, P.A. (1959) Studies on carbohydrate metabolism in patients with neoplastic disease. II. Response to insulin administration. *Journal of Clinical Investigation* 38, 668–672.

Björck, I., Granfeldt, Y., Liljeberg, H., Tovar, J. and Asp, N.G. (1994) Food properties affecting the digestion and absorption of carbohydrates. *American Journal of Clinical Nutrition* 59 (Suppl. 3), 699S–705S.

Björck, I., Liljeberg, H. and Östman, E. (2000) Low glycaemic-index foods. *British Journal of Nutrition* 83 (Suppl. 1), S149–S155.

Black, D.D. (1995) Intestinal lipoprotein metabolism. *Journal of Pediatric Gastroenterology and Nutrition* 20, 125–147.

Black, A.E., Prentice, A.M., Goldberg, G.R., Jebb, S.A., Livingston, M.B.E. and Coward, W.A. (1993) Measurements of total energy expenditure provide insights into the validity of dietary measurements of energy intake. *Journal of the American Dietetic Association* 93, 572–579.

Blackburn, N.A., Redfern, J.S., Jarjis, H., Holgate, A.M., Hanning, I., Scarpello, J.H.B., Johnson, I.T. and Read, N.W. (1984) The mechanism of action of guar gum in improving glucose tolerance in man. *Clinical Science* 66, 329–336.

Block, G., Hartman, A.M., Dresser, C.M., Carroll, M.D., Gannon, J. and Gardner, L. (1986) A data-bases approach to diet questionnaire design and testing. *American Journal of Epidemiology* 124, 453–469.

Block, G., Woods, M., Potosky, A. and Clifford, C. (1990) Validation of a self-administered diet history questionnaire using multiple diet records. *Journal of Clinical Epidemiology* 43, 1327–1335.

Bloom, S.R. and Polak, J.M. (1981) *Gut Hormones*, 2nd edn. Churchill Livingstone, Edinburgh, London, 664 pp.

Boden, G. and Tappy, L. (1990) Effects of amino acids on glucose disposal. *Diabetes* 39, 1079–1084.

Boden, G., Chen, X., Ruiz, J., White, J.V. and Rossetti, L. (1994) Mechanisms of fatty acid-induced inhibition of glucose uptake. *Journal of Clinical Investigation* 93, 2438–2446.

Boekema, P.J., Samson, M., van Berge Henegouwen, G.P. and Smout, A.J. (1999) Coffee and gastrointestinal function: facts and fiction. A review. *Scandinavian Journal of Gastroenterology Supplement* 230, 35–39.

Bolton, R.P., Heaton, K.W. and Burroughs, L.F. (1981) The role of dietary fiber in satiety, glucose, and insulin: studies with fruit and fruit juice. *American Journal of Clinical Nutrition* 34, 211–217.

Bond, J.H. Jr and Levitt, M.D. (1972) Use of pulmonary hydrogen ($H_2$) measurements to quantitate carbohydrate absorption. Study of partially gastrectomized patients. *Journal of Clinical Investigation* 51, 1219–1225.

Bond, J.H. Jr and Levitt, M.D. (1975) Factors affecting the concentration of combustible gases in the colon during colonoscopy. *Gastroenterology* 68, 1445–1448.

Bond, J.H. Jr, Levitt, M.D. and Prentiss, R. (1975) Investigation of small bowel transit time in man utilizing pulmonary hydrogen ($H_2$) measurements. *Journal of Laboratory and Clinical Medicine* 85, 546–555.

Bond, J.H., Levy, M. and Levitt, M.D. (1976) Explosion of hydrogen gas in the colon during proctosigmoidoscopy. *Gastrointestinal Endoscopy* 23, 41–42.

Bonora, E., Moghetti, P., Zancanaro, C., Cigolini, M., Querena, M., Cacciatori, V., Corgnati, A. and Muggeo, M. (1989) Estimates of *in-vivo* insulin action in man: comparison of insulin tolerance tests with euglycemic and hyperglycemic glucose clamp studies. *Journal of Clinical Endocrinology and Metabolism* 68, 374–378.

Borghouts, L.B. and Keizer, H.A. (2000) Exercise and insulin sensitivity: a review. *International Journal of Sports Medicine* 21, 1–12.

Bornet, F.R.J., Costagliola, D., Rizkalla, S.W., Blayo, A., Fontvieille, A.-M., Haardt, M.-J., Letanoux, M., Tchobroutsky, G. and Slama, G. (1987) Insulinemic and glycemic indexes of six starch-rich foods taken alone and in a mixed meal by type 2 diabetics. *American Journal of Clinical Nutrition* 45, 588–595.

Bornet, F.R.J., Fontvieille, A.M., Rizkalla, S., Colonna, P., Blayo, A., Mercier, C. and Slama, G. (1989) Insulin and glycemic responses in healthy humans to native starches processed in different ways: correlation with *in vitro* alpha-amylase hydrolysis. *American Journal of Clinical Nutrition* 50, 315–323.

Bornet, F.R.J., Bizais, Y., Varannes, S.B.D., Pouliquen, B., Laval, J.D. and Galmiche, J.P. (1990) Alpha-amylase (EC 3.2.1.1) susceptibility rather than viscosity or gastric emptying rate controls plasma responses to starch in healthy humans. *British Journal of Nutrition* 63, 207–220.

Bouché, C., Rizkalla, S.W., Luo, J., Vidal, H., Veronese, A., Pacher, N., Fouquet, C., Lang, V. and Slama, G. (2002) Five-week, low-glycemic index diet decreases total fat mass and improves plasma lipid profile in moderately overweight nondiabetic men. *Diabetes Care* 25, 822–828.

Bouhnik, Y., Raskine, L., Simoneau, G., Vicaut, E., Neut, C., Flourie, B., Brouns, F. and Bornet, F.R. (2004) The capacity of nondigestible carbohydrates to stimulate fecal bifidobacteria in healthy humans: a double-blind, randomized, placebo-controlled, parallel-group, dose–response relation study. *American Journal of Clinical Nutrition* 80, 1658–1664.

Bourdon, I., Yokoyama, W., Davis, P., Hudson, C., Backus, R., Richter, D., Knuckles, B. and Schneeman, B.O. (1999) Postprandial lipid, glucose, insulin, and cholecystokinin responses in men fed barley pasta enriched with beta-glucan. *American Journal of Clinical Nutrition* 69, 55–63.

Bourdon, I., Olson, B., Backus, R., Richter, B.D., Davis, P.A. and Schneeman, B.O. (2001) Beans, as a source of dietary fiber, increase cholecystokinin and apolipoprotein b48 response to test meals in men. *Journal of Nutrition* 131, 1485–1490.

Boushey, C.J., Beresford, S.A., Omenn, G.S. and Motulsky, A.G. (1995) A quantitative assessment of plasma homocysteine as a risk factor for vascular disease. Probable benefits of increasing folic acid intakes. *Journal of the American Medical Association* 274, 1049–1057.

Brand, J.C., Nicholson, P.L., Thorburn, A.W. and Truswell, A.S. (1985) Food processing and the glycemic index. *American Journal of Clinical Nutrition* 42, 1192–1196.

Brand, J.C., Colagiuri, S., Crossman, S., Allen, A., Roberts, D.C.K. and Truswell, A.S. (1991) Low-glycemic index foods improve long-term glycemic control in NIDDM. *Diabetes Care* 14, 95–101.

Brand Miller, J.C. and Foster-Powell, K. (1999) Diets with a low glycemic index: from theory to practice. *Nutrition Today* 34, 64–72.

Brand-Miller, J. and Holt, S. (2004) Testing the glycaemic index of foods: *in vivo*, not *in vitro*. *European Journal of Clinical Nutrition* 58, 700–701.

Brand Miller, J.C. and Lobbesoo, I. (1994) Replacing starch with sucrose in a high glycaemic index breakfast cereal lowers glycaemic and insulin responses. *European Journal of Clinical Nutrition* 48, 749–752.

Brand Miller, J. and Wolever, T.M.S. (2005) The use of glycaemic index tables to predict glycaemic index of breakfast meals. *British Journal of Nutrition* 94, 133–134.

Brand Miller, J., Pang, E. and Bramall, L. (1992) Rice: a high or low glycemic index food? *American Journal of Clinical Nutrition* 56, 1034–1036.

Brand Miller, J., Pang, E. and Broomhead, L. (1995) The glycaemic index of foods containing sugars: comparison of foods with naturally-occurring v. added sugars. *British Journal of Nutrition* 73, 613–623.

Brand-Miller, J.C., McVeagh, P., McNeil, Y. and Messer, M. (1998) Digestion of human milk oligosaccharides by healthy infants evaluated by the lactulose hydrogen breath test. *Journal of Pediatrics* 133, 95–98.

Brand-Miller, J.C., Colagiuri, S. and Gan, S.T. (2000) Insulin sensitivity predicts glycemia after a protein load. *Metabolism: Clinical and Experimental* 49, 1–5.

Brand-Miller, J.C., Thomas, M., Swan, V., Ahmad, Z.I., Petocz, P. and Colagiuri, S. (2003a) Physiological validation of the concept of glycemic load in lean young men. *Journal of Nutrition* 133, 2728–2732.

Brand-Miller, J., Hayne, S., Petocz, P. and Colagiuri, S. (2003b) Low-glycemic index diets in the management of diabetes: a meta-analysis of randomized controlled trials. *Diabetes Care* 26, 2261–2267.

Brief, D.J. and Davis, J.D. (1984) Reduction of food intake and body weight by chronic intraventricular insulin infusion. *Brain Research Bulletin* 12, 571–575.

Brighenti, F., Castellani, G., Benini, L., Casiraghi, M.C., Leopardi, E., Crovetti, R. and Testolin, G. (1995) Effect of neutralized and native vinegar on blood glucose and acetate responses to a mixed meal in healthy subjects. *European Journal of Clinical Nutrition* 49, 242–247.

Brighenti, F., Casiraghi, M.C., Canzi, E. and Ferrari, A. (1999) Effect of consumption of a ready-to-eat breakfast cereal containing inulin on the intestinal milieu and blood lipids in healthy male volunteers. *European Journal of Clinical Nutrition* 53, 726–733.

Brouns, F., Senden, J., Beckers, E.J. and Saris, W.H. (1995) Osmolarity does not affect the gastric emptying rate of oral rehydration solutions. *Journal of Parenteral and Enteral Nutrition* 19, 403–406.

Brown, R.C., Kelleher, J. and Losowsky, M.S. (1979) The effect of pectin on the structure and function of the rat small intestine. *British Journal of Nutrition* 42, 357–365.

Brubaker, P.L. (1991) Regulation of intestinal proglucagon-derived peptide secretion by intestinal regulatory peptides. *Endocrinology* 128, 3175–3182.

Bruce, W.R., Wolever, T.M.S. and Giacca, A. (2000) Mechanisms linking diet and colorectal cancer: the possible role of insulin resistance. *Nutrition and Cancer* 37, 19–26.

Brynes, A.E., Lee, J.L., Brighton, R.E., Leeds, A.R., Dornhorst, A. and Frost, G.S. (2003) A low glycemic diet significantly improves the 24-h blood glucose profile in people with type 2 diabetes, as assessed using the continuous glucose MiniMed monitor. *Diabetes Care* 26, 548–549.

Brynes, A.E., Adamson, J., Dornhorst, A. and Frost, G.S. (2005) The beneficial effect of a diet with low glycaemic index on 24 h glucose profiles of healthy young people as assessed by continuous glucose monitoring. *British Journal of Nutrition* 93, 179–182.

Burke, L.M., Collier, G.R. and Hargreaves, M. (1993) Muscle glycogen storage after prolonged exercise: effect of the glycemic index of carbohydrate feedings. *Journal of Applied Physiology* 75, 1019–1023.

Burke, L.M., Kiens, B. and Ivy, J.L. (2004) Carbohydrates and fat for training and recovery. *Journal of Sports Sciences* 22, 15–30.

Burkitt, D.P. (1971) Epidemiology of cancer of the colon and rectum. *Cancer* 28, 3–13.

Burkitt, D.P. and Trowell, H.C. (1975) *Refined Carbohydrate Foods and Disease.* Academic Press, London.

Burrin, J.M. and Alberti, K.G.M.M. (1990) What is blood glucose: can it be measured? *Diabetic Medicine* 7, 199–206.

Buyken, A.E., Toeller, M., Heitkamp, G., Karamanos, B., Rottiers, R., Muggeo, M., Fuller, J.H. and the EURODIAB IDDM Complications Study Group (2001) Glycemic index in the diet of European outpatients with type 1 diabetes: relations to glycated hemoglobin and serum lipids. *American Journal of Clinical Nutrition* 73, 574–581.

Cai, W., He, J.C., Zhu, L., Peppa, M., Lu, C., Uribarri, J. and Vlassara, H. (2004) High levels of dietary advanced glycation end products transform low-density lipoprotein into a potent redox-sensitive mitogen-activated protein kinase stimulant in diabetic patients. *Circulation* 110, 285–291.

Calle-Pascual, A.L., Bordiu, E., Romeo, S., Romero, C., Martin-Alvarez, P.J. and Marañes, J.P. (1987) Food glycaemic index of meal glycaemic response. *Human Nutrition: Applied Nutrition* 40A, 282–286.

Calloway, D.H. (1972) End products of human metabolism as affected by diet and space conditions. *Environmental Biology and Medicine* 1, 197–202.

Calloway, D.H. and Burroughs, S.E. (1969) Effect of dried beans and silicone on intestinal hydrogen and methane production in man. *Gut* 10, 180–184.

Calloway, D.H. and Murphy, E.L. (1969) Intestinal hydrogen and methane of men fed space diet. *Life Science and Space Research* 7, 102–109.

Calloway, D.H., Murphy, E.L. and Bauer, D. (1969) Determination of lactose intolerance by breath analysis. *American Journal of Digestive Diseases* 14, 811–815.

Calloway, D.H., Hickey, C.A. and Murphy, E.L. (1971) Reduction of intestinal gas-forming properties of legumes by traditional and experimental food processing methods. *Journal of Food Science* 36, 251–255.

Campbell, J.E., Glowczewski, T. and Wolever, T.M.S. (2003) Controlling subjects' prior diet and activities does not reduce within-subject variation of postprandial glycemic responses to foods. *Nutrition Research* 23, 621–629.

Campfield, L.A., Brandon, P. and Smith, F.J. (1985) On-line continuous measurement of blood glucose and meal pattern in free-feeding rats: the role of glucose in meal initiation. *Brain Research Bulletin* 14, 605–616.

Campfield, L.A., Smith, F.J., Rosenbaum, M. and Hirsch, J. (1996) Human eating: evidence for a physiological basis using a modified paradigm. *Neuroscience and Biobehavioural Reviews* 20, 133–137.

Canadian Diabetes Association Clinical Practice Guidelines Expert Committee (2003) Canadian Diabetes Association 2003 Clinical Practice Guidelines for the Prevention and Management of Diabetes in Canada. *Canadian Journal of Diabetes* 27 (Suppl. 2), S1–S152.

Canadian Pharmacists Association (2003) *Compendium of Pharmaceuticals and Specialities: The Canadian Drug Reference for Health Professionals.* Ottawa, Ontario.

Carlsson, S., Persson, P.G., Alvarsson, M., Efendic, S., Norman, A., Svanstrom, L., Ostenson, C.G. and Grill, V. (1999) Low birth weight, family history of diabetes, and glucose intolerance in Swedish middle-aged men. *Diabetes Care* 22, 1043–1047.

Carpentier, A., Mittelman, S.D., Lamarche, B., Bergman, R.N., Giacca, A. and Lewis, G.F. (1999) Acute enhancement of insulin secretion by FFA in humans is lost with prolonged FFA elevation. *American Journal of Physiology* 276, E1055–E1066.

Caspary, W.F. (1972) On the mechanism of D-xylose absorption from the intestine. *Gastroenterology* 63, 531–532.

Castro, A., Scott, J.P., Grettie, D.P., Macfarlane, D. and Bailey, R.E. (1970) Plasma insulin and glucose responses of healthy subjects to varying glucose loads during three-hour oral glucose tolerance tests. *Diabetes* 19, 842–851.

Catalano, P.M., Tyzbir, E.D., Wolfe, R.R., Calles, J., Roman, N.M., Amini, S.B. and Sims, E.A. (1993) Carbohydrate metabolism during pregnancy in control subjects and women with gestational diabetes. *American Journal of Physiology* 264, E60–E67.

Catalano, P.M., Huston, L., Amini, S.B. and Kalhan, S.C. (1999) Longitudinal changes in glucose metabolism during pregnancy in obese women with normal glucose tolerance and gestational diabetes mellitus. *American Journal of Obstetrics and Gynecology* 180, 903–916.

Caumo, A., Bergman, R.N. and Cobelli, C. (2000) Insulin sensitivity from meal tolerance tests in normal subjects: a minimal model index. *Journal of Clinical Endocrinology and Metabolism* 85, 4396–4402.

Cavaghan, M.K., Ehrmann, D.A. and Polonsky, K.S. (2000) Interactions between insulin resistance and insulin secretion in the development of glucose intolerance. *Journal of Clinical Investigation* 106, 329–333.

Ceriello, A. (1998) The emerging role of post-prandial hyperglycaemic spikes in the pathogenesis of diabetic complications. *Diabetic Medicine* 15, 188–193.

Ceriello, A., Piconi, L., Quagliaro, L., Wang, Y., Schnabel, C.A., Ruggles, J.A., Gloster, M.A., Maggs, D.G., and Weyer, C. (2005) Effects of pramlintide on postprandial glucose excursions and measures of oxidative stress in patients with type 1 diabetes. *Diabetes Care* 28, 632–637.

Champ, M.M., Molis, C., Flourie, B., Bornet, F., Pellier, P., Colonna, P., Galmiche, J.P. and Rambaud, J.C. (1998) Small-intestinal digestion of partially resistant cornstarch in healthy subjects. *American Journal of Clinical Nutrition* 68, 705–710.

Champ, M., Langkilde, A.M., Brouns, F., Kettlitz, B. and Le Bail-Collet, Y. (2003) Advances in dietary fibre characterization II: consumption, chemistry, physiology and measurement of resistant starch: implications for health and food labeling. *Nutrition Research Reviews* 16, 143–161.

Chapman, I.M., Goble, E.A., Wittert, G.A., Morley, J.E. and Horowitz, M. (1998) Effect of intravenous glucose and euglycemic insulin infusions on short-term appetite and food intake. *American Journal of Physiology* 274, R596–R603.

Chen, M. and Porte, D. Jr (1975) The effect of rate and dose of glucose infusion on the acute insulin response in man. *Journal of Clinical Endocrinology and Metabolism* 42, 1168–1175.

Chen, Y.-D.I., Coulston, A.M., Zhou, M.-Y., Hollenbeck, C.B. and Reaven, G.M. (1995) Why do low-fat high-carbohydrate diets accentuate postprandial lipemia in patients with NIDDM? *Diabetes Care* 18, 10–16.

Cherbut, C., des Varannes, S., Schnee, M., Rival, M., Galmiche, J.-P. and Delort-Laval, J. (1994) Involvement of small intestinal motility in blood glucose response to dietary fibre in man. *British Journal of Nutrition* 71, 675–685.

Chew, I., Brand, J.C., Thorburn, A.W. and Truswell, A.S. (1988) Application of the glycemic index to mixed meals. *American Journal of Clinical Nutrition* 47, 53–56.

Chiasson, J.-L., Josse, R.G., Hunt, J.A., Palmason, C., Rodger, N.W., Ross, S.A., Ryan, E.A., Tan, M.H. and Wolever, T.M.S. (1994) The efficacy of acarbose in the treatment of patients with non-insulin-dependent diabetes mellitus. A multicenter controlled clinical trial. *Annals of Internal Medicine* 121, 928–935.

Chiasson, J-L., Josse, R.G., Leiter, L.A., Mihic, M., Nathan, D.M., Palmason, C., Cohen, R.M. and Wolever, T.M.S. (1996) The effect of acarbose on insulin sensitivity in subjects with impaired glucose tolerance. *Diabetes Care* 19, 1190–1193.

Chiasson, J.-L., Naditch, L. and Miglitol Canadian University Investigator Group (2001) The synergistic effect of miglitol plus metformin combination therapy in the treatment of type 2 diabetes. *Diabetes Care* 24, 989–994.

Chiasson, J.-L., Josse, R.G., Gomis, R., Hanefeld, M., Karasik, A., Laakso, M. and the STOP-NIDDM Trial Research Group (2002) Acarbose for prevention of type 2 diabetes mellitus: the STOP-NIDDM randomised trial. *Lancet* 359, 2072–2077.

Chiasson, J.-L., Josse, R.G., Gomis, R., Hanefeld, M., Karasik, A., Laakso, M. and the STOP-NIDDM Trial Research Group (2003) Acarbose treatment and the risk of cardiovascular disease and hypertension in patients with impaired glucose tolerance: the STOP-NIDDM trial. *Journal of the American Medical Association* 290, 486–494.

Christensen, N.J., Ørskov, H. and Hansen, A.P. (1972) Significance of glucose load in oral glucose tolerance tests. *Acta Medica Scandinavica* 192, 337–342.

Christie, M.R., Molvig, J., Hawkes, C.J., Carstensen, B., Mandrup-Poulsen, T. and the Canadian-European Randomized Control Trial Group (2002) IA-2 antibody-negative status predicts remission and recovery of C-peptide levels in type 1 diabetic patients treated with cyclosporin. *Diabetes Care* 25, 1192–1197.

Clapp, J.F. III (2002) Maternal carbohydrate intake and pregnancy outcome. *Proceedings of the Nutrition Society* 61, 45–50.

Clausen, J.O., Borch-Johnsen, K., Ibsen, H., Bergman, R.N., Hougaard, P., Winther, K. and Pedersen, O. (1996) Insulin sensitivity index, acute insulin response, and glucose effectiveness in a population-based sample of 380 young healthy Caucasians: analysis of the impact of gender, body fat, physical fitness and life-style factors. *Journal of Clinical Investigation* 98, 1195–1209.

Clissold, S.P. and Edwards, C. (1988) Acarbose: a preliminary review of its pharmacodynamic and pharmacokinetic properties, and therapeutic potential. *Drugs* 35, 214–243.

Coffey, R.J., Go, G.L., Zinsmeister, A.R. and DiMagno, E.P. (1986) The acute effects of coffee and caffeine on human interdigestive exocrine pancreatic secretion. *Pancreas* 1, 55–61.

Cohen, M.A., Ellis, S.M., Le Roux, C.W., Batterham, R.L., Park, A., Patterson, M., Frost, G.S., Ghatei, M.A. and Bloom, S.R. (2003) Oxyntomodulin suppresses appetite and reduces food intake in humans. *Journal of Clinical Endocrinology and Metabolism* 88, 4696–4701.

Colagiuri, S., Miller, J.J., Holliday, J.L. and Phelan, E. (1986) Comparison of plasma glucose, serum insulin, and c-peptide responses to three isocaloric breakfasts in non-insulin-dependent diabetic subjects. *Diabetes Care* 9, 250–254.

Collier, G.R. and O'Dea, K. (1983) The effect of coingestion of fat on the glucose, insulin and gastric inhibitory polypeptide responses to carbohydrate and protein. *American Journal of Clinical Nutrition* 37, 941–944.

Collier, G.R., McLean, A. and O'Dea, K. (1984) Effect of co-ingestion of fat on the metabolic responses to slowly and rapidly absorbed carbohydrates. *Diabetologia* 26, 50–54.

Collier, G.R., Wolever, T.M.S., Wong, G.S. and Josse, R.G. (1986) Prediction of glycemic response to mixed meals in non-insulin dependent diabetic subjects. *American Journal of Clinical Nutrition* 44, 349–352.

Collier, G.R., Wolever, T.M.S. and Jenkins, D.J.A. (1987) Concurrent ingestion of fat and reduction in starch content impairs carbohydrate tolerance to subsequent meals. *American Journal of Clinical Nutrition* 45, 963–969.

Collier, G.R., Greenberg, G.R., Wolever, T.M.S. and Jenkins, D.J.A. (1988) The acute effect of fat on insulin secretion. *Journal of Clinical Endocrinology and Metabolism* 66, 323–326.

Conn, J.W. and Newburgh, L.H. (1936) The glycemic response to isoglucogenic quantities of protein and carbohydrate. *Journal of Clinical Investigation* 15, 665–671.

Copeland, G.P., Leinster, S.J., Davis, J.C. and Hipkin, L.J. (1987) Insulin resistance in patients with colorectal cancer. *British Journal of Surgery* 74, 1031–1035.

Coppack, S.W., Fisher, R.M., Gibbons, G.F., Humphreys, S.M., McDonough, M.J., Potts, J.L. and Frayn, K.N. (1990) Postprandial substrate deposition in human forearm and adipose tissue *in vivo*. *Clinical Science* 79, 339–348.

Corpe, C.P., Burant, C.F. and Hoekstra, J.H. (1999) Intestinal fructose absorption: clinical and molecular aspects. *Journal of Pediatric Gastroenterology and Nutrition* 28, 364–374.

Coulston, A.M., Greenfield, M.S., Kraemer, F.B., Tobey, T.A. and Reaven, G.M. (1980) Effect of source of dietary carbohydrate on plasma glucose and insulin responses to test meals in normal subjects. *American Journal of Clinical Nutrition* 33, 1279–1282.

Coulston, A.M., Greenfield, M.S., Kraemer, F.B., Tobey, T.A. and Reaven, G.M. (1981) Effect of difference in source of dietary carbohydrate on plasma glucose and insulin responses to meals in patients with impaired carbohydrate tolerance. *American Journal of Clinical Nutrition* 34, 2716–2720.

Coulston, A.M., Liu, G.C. and Reaven, G.M. (1983) Plasma glucose, insulin and lipid responses to high-carbohydrate low-fat diets in normal humans. *Metabolism: Clinical and Experimental* 32, 52–56.

Coulston, A.M., Hollenbeck, C.B., Liu, G.C., Williams, R.A., Starich, G.H., Mazzaferri, E.L. and Reaven, G.M. (1984a) Effect of source of dietary carbohydrate on plasma glucose, insulin, and gastric inhibitory polypeptide responses to test meals in subjects with noninsulin-dependent diabetes mellitus. *American Journal of Clinical Nutrition* 40, 965–970.

Coulston, A.M., Hollenbeck, C.B. and Reaven, G.M. (1984b) Utility of studies measuring glucose and insulin responses to various carbohydrate-containing foods. *American Journal of Clinical Nutrition* 39, 163–165.

Coulston, A.M., Hollenbeck, C.B., Swislocki, A.L. and Reaven, G.M. (1987) Effect of source of dietary carbohydrate on plasma glucose, insulin responses to mixed meals in subjects with NIDDM. *Diabetes Care* 10, 395–400.

Coutinho, M., Gerstein, H.C., Wang, Y. and Yusef, S. (1999) The relationship between glucose and incident cardiovascular events. A metaregression analysis of published data from 20 studies of 95,783 individuals followed for 12.4 years. *Diabetes Care* 22, 233–240.

Crapo, P.A., Reaven, G. and Olefsky, J. (1976) Plasma glucose and insulin responses to orally administered simple and complex carbohydrates. *Diabetes* 25, 741–747.

Crapo, P.A., Reaven, G. and Olefsky, J. (1977) Post-prandial plasma-glucose and -insulin responses to different complex carbohydrates. *Diabetes* 26, 1178–1183.

Crapo, P.A., Kolterman, O.G., Waldeck, N., Reaven, G. and Olefsky, J. (1980) Postprandial hormonal responses to different types of complex carbohydrate in individuals with impaired glucose tolerance. *American Journal of Clinical Nutrition* 33, 1723–1728.

Crapo, P.A., Insel, J., Sperling, M. and Kolterman, O.G. (1981) Comparison of serum glucose, insulin, and glucagon responses to different types of complex carbohydrate in noninsulin-dependent diabetic patients. *American Journal of Clinical Nutrition* 34, 184–190.

Crespo, C.J., Smit, E., Troiano, R., Barlett, S.J., Macera, C. and Andersen, R.E. (2001) Television watching, energy intake and obesity in US children: results from the third National Health and Nutrition Examination Survey, 1988–1994. *Archives of Pediatric and Adolescent Medicine* 155, 360–365.

Cummings, J.H. and Englyst, H.N. (1995) Gastrointestinal effects of food carbohydrates. *American Journal of Clinical Nutrition* 61(Suppl.), 938S–945S.

Cummings, J.H. and MacFarlane, G.T. (1991) The control and consequences of bacterial fermentation in the human colon. *Journal of Applied Bacteriology* 70, 443–459.

Cunningham, K.M. and Read, N.W. (1989) The effect of incorporating fat into different components of a meal on gastric emptying and postprandial blood glucose and insulin response. *British Journal of Nutrition* 61, 285–290.

Cunningham, K.M., Daly, J., Horowitz, M. and Read, N.W. (1991) Gastrointestinal adaptation to diets of differing fat composition in human volunteers. *Gut* 32, 483–486.

Cusin, I., Rohner-Jeanrenaud, F., Terrettaz, J. and Jeanrenaud, B. (1992) Hyperinsulinemia and its impact on obesity and insulin resistance. *International Journal of Obesity* 16 (Suppl. 4), S1–S11.

Dahlqvist, A. and Borgstrom, B. (1961) Digestion and absorption in man. *Biochemical Journal* 81, 411–418.

D'Alessio, D.D., Thirlby, R., Laschansky, E., Zebroski, H. and Ensinck, J. (1993) Response of tGLP-1 to nutrients in humans. *Digestion* 54, 377–379.

Daly, M.E., Vale, C., Walker, M., Littlefield, A., Alberti, K.G.M.M. and Mathers, J. (1998) Acute effects on insulin sensitivity and diurnal metabolic profiles of a high-sucrose compared with a high-starch diet. *American Journal of Clinical Nutrition* 67, 1186–1196.

Daly, M.E., Vale, C., Walker, M., Littlefield, A., Alberti, K.G.M.M. and Mathers, J. (2000) Acute fuel selection in response to high-sucrose and high-starch meals in healthy men. *American Journal of Clinical Nutrition* 71, 1516–1524.

Danjo, K., Nakaji, S., Fukuda, S., Shinoyama, T., Sakamoto, J. and Sugawara, K. (2003) The resistant starch level of health moisture-treated high amylose cornstarch is much lower when measured in the human terminal ileum than when estimated *in vitro*. *Journal of Nutrition* 133, 2218–2221.

Dansinger, M.L., Gleason, J.A., Griffith, J.L., Selker, H.P. and Schaefer, E.J. (2005) Comparison of the Atkins, Ornish, Weight Watchers, and Zone diets for weight loss and heart disease risk reduction: a randomized trial. *Journal of the American Medical Association* 293, 43–53.

de Castro, J.M. (2004) Genes, the environment and the control of food intake. *British Journal of Nutrition* 92 (Suppl. 1), S59–S62.

DECODE Study Group on behalf of the European Diabetes Epidemiology Group (2001) Glucose tolerance and cardiovascular mortality: comparison of fasting and 2-hour diagnostic criteria. *Archives of Internal Medicine* 161, 397–404.

Deeb, S.S., Zambon, A., Carr, M.C., Ayyobi, A.F. and Brunzell, J.D. (2003) Hepatic lipase and dyslipidemia: interactions among genetic variants, obesity, gender, and diet. *Journal of Lipid Research* 44, 1279–1286.

DeFronzo, R.A. (1988) Lilly Lecture 1987. The triumvirate: β-cell, muscle, liver: a collision responsible for NIDDM. *Diabetes* 37, 667–687.

DeFronzo, R.A. and Ferrannini, E. (1991) Insulin resistance: a multifaceted syndrome responsible for NIDDM, obesity, hypertension, dyslipidemia, and atherosclerotic cardiovascular disease. *Diabetes Care* 14, 173–194.

DeFronzo, R.A., Tobin, J.D. and Andres, R. (1979) Glucose clamp technique: a method for quantifying insulin secretion and resistance. *American Journal of Physiology* 237, E214–E223.

de Kalbermatten, N., Ravussin, E., Maeder, E., Geser, C., Jéquier, E. and Felber, J.P. (1980) Comparison of glucose, fructose, sorbitol and xylitol utilization in humans during insulin suppression. *Metabolism: Clinical and Experimental* 29, 62–66.

Delarue, J., Normand, S., Pachiaudi, C., Beylot, M., Lamisse, F. and Riou, J.P. (1993) The contribution of naturally labelled 13C fructose to glucose appearance in humans. *Diabetologia* 36, 338–345.

Della Man, C., Caumo, A. and Cobelli, C. (2002) The oral glucose minimal model: estimation of insulin sensitivity from a meal test. *IEEE Transactions on Biomedical Engineering* 49, 419–429.

Della Man, C., Caumo, A., Basu, R., Rizza, R., Toffolo, G. and Cobelli, C. (2004) Minimal model estimation of glucose absorption and insulin sensitivity from oral test: validation with a tracer method. *American Journal of Physiology – Endocrinology and Metabolism* 287, E637–E643.

de Lorgeril, M., Salen, P., Martin, J.-L., Monjaud, I., Delaye, J. and Mamelle, N. (1999) Mediterranean diet, traditional risk factors, and the rate of cardiovascular complications after myocardial infarction. *Circulation* 99, 779–785.

Del Prato, S., Leonetti, F., Simonson, D.C., Sheehan, P., Matsuda, M. and DeFronzo, R.A. (1994) Effect of sustained physiologic hyperinsulinaemia and hyperglycaemia on insulin secretion and insulin sensitivity in man. *Diabetologia* 37, 1025–1035.

Delzenne, N.M., Daubioul, C., Neyrinck, A., Lasa, M. and Taper, H.S. (2002) Inulin and oligofructose modulate lipid metabolism in animals: review of biochemical events and future prospects. *British Journal of Nutrition* 87 (Suppl. 2), S255–S259.

DeMarco, H.M., Sucher, K.P., Cisar, C.J. and Butterfield, G.E. (1999) Pre-exercise carbohydrate meals: application of glycemic index. *Medicine and Science in Sports and Exercise* 31, 164–170.

Demigné, C. and Rémésy, C. (1985) Stimulation of absorption of volatile fatty acids and minerals in the cecum of rats adapted to a very high fiber diet. *Journal of Nutrition* 115, 53–60.

de Nobel, E. and van't Laar, A. (1978) The size of the loading dose as an important determinant of the results of the oral glucose tolerance test: a study in subjects with slightly impaired glucose tolerance. *Diabetes* 27, 42–48.

Després, J.P. (1998) The insulin resistance-dyslipidemic syndrome of visceral obesity: effect on patients' risk. *Obesity Research* 6 (Suppl. 1), 8S–17S.

Després, J.-P., Lemieux, I. and Prud'homme, D. (2001) Treatment of obesity: need to focus on high risk abdominally obese patients. *British Medical Journal* 322, 716–720.

Diabetes Prevention Trial Type 1 Diabetes Study Group (2002) Effects of insulin in relatives of patients with type 1 diabetes mellitus. *New England Journal of Medicine* 346, 1685–1691.

Díaz, E.O., Galgani, J.E., Aguiree, C.A., Atwater, I.J. and Burrows, R. (2005) Effect of glycemic index on whole-body substrate oxidation in obese women. *International Journal of Obesity* 29, 108–114.

Dickson, B.C. and Gotlieb, A.I. (2003) Towards understanding acute destabilization of vulnerable atherosclerotic plaques. *Cardiovascular Pathology* 12, 237–248.

Dikeman, C.L., Bauer, L.L. and Fahey, G.C. Jr (2004) Carbohydrate composition of selected plum/prune preparations. *Journal of Agricultural and Food Chemistry* 52, 853–859.

Di Lorenzo, C., Williams, C.M., Hajnal, F. and Valenzuela, J.E. (1988) Pectin delays gastric emptying and satiety in obese subjects. *Gastroenterology* 95, 1211–1215.

Donovan, J.L. and DeVane, C.L. (2001) A primer on caffeine pharmacology and its drug interactions in clinical psychopharmacology. *Psychopharmacology Bulletin* 35, 30–48.

Drucker, D.J. (1998) Glucagon-like peptides. *Diabetes* 47, 159–169.

Dubey, P., Dundram, K.R. and Nundy, S. (1984) Effect of tea on gastric acid secretion. *Digestive Diseases and Sciences* 29, 202–206.

Ducimetiere, P., Eschwege, E., Papoz, L., Richard, J.L., Claude, J.R. and Rosselin, G. (1980) Relationship of plasma insulin levels to the incidence of myocardial infarction and coronary heart disease mortality in a middle-aged population. *Diabetologia* 19, 205–210.

Ducros, V., Arnaud, J., Tahiri, M., Coudray, C., Bornet, F., Bouteloup-Demange, C., Brouns, F., Rayssiguier, Y. and Roussel, A.M. (2005) Influence of short-chain fructo-oligosaccharides (sc-FOS) on absorption of Cu, Zn, and Se in healthy postmenopausal women. *Journal of the American College of Nutrition* 24, 30–37.

Dukas, L., Willett, W.C. and Giovannucci, E.L. (2003) Association between physical activity, fiber intake, and other lifestyle variables and constipation in a study of women. *American Journal of Gastroenterology* 98, 1790–1796.

Dumesnil, J.G., Turgeon, J., Tremblay, A., Poirier, P., Gilbert, M., Gagnon, L., St-Pierre, S., Gerneau, C., Lemieux, I., Pascot, A., Bergeron, J. and Després, J.-P. (2001) Effect of a low-glycaemic index-low-fat-high protein diet on the atherogenic metabolic risk profile of abdominally obese men. *British Journal of Nutrition* 86, 557–568.

Durrington, P. (2003) Dyslipidemia. *Lancet* 362, 717–731.

Dworatzek, P.N., Hegele, R.A. and Wolever, T.M.S. (2004) Postprandial lipemia in subjects with the threonine 54 variant of fatty acid-binding protein 2 gene is dependent on the type of fat ingested. *American Journal of Clinical Nutrition* 79, 1110–1117.

Ebbeling, C.B., Leidig, M.M., Sinclair, K.B., Hangen, J.P. and Ludwig, D.S. (2003) A reduced-glycemic load diet in the treatment of adolescent obesity. *Archives of Pediatrics and Adolescent Medicine* 157, 773–779.

Ebbeling, C.B., Leidig, M.M., Sinclair, K.B., Seger-Shippee, L.G., Feldman, H.A. and Ludwig, D.S. (2005) Effects of an *ad libitum* low-glycemic load diet on cardiovascular disease risk factors in obese young adults. *American Journal of Clinical Nutrition* 81, 976–982.

Eckel, R.H., Yost, T.J. and Jensen, D.R. (1995) Alteration in lipoprotein lipase in insulin resistance. *International Journal of Obesity* 19, S16–S23.

Eliasson, A.-C., Carlson, T.L.-G., Larsson, K. and Miezis, Y. (1981) Some effects of starch lipids on the thermal and rheological properties of wheat starch. *Starch/Stärke* 33, 130–134.

Elliott, R.M., Morgan, L.M., Tredger, J.A., Deacon, S., Wright, J. and Marks, V. (1993) Glucagon-like peptide-1 (7–36) amide and glucose-dependent insulinotropic polypeptide secretion in response to nutrient ingestion in man: acute post-prandial and 24-h secretion patterns. *Journal of Endocrinology* 138, 159–166.

Ellison, J.M., Stegmann, J.M., Colner, S.L., Michael, R.H., Sharma, M.K., Ervin, K.R. and Horwitz, D.L. (2002) Rapid changes in postprandial blood glucose produce concentration differences at finger, forearm, and thigh sampling sites. *Diabetes Care* 25, 961–964.

Elsenhaus, B., Sufkë, U., Blume, R. and Caspary, W.F. (1980) The influence of carbohydrate gelling agents on rat intestinal transport of monosaccharides and neutral amino acids *in vitro*. *Clinical Science* 59, 373–380.

Emberson, J.R., Whincup, P.H., Walker, M., Thomas, M. and Albert, K.G.M.M. (2002) Biochemical measures in a population-based study: effect of fasting duration and time of day. *Annals of Clinical Biochemistry* 39, 493–501.

Engel, L., Delaney, C. and Cohen, M. (1998) Blood glucose meters: an independent head-to-head comparison. *Practical Diabetes International* 15, 15–18.

Englyst, H.N. and Cummings, J.H. (1984) Simplified method for measurement of total non-starch polysaccharides by gas–liquid chromatography of constituent sugars as alditol acetates. *Analyst* 109, 937–942.

Englyst, H.N. and Cummings, J.H. (1985) Digestion of the polysaccharides of some cereal foods in the human small intestine. *American Journal of Clinical Nutrition* 42, 778–787.

Englyst, H.N. and Cummings, J.H. (1986) Digestion of the carbohydrates of banana (*Musa paradisiacal sapientum*) in the human small intestine. *American Journal of Clinical Nutrition* 44, 42–50.

Englyst, H.N. and Cummings, J.H. (1987) Digestion of polysaccharides of potato in the small intestine of man. *American Journal of Clinical Nutrition* 45, 423–431.

Englyst, H.N., Wiggins, H.S. and Cummings, J.H. (1982) Determination of the non-starch polysaccharides in plant foods by gas–liquid chromatography of constituent sugars as alditol acetates. *Analyst* 107, 307–318.

Englyst, H.N., Kingman, S.M. and Cummings, J.H. (1992) Classification and measurement of nutritionally important starch fractions. *European Journal of Clinical Nutrition* 46 (Suppl. 2), S33–S50.

Englyst, H.N., Kingman, S.M., Hudson, G.J. and Cummings, J.H. (1996a) Measurement of resistant starch *in vitro* and *in vivo*. *British Journal of Nutrition* 75, 749–755.

Englyst, H.N., Veenstra, J. and Hudson, G.J. (1996b) Measurement of rapidly available glucose (RAG) in plant foods: a potential *in vitro* predictor of the glycaemic response. *British Journal of Nutrition* 75, 327–337.

Englyst, K.N., Englyst, H.N., Hudson, G.J., Cole, T.J. and Cummings, J.H. (1999) Rapidly available glucose in foods: an *in vitro* measurement that reflects glycemic response. *American Journal of Clinical Nutrition* 69, 448–454.

Englyst, K.N., Vinoy, S., Englyst, H.N. and Lang, V. (2003) Glycaemic index of cereal products explained by their content of rapidly and slowly available glucose. *British Journal of Nutrition* 89, 329–340.

Ercan, N., Nuttall, F.Q., Gannon, M.C., Lane, J.T., Burmeister, L.A. and Westphal, S.A. (1993) Plasma glucose and insulin responses to bananas of varying ripeness in persons with noninsulin-dependent diabetes mellitus. *Journal of the American College of Nutrition* 12, 703–709.

Ercan, N., Gannon, M.C. and Nuttall, F.Q. (1994) Effect of added fat on the plasma glucose and insulin response to ingested potato given in various combinations as two meals in normal individuals. *Diabetes Care* 17, 1453–1459.

Evans, K., Kuusela, P.J., Cruz, M.L., Wilhelmova, I., Fielding, B.A. and Frayn, K.N. (1998) Rapid chylomicron appearance following sequential meals: effects of second meal composition. *British Journal of Nutrition* 79, 425–429.

Expert Committee on the Diagnosis and Classification of Diabetes Mellitus (2003) Report of the expert committee on the diagnosis and classification of diabetes mellitus. *Diabetes Care* 26 (Suppl. 1), S5–S20.

Expert Panel on Detection, Evaluation, and Treatment of High Blood Cholesterol in Adults (2001) Executive summary of the Third Report of the National Cholesterol Education Program (NCEP) Expert Panel on detection, evaluation, and treatment of high blood cholesterol in adults (Adult Treatment Panel III). *Journal of the American Medical Association* 285, 2486–2497.

Food and Agriculture Organization of the United Nations (1998) FAO food and nutrition paper 66. Carbohydrates in human nutrition.Report of an FAO/WHO Expert Consultation on Carbohydrates, 14–18 April, 1997, Rome, Italy. FAO, Rome.

Farquhar, J.W., Frank, A., Gross, R.C. and Reaven, G.M. (1966) Glucose, insulin and triglyceride responses to high and low carbohydrate diets in man. *Journal of Clinical Investigation* 45, 1648–1656.

Febbraio, M.A. and Stewart, K.L. (1996) CHO feeding before prolonged exercise: effects of glycemic index on muscle glycogenolysis and exercise performance. *Journal of Applied Physiology* 81, 1115–1120.

Feig, D.S. and Naylor, C.D. (1998) Eating for two: are guidelines for weight gain during pregnancy too liberal? *Lancet* 351, 1054–1055.

Felber, J.P., Tappy, L., Vouillamoz, D., Randin, J.P. and Jéquier, E. (1987) Comparative study of maltitol and sucrose by means of continuous indirect calorimetry. *Journal of Parenteral Enteral Nutrition* 11, 250–254.

Fernandes, G., Velangi, A. and Wolever, T.M.S. (2005) Glycemic index of potatoes commonly consumed in North America. *Journal of the American Dietetic Association*, 105, 557–562.

Fernstrom, M.H. and Fernstrom, J.D. (1995) Brain tryptophan concentrations and serotonin synthesis remain responsive to food consumption after the ingestion of sequential meals. *American Journal of Clinical Nutrition* 61, 312–319.

Ferrannini, E. (1998) Insulin resistance versus insulin deficiency in non-insulin-dependent diabetes mellitus: problems and prospects. *Endocrine Reviews* 19, 477–490.

Ferrannini, E. and Balkau, B. (2002) Insulin: in search of a syndrome. *Diabetic Medicine* 19, 724–729.

Ferrannini, E., Barrett, E.J., Beviacqua, S. and DeFronzo, R.A. (1983) Effect of fatty acids on glucose production and utilization in man. *Journal of Clinical Investigation* 72, 1737–1747.

Fielding, B.A., Callow, J., Owen, R.M., Samra, J.S., Matthews, D.R. and Frayn, K.N. (1996) Postprandial lipemia: the origin of an early peak studied by specific dietary fatty acid intake during sequential meals. *American Journal of Clinical Nutrition* 63, 36–41.

Finegood, D.T. and Topp, B.G. (2001) β-cell deterioration – prospects for reversal or prevention. *Diabetes, Obesity and Metabolism* 3 (Suppl. 1), S20–S27.

Finegood, D.T. and Tzur, D. (1996) Reduced glucose effectiveness associated with reduced insulin release: an artifact of the minimal-model method. *American Journal of Physiology* 271, E485–E495.

Finegood, D.T., Pacini, G. and Bergman, R.N. (1984) The insulin sensitivity index. Correlation in dogs between values determined from the intravenous glucose tolerance test and the euglycemic glucose clamp. *Diabetes* 33, 362–368.

Finegood, D.T., Hramiak, I.M. and Dupre, J. (1990) A modified protocol for estimation of insulin sensitivity with the minimal model of glucose kinetics in patients with insulin-dependent diabetes. *Journal of Clinical Endocrinology and Metabolism* 70, 1538–1549.

Fischer, U., Ertle, R., Abel, P., Rebrin, K., Brunstein, E., Hahn von Dorsche, H. and Freyse, E.J. (1987) Assessment of subcutaneous glucose concentration: validation of the wick technique as a reference for implanted electrochemical sensors in normal and diabetic dogs. *Diabetologia* 30, 940–945.

Fischer, K., Colombani, P.C., Langhans, W. and Wenk, C. (2001) Cognitive performance and its relationship with postprandial metabolic changes after ingestion of different macronutrients in the morning. *British Journal of Nutrition* 85, 393–405.

Flakoll, P.J., Kulaylat, M., Frexes-Steed, M., Hill, J.O. and Abumrad, N.N. (1991) Amino acids enhance insulin resistance to exogenous glucose infusion in overnight-fasted humans. *Journal of Parenteral and Enteral Nutrition* 15, 123–127.

Flatt, J.P. (1995) McCollum Award Lecture, 1995: diet, lifestyle, and weight maintenance. *American Journal of Clinical Nutrition* 62, 820–836.

Flint, A., Moller, B.K., Raben, A., Pedersen, D., Tetens, I., Holst, J.J. and Astrup, A. (2004) The use of glycaemic index tables to predict glycaemic index of composite breakfast meals. *British Journal of Nutrition* 91, 979–989.

Florent, C., Flourie, B., Leblond, A., Rautureau, M., Bernier, J.-J. and Rambaud, J.-C. (1985) Influence of chronic lactulose ingestion on the colonic metabolism of lactulose in man (an *in vivo* study). *Journal of Clinical Investigation* 75, 608–613.

Flourié, B., Florent, C., Etanchaud, F., Evard, D., Franchisseur, C. and Rambaud, J.-C. (1988a) Starch absorption by healthy man evaluated by lactulose hydrogen breath test. *American Journal of Clinical Nutrition* 47, 61–66.

Flourié, B., Leblond, A., Florent, C., Rautureau, M., Bisalli, A. and Rambaud, J.-C. (1988b) Starch malabsorption and breath gas excretion in healthy humans consuming low- and high-starch diets. *Gastroenterology* 95, 356–363.

Floyd, J.C. Jr, Fajans, S.S., Conn, J.W., Thiffault, C., Knopf, R.F. and Guntsche, E. (1968) Secretion of insulin induced by amino acids and glucose in diabetes mellitus. *Journal of Clinical Endocrinology* 28, 266–276.

Fogel, M.R. and Gray, G.M. (1973) Starch hydrolysis in man: an intraluminal process not requiring membrane digestion. *Journal of Applied Physiology* 35, 236–267.

Foley, J.E., Chen, Y.D., Lardinois, C.K., Hollenbeck, C.B., Liu, G.C. and Reaven, G.M. (1985) Estimates of *in vivo* insulin action in humans: comparison of the insulin clamp and the minimal model techniques. *Hormone and Metabolic Research* 17, 406–409.

Folin, O. and Berglund, H. (1922) Some new observations and interpretations with reference to transportation, retention, and excretion of carbohydrates. *Journal of Biological Chemistry* 51, 213–273.

Fontbonne, A. (1994) Why can high insulin levels indicate a risk for coronary heart disease? *Diabetologia* 37, 953–955.

Fontvieille, A.M., Acosta, M., Rizkalla, S.W., Bornet, F., David, P., Letanoux, M., Tchobroutsky, G. and Slama, G. (1988) A moderate switch from high to low glycaemic-index foods for 3 weeks improves the metabolic control of type I (IDDM) diabetic subjects. *Diabetes Nutrition and Metabolism* 1, 139–143.

Fontvieille, A.M., Rizkalla, S.W., Penfornis, M., Acosta, M., Bornet, F. and Slama, G. (1992) The use of low glycaemic index foods improves metabolic control of diabetic patients over five weeks. *Diabetic Medicine* 9, 444–450.

Ford, E.S. and Liu, S. (2001) Glycemic index and serum high-density lipoprotein cholesterol concentration among US adults. *Archives of Internal Medicine* 161, 572–576.

Foster, L.A., Ames, N.K., and Emery, R.S. (1991) Food intake and serum insulin responses to intraventricular infusions of insulin and IGF-1. *Physiolology and Behaviour* 50, 743–749.

Foster, G.D., Wyatt, H.R., Hill, J.O., McGuckin, B.G., Brill, C., Mohammed, B.S., Szapary, P.O., Rader, D.J., Edman, J.S. and Klein, S. (2003) A randomized trial of a low-carbohydrate diet for obesity. *New England Journal of Medicine* 348, 2082–2090.

Foster-Powell, K. and Brand Miller, J. (1995) International tables of glycemic index. *American Journal of Clinical Nutrition* 62, 871S–893S.

Foster-Powell, K., Holt, S.H. and Brand-Miller, J.C. (2002) International table of glycemic index and glycemic load values: 2002. *American Journal of Clinical Nutrition* 76, 5–56.

Franceschi, S., Dal Maso, L., Augustin, L., Negri, E., Parpinel, M., Boyle, P., Jenkins, D.J.A. and La Vecchia, C. (2001) Dietary glycemic load and colorectal cancer risk. *Annals of Oncology* 12, 1–6.

Franz, M.J., Horton, E.S., Bantle, J.P., Beebe, C.A., Brunzell, J.D., Coulston, A.M., Henry, R.R., Hoogwerf, B.J. and Stacpoole, P.W. (1994) Nutrition principles for the management of diabetes and related complications. *Diabetes Care* 17, 490–518.

Franz, M.J., Bantle, J.P., Beebe, C.A., Chiasson, J.-L., Garg, A., Holzmeister, L.A., Hoogwerf, B., Mayer-Davis, E., Mooradian, A.D., Purnell, J.Q. and Wheeler, M. (2002) Evidence-based nutrition principles and recommendations for the treatment and prevention of diabetes and related complications. *Diabetes Care* 25, 148–198.

Frati, A.C., Iniestra, F. and Ariza, C.R. (1996) Acute effect of cigarette smoking on glucose tolerance and other cardiovascular risk factors. *Diabetes Care* 19, 112–118.

Frayn, K.N., Whyte, P.L., Benson, H.A., Earl, D.J. and Smith, H.A. (1989) Changes in forearm blood flow at elevated ambient temperature and their role in the apparent impairment of glucose tolerance. *Clinical Science* 76, 323–328.

Freeland, K.R. and Wolever, T.M.S. (2002) Effect of cereal fiber compared to glycemic carbohydrate on appetite, short-term food intake, orocecal transit time and blood glucose. *American Journal of Clinical Nutrition* 75, 379S–380S.

Frost, G., Wilding, J. and Beecham, J. (1994) Dietary advice based on the glycaemic index improves dietary profile and metabolic control in type 2 diabetic patients. *Diabetic Medicine* 11, 397–401.

Frost, G., Keogh, B., Smith, D., Akinsanya, K. and Leeds, A. (1996) The effect of low-glycemic carbohydrate on insulin and glucose response *in vivo* and *in vitro* in patients with coronary heart disease. *Metabolism: Clinical and Experimental* 45, 669–672.

Frost, G., Leeds, A., Trew, G., Margara, R. and Dornhorst, A. (1998) Insulin sensitivity in women at risk of coronary heart disease and the effect of a low glycemic diet. *Metabolism: Clinical and Experimental* 47, 1245–1251.

Frost, G., Leeds, A., Doré, C.J., Madeiros, S., Brading, S. and Dornhorst, A. (1999) Glycaemic index as a determinant of serum HDL-cholesterol concentration. *Lancet* 353, 1045–1048.

Frost, G.S., Brynes, A.E., Bovill-Taylor, C. and Dornhorst, A. (2004) A prospective randomised trial to determine the efficacy of a low glycaemic index diet given in addition to healthy eating and weight loss advice in patients with coronary heart disease. *European Journal of Clinical Nutrition* 58, 121–127.

Furtado, L.M., Somwar, R., Sweeney, G., Niu, W. and Klip, A. (2002) Activation of the glucose transporter GLUT4 by insulin. *Biochemistry and Cell Biology* 80, 569–578.

Ganda, O.P., Soeldner, J.S., Gleason, R.E., Cleator, I.G.M. and Reynolds, C. (1979) Metabolic effects of glucose, mannose, galactose, and fructose in man. *Journal of Clinical Endocrinology and Metabolism* 49, 616–622.

Gannon, M.C., Nuttal, F.Q., Westphal, S.A., Neil, B.J. and Westphal, S.A. (1988) The insulin and glucose responses to meals of glucose plus various proteins in type II diabetic subjects. *Metabolism: Clinical and Experimental* 37, 1081–1088.

Gannon, M.C., Nuttal, F.Q., Westphal, S.A., Neil, B.J. and Seaquist, E.R. (1989) Effects of dose of ingested glucose on plasma metabolite and hormone responses in type II diabetic subjects. *Diabetes Care* 12, 544–552.

Gannon, M.C., Ercan, N., Westphal, S.A. and Nuttall, F.Q. (1993) Effect of added fat on plasma glucose and insulin response to ingested potato in individuals with NIDDM. *Diabetes Care* 16, 874–880.

Gannon, M.C., Nuttall, J.A., Damberg, G., Gupta, V. and Nuttall, F.Q. (2001a) Effect of protein ingestion on the glucose appearance rate in people with type 2 diabetes. *The Journal of Clinical Endocrinology and Metabolism* 86, 1040–1047.

Gannon, M.C., Khan, M.A. and Nuttall, F.Q. (2001b) Glucose appearance rate after the ingestion of galactose. *Metabolism: Clinical and Experimental* 50, 93–98.

Gannon, M.C., Nuttall, J.A. and Nuttall, F.Q. (2002) The metabolic response to ingested glycine. *American Journal of Clinical Nutrition* 76, 1302–1307.

Garg, A. (1998) High-monounsaturated-fat diets for patients with diabetes mellitus: a meta-analysis. *American Journal of Clinical Nutrition* 67 (Suppl.), 577S–582S.

Gatti, E., Noè, D., Pazzucconi, F., Gianfranceschi, G., Porrini, M., Testolin, G. and Sirtori, C.R. (1992) Differential effect of unsaturated oils and butter on blood glucose and insulin response to carbohydrate in normal volunteers. *European Journal of Clinical Nutrition* 46, 161–166.

Genuth, S.M. (1973) Plasma insulin and glucose profiles in normal, obese and diabetic persons. *Annals of Internal Medicine* 79, 812–822.

Gerich, J.E. (1998) The genetic basis of type 2 diabetes mellitus: impaired insulin secretion versus impaired insulin sensitivity. *Endocrine Reviews* 19, 491–503.

Gerich, J.E. (2003) Clinical significance, pathogenesis, and management of postprandial hyperglycemia. *Archives of Internal Medicine* 163, 1306–1316.

Gielkens, H.A.J., Verkijk, M., Lam, W.F., Lamers, C.G.H.W. and Masclee, A.A.M. (1998) Effects of hyperglycemia and hyperinsulinemia on satiety in humans. *Metabolism: Clinical and Experimental* 47, 321–324.

Gilat, T., Ben Hur, H., Gelman-Malachi, E., Terdiman, R. and Peled, Y. (1978) Alterations of the colonic flora and their effect on the hydrogen breath test. *Gut* 19, 602–605.

Giles, G.G., Simpson, J.A., English, D.R., Hodge, A.M., Gertig, D.M., Macinnis, R.J. and Hopper, J.L. (2005) Dietary carbohydrate, fibre, glycaemic index, glycaemic load and the risk of postmenopausal breast cancer. *International Journal of Cancer* Published Online: 10 Oct 2005 DOI: 10.1002/ijc.21548.

Gionchetti, P., Rizzello, F., Venturi, A., Brigidi, P., Matteuzzi, D., Bazzocchi, G., Poggioli, G., Miglioli, M. and Campieri, M. (2000) Oral bacteriotherapy as maintenance treatment for patients with chronic pouchitis: a double-blind, placebo-controlled trial. *Gastroenterology* 119, 305–309.

Giovannucci, E. (1995) Insulin and colon cancer. *Cancer Causes and Control* 6, 164–179.

Glicksman, A.S. and Rawson, R.W. (1956) Diabetes and altered carbohydrate metabolism in patients with cancer. *Cancer* 9, 1127–1134.

Goodfellow, J., Bellamy, M.F., Ramsey, M.W., Jones, C.J.H. and Lewis, M.J. (2000) Dietary supplementation with omega–3 fatty acids improve systemic large artery function in subjects with hypercholesterolemia. *Journal of the American College of Cardiology* 35, 265–270.

Goodyear, L.J. and Kahn, B.B. (1998) Exercise, glucose transport, and insulin sensitivity. *Annual Review of Medicine* 49, 235–261.

Graham, T.E., Sathasivam, P., Rowland, M., Marko, N., Greer, F. and Battram, D. (2001) Caffeine ingestion elevates plasma insulin response in humans during an oral glucose tolerance test. *Canadian Journal of Physiology and Pharmacology* 79, 559–565.

Granfeldt, Y., Björk, I., Drews, A. and Tovar, J. (1992) An *in vitro* procedure based on chewing to predict the metabolic responses to starch in cereal and legume products. *European Journal of Clinical Nutrition* 46, 649–660.

Granfeldt, Y., Hagander, B. and Björck, I. (1995) Metabolic responses to starch in oat and wheat products. On the importance of food structure, incomplete gelatinization or presence of viscous dietary fibre. *European Journal of Clinical Nutrition* 49, 189–199.

Gray, H. (1923) Blood sugar standards. Part I. Normal and diabetic persons. *Archives of Internal Medicine* 39, 241–261.

Greenwood, C.E. (2003) Dietary carbohydrate, glucose regulation, and cognitive performance in elderly persons. *Nutrition Reviews* 61, S68–S74.

Greenwood, C.E., Kaplan, R.J., Hebblethwaite, S. and Jenkins, D.J.A. (2003) Carbohydrate-induced memory impairment in adults with type 2 diabetes. *Diabetes Care* 26, 1961–1966.

Gregerson, S., Rasmussen, O., Winther, E. and Hermansen, K. (1990) Water volume and consumption time: influence on the glycemic and insulinemic responses in non-insulin-dependent diabetic subjects. *American Journal of Clinical Nutrition* 52, 515–518.

Gulliford, M.C., Bicknell, E.J. and Scarpello, J.H. (1989) Differential effect of protein and fat ingestion on blood glucose responses to high- and low-glycemic-index carbohydrates in noninsulin-dependent diabetic subjects. *American Journal of Clinical Nutrition* 50, 773–777.

Gustafsson, K., Asp, N.-G., Hagander, B., Nyman, M. and Schweizer, T. (1995a) Influence of processing and cooking of carrots in mixed meals on satiety, glucose and hormonal response. *International Journal of Food Sciences and Nutrition* 46, 3–12.

Gustafsson, K., Asp, N.-G., Hagander, B. and Nyman, M. (1995b) Satiety effects of spinach in mixed meals: comparison with other vegetables. *International Journal of Food Sciences and Nutrition* 46, 327–334.

Guthrie, J.F. and Morton, J.F. (2000) Food sources of added sweeteners in the diets of Americans. *Journal of the American Dietetic Association* 100, 43–51.

Ha, M.-A., Mann, J.I., Melton, L.D. and Lewis-Barned, N.J. (1992) Calculation of the glycaemic index. *Diabetes Nutrition and Metabolism* 5, 137–139.

Haber, G.B., Heaton, K.W., Murphy, D. and Burroughs, L.F. (1977) Depletion and disruption of dietary fibre: effects on satiety, plasma-glucose, and serum-insulin. *Lancet* ii, 679–682.

Hamberg, O., Rumessen, J.J. and Gudmand-Høyer, E. (1989) Inhibition of starch absorption by dietary fibre. A comparative study of wheat bran, sugar-beet fibre, and pea fibre. *Scandinavian Journal of Gastroenterology* 24, 103–109.

Hankey, G.J. and Eikelboom, J.W. (1999) Homocysteine and vascular disease. *Lancet* 354, 407–413.

Hassinger, W., Sauer, G., Cordes, U., Krause, U., Beyer, J. and Baessler, K.H. (1981) The effects of equal caloric amounts of xylitol, sucrose and starch on insulin requirements and blood glucose levels in insulin-dependent diabetics. *Diabetologia* 21, 37–40.

Heaney, R.P. (2002) Effects of caffeine on bone and the calcium economy. *Food and Chemical Toxicology* 40, 1263–1270.

Heaton, K.W. (1973) Food fibre as an obstacle to energy intake. *Lancet* ii, 1418–1421.

Heaton, K.W., Marcus, S.N., Emmett, P.M. and Bolton, C.H. (1988) Particle size of wheat, maize, and oat test meals: effects on plasma glucose and insulin responses and on the rate of starch digestion *in vitro*. *American Journal of Clinical Nutrition* 47, 675–682.

Heilbronn, L.K., Noakes, M. and Clifton, P.M. (2002) The effect of high- and low-glycemic index energy restricted diets on plasma lipid and glucose profiles in type 2 diabetic subjects with varying glycemic control. *Journal of the American College of Nutrition* 21, 120–127.

Heine, R.J., Hanning, I., Morgan, L. and Alberti, K.G.M.M. (1983) The oral glucose tolerance test (OGTT): effect of rate of ingestion of carbohydrate and different carbohydrate preparations. *Diabetes Care* 6, 441–445.

Heine, R.J., Balkau, B., Ceriello, A., Del Prato, S., Horton, E.S. and Taskinen, M.-R. (2004) What does postprandial hyperglycaemia mean? *Diabetic Medicine* 21, 208–213.

Heini, A.F. and Weinsier, R.L. (1997) Divergent trends in obesity and fat intake patterns: the American Paradox. *American Journal of Medicine* 102, 259–264.

Hellerstein, M.K. (2002) Carbohydrate-induced hypertriglyceridemia: modifying factors and implications for cardiovascular risk. *Current Opinion in Lipidology* 13, 33–40.

Hermansen, K., Rasmussen, O., Arnfred, J., Winther, E. and Schmitz, O. (1987) Glycemic effects of spaghetti and potato consumed as part of a mixed meal on IDDM patients. *Diabetes Care* 10, 401–406.

Hermansen, K., Rasmussen, O., Gregersen, S. and Larsen, S. (1992) Influence of ripeness of banana on the blood glucose and insulin response in type 2 diabetic subjects. *Diabetic Medicine* 9, 730–743.

Herrmann, C., Göke, R., Richter, G., Fehmann, H.-C., Arnold, R. and Göke, B. (1995) Glucagon-like peptide-1 and glucose-dependent insulin-releasing polypeptide plasma levels in response to nutrients. *Digestion* 56, 117–126.

Hertzler, S. (2000) Glycemic index of "energy" snack bars in normal volunteers. *Journal of the American Dietetic Association* 100, 97–100.

Hertzler, S.R. and Kim, Y. (2003) Glycemic and insulinemic responses to energy bars of differing macronutrient composition in healthy adults. *Medical Science Monitor* 9, CR84–CR90.

Hickey, C.A., Calloway, D.H. and Murphy, E.L. (1972a) Intestinal gas production following ingestion of fruits and fruit juices. *American Journal of Digestive Diseases* 17, 383–389.

Hickey, C.A., Murphy, E.L. and Calloway, D.H. (1972b) Intestinal gas production following ingestion of commercial wheat cereals and milling fractions. *American Association of Cereal Chemists* 49, 276–283.

Higginbotham, S., Zhang, Z.-F., Lee, I.-M., Cook, N.R., Giovannucci, E., Buring, J.E. and Liu, S. (2004) Dietary glycemic load and risk of colorectal cancer in the Women's Health Study. *Journal of the National Cancer Institute* 96, 229–233.

Hill, J.H. and Fernandez, F. (1986) Bacterial metabolism, fiber and colorectal cancer. In: Kritchevsky, D., Bonfield, C. and Anderson, J.W. (eds) *Dietary Fiber: Chemistry, Physiology and Health Effects.* Plenum Press, New York, pp. 417–429.

Hill, J.O. and Prentice, A.M. (1995) Sugars and body weight regulation. *American Journal of Clinical Nutrition* 62 (Suppl.), 264S–274S.

Himsworth, H.P. (1932) The activation of insulin. *Lancet* 2, 935–936.

Himsworth, H.P. (1935) The dietetic factor determining the glucose tolerance and sensitivity to insulin of healthy men. *Clinical Science* 2, 67–94.

Himsworth, H.P. (1936) Diabetes mellitus. Its differentiation into insulin-sensitive and insulin-insensitive types. *Lancet* 1, 127–130.

Hoag, S., Marshall, J.A., Jones, R.H. and Hamman, R.F. (1995) High fasting insulin levels associated with lower rates of weight gain in persons with normal glucose tolerance: the San Luis Valley diabetes study. *International Journal of Obesity* 19, 175–180.

Hodge, A.M., English, D.R., O'Dea, K. and Giles, G.G. (2004) Glycemic index and dietary fiber and the risk of type 2 diabetes. *Diabetes Care* 27, 2701–2706.

Hoebler, C., Karinthi, A., Chiron, H., Champ, M. and Barry, J.L. (1999) Bioavailability of starch in bread rich in amylose: metabolic responses in healthy subjects and starch structure. *European Journal of Clinical Nutrition* 53, 360–366.

Hoekstra, J.H. and van den Aker, J.H.L. (1996) Facilitating effect of amino acids on fructose and sorbitol absorption in children. *Journal of Pediatric Gastroenterology and Nutrition* 23, 118–124.

Hollenbeck, C.B., Coulston, A.M., Donner, C., Williams, R.A. and Reaven, G.M. (1985) The effects of variations in percent of naturally occurring complex and simple carbohydrates on plasma glucose and insulin responses in individuals with non-insulin-dependent diabetes mellitus. *Diabetes* 34, 151–155.

Hollenbeck, C.B., Coulston, A.M. and Reaven, G.M. (1986) Glycemic effects of carbohydrates: a different perspective. *Diabetes Care* 9, 641–647.

Hollenbeck, C.B., Coulston, A.M. and Reaven, G.M. (1988) Comparison of plasma glucose and insulin responses to mixed meals of high-, intermediate- and low-glycemic potential. *Diabetes Care* 11, 323–329.

Holm, J., Lundquist, I., Bjorck, I., Eliasson, A.C. and Asp, N.G. (1988) Degree of starch gelatinization, digestion rate of starch *in vitro*, and metabolic response in rats. *American Journal of Clinical Nutrition* 47, 1010–1016.

Holm, J., Hagander, B., Bjorck, I., Eliasson, A.C. and Lundquist, I. (1989) The effect of various thermal processes on the glycemic response to whole grain wheat products in humans and rats. *Journal of Nutrition* 119, 1631–1638.

Holt, S.H.A. and Brand Miller, J. (1994) Particle size, satiety and the glycemic response. *European Journal of Clinical Nutrition* 48, 496–502.

Holt, S.H.A. and Brand Miller, J. (1995) Increased insulin responses to ingested foods are associated with lessened satiety. *Appetite* 24, 43–54.

Holt, S., Heading, R.C., Carter, D.C., Prescott, L.F. and Tothill, P. (1979) Effect of gel fibre on gastric emptying and absorption of glucose and paracetamol. *Lancet* i, 636–639.

Holt, S.H.A., Brand Miller, J., Soveny, C. and Hansky, J. (1992) Relationship of satiety to postprandial glycaemic, insulin and cholecystokinin responses. *Appetite* 18, 129–141.

Holt, S.H.A., Brand Miller, J.C. and Petocz, P. (1996) Interrelationships among postprandial satiety, glucose and insulin responses and changes in subsequent food intake. *European Journal of Clinical Nutrition* 50, 788–797.

Holt, S.H.A., Brand Miller, J.C. and Petocz, P. (1997) An insulin index of foods: the insulin demand generated by 1000-kJ portions of common foods. *American Journal of Clinical Nutrition* 66, 1264–1276.

Hong, Y., Rice, T., Gagnon, J., Després, J.P., Nadeau, A., Perusse, L., Bouchard, C., Leon, A.S., Skinner, J.S., Wilmore, J.H. and Rao, D.C. (1998) Familial clustering of insulin and abdominal visceral fat: the HERITAGE Family Study. *Journal of Clinical Endocrinology and Metabolism: Clinical and Experimental* 83, 4239–4245.

Horton, R. (2005) Expression of concern: Indo-Mediterranean Diet Heart Study. *Lancet* 366, 354–356.

Horton, T.J. and Hill, J.O. (2001) Prolonged fasting significantly changes nutrient oxidation and glucose tolerance after a normal mixed meal. *Journal of Applied Physiology* 90, 155–163.

Houghton, L.A., Green, T.J., Donovan, U.M., Gibson, R.S., Stephen, A.M. and O'Connor, D.L. (1997) Association between dietary fiber intake and the folate status of a group of female adolescents. *American Journal of Clinical Nutrition* 66, 1414–1421.

Hoyt, G., Hickey, M.S. and Cordain, L. (2005) Dissociation of the glycaemic and insulinaemic responses to whole and skimmed milk. *British Journal of Nutrition* 93, 175–177.

Hudgins, L.C., Hellerstein, M.K., Seidman, C.E., Neese, R.A., Tremaroli, J.D. and Hirsch, J. (2000) Relationship between carbohydrate-induced hypertriglyceridemia and fatty acid synthesis in lean and obese subjects. *Journal of Lipid Research* 41, 595–604.

Hunt, J.N., Smith, J.L. and Jiang, C.L. (1985) Effect of meal volume and energy density on the gastric emptying of carbohydrates. *Gastroenterology* 89, 1326–1330.

Hylla, S., Gostner, A., Dusel, G., Anger, H., Bartram, H.P., Christl, S.U., Kasper, H. and Scheppach, W. (1998) Effects of resistant starch on the colon in healthy volunteers: possible implications for cancer prevention. *American Journal of Clinical Nutrition* 67, 136–142.

Inan, M.S., Rasoulpour, R.J., Yin, L., Hubbard, A.K., Rosenberg, D.W. and Giardina, C. (2000) The luminal short-chain fatty acid butyrate modulates NF-kappaB activity in human colonic epithelial cell line. *Gastroenterology* 118, 724–734.

Indar-Brown, K., Norenberg, C. and Madar, Z. (1992) Glycemic and insulinemic responses after ingestion of ethnic foods by NIDDM and healthy subjects. *American Journal of Clinical Nutrition* 55, 89–95.

International Diabetes Federation (2005) The IDF consensus worldwide definition of the metabolic syndrome. Available at: *www.idf.org/webdata/docs/Metabolic_syndromedefinition.pdf* Accessed on 19 September, 2005.

Ireland, P., O'Dea, K. and Nankervis, A. (1992) How important is a high carbohydrate, high fiber diet in the management of insulin-dependent diabetes mellitus? *Diabetes Nutrition and Metabolism: Clinical and Experimental* 5, 113–120.

Iso, H., Stampfer, M.J., Manson, J.E., Rexrode, K., Hennekens, C.H., Colditz, G.A., Speizer, F.E. and Willett, W.C. (1999) Prospective study of calcium, potassium, and magnesium intake and risk of stroke in women. *Stroke* 30, 1772–1779.

Isomaa, B., Almgren, P., Tuomi, T., Forsen, B., Lahti, K., Missen, M., Tasknien, M.-R. and Groop, L. (2001) Cardiovascular morbidity and mortality associated with the metabolic syndrome. *Diabetes Care* 24, 683–689.

Jackson, R.A., Peters, N., Advani, U., Perry, G., Rogers, J., Brough, W.H. and Pilkington, T.R.E. (1973) Forearm glucose uptake during the oral glucose tolerance test in normal subjects. *Diabetes* 22, 442–458.

Jackson, K.G., Robertson, M.D., Fielding, B.A., Frayn, K.N. and Williams, C.M. (2001) Second meal effect: modified sham feeding does not provoke the release of stored triacylglycerol from a previous high-fat meal. *British Journal of Nutrition* 85, 149–156.

Jackson, K.G., Robertson, M.D., Fielding, B.A., Frayn, K.N. and Williams, C.M. (2002) Olive oil increases the number of triacylglycerol-rich chylomicron particles compared with other oils: an effect retained when a second standard meal is fed. *American Journal of Clinical Nutrition* 76, 942–949.

Jarrett, R.J. (1994) Why is insulin not a risk factor for coronary heart disease? *Diabetologia* 37, 945–947.

Järvi, A.E., Karlström, B.E., Granfeldt, Y.E., Björck, I.E., Asp, N.-E.L. and Vessby, B.O.H. (1999) Improved glycemic control and lipid profile and normalized fibrinolytic activity on a low-glycemic index diet in type 2 diabetic patients. *Diabetes Care* 22, 10–18.

Jenkins, D.J.A. and Wolever, T.M.S. (1981) Slow release carbohydrate in the treatment of diabetes. *Proceedings of the Nutrition Society* 40, 227–235.

Jenkins, D.J.A., Leeds, A.R., Gassull, M.A., Wolever, T.M.S., Goff, D.V., Alberti, K.G.M.M. and Hockaday, T.D.R. (1976) Unabsorbable carbohydrates and diabetes: decreased postprandial hyperglycaemia. *Lancet* 2, 172–174.

Jenkins, D.J.A., Wolever, T.M.S., Hockaday, T.D.R., Leeds, A.R., Haworth, R., Bacon, S., Apling, E.C. and Dilawari, J. (1977) Treatment of diabetes with guar gum. *Lancet* 2, 779–780.

Jenkins, D.J.A., Wolever, T.M.S., Nineham, R., Taylor, R.H., Metz, G.L., Bacon, S. and Hockaday, T.D.R. (1978a) Guar crispbread in the diabetic diet. *British Medical Journal* 2, 1744–1746.

Jenkins, D.J.A., Wolever, T.M.S., Leeds, A.R., Gassull, M.A., Dilawari, J.B., Goff, D.V., Metz, G.L. and Alberti, K.G.M.M. (1978b) Dietary fibres, fibre analogues and glucose tolerance: importance of viscosity. *British Medical Journal* 1, 1392–1394.

Jenkins, D.J.A., Wolever, T.M.S., Taylor, R.H., Ghafari, H., Jenkins, A.L., Barker, H. and Jenkins, M.J.A. (1980a) Rate of digestion of foods and postprandial glycaemia in normal and diabetic subjects. *British Medical Journal* 2, 14–17.

Jenkins, D.J.A., Wolever, T.M.S., Nineham, R., Sarson, D.L., Bloom, S.R., Ahern, J., Alberti, K.G.M.M. and Hockaday, T.D.R. (1980b) Improved glucose tolerance four hours after taking guar with glucose. *Diabetologia* 19, 21–24.

Jenkins, D.J.A., Wolever, T.M.S., Taylor, R.H., Reynolds, D., Nineham, R. and Hockaday, T.D.R. (1980c) Diabetic glucose control, lipids, and trace elements on long term guar. *British Medical Journal* 1, 1353–1354.

Jenkins, D.J.A., Wolever, T.M.S., Taylor, R.H., Barker, H.M. and Fielden, H. (1980d) Exceptionally low blood glucose response to dried beans: comparison with other carbohydrate foods. *British Medical Journal* 2, 578–580.

Jenkins, D.J.A., Wolever, T.M.S., Taylor, R.H., Barker, H.M., Fielden, H., Baldwin, J.M., Bowling, A.C., Newman, H.C., Jenkins, A.L. and Goff, D.V. (1981a) Glycemic index of foods: a physiological basis for carbohydrate exchange. *American Journal of Clinical Nutrition* 34, 362–366.

Jenkins, D.J.A., Taylor, R.H., Goff, D.V., Fielden, J., Misiewicz, J.J., Sarson, D.L., Bloom, S.R. and Alberti, K.G.M.M. (1981b) Scope and specificity of acarbose in slowing carbohydrate absorption in man. *Diabetes* 30, 951–954.

Jenkins, D.J.A., Wolever, T.M.S., Taylor, R.H., Barker, H.M., Fielden, H. and Gassull, M.A. (1981c) Lack of effect of refining on the glycemic response to cereals. *Diabetes Care* 4, 509–513.

Jenkins, D.J.A., Ghafari, H., Wolever, T.M.S., Taylor, R.H., Barker, H.M., Fielden, H., Jenkins, A.L. and Bowling, A.C. (1982a) Relationship between the rate of digestion of foods and postprandial glycaemia. *Diabetologia* 22, 450–455.

Jenkins, D.J.A., Wolever, T.M.S., Taylor, R.H., Griffiths, C., Krzeminska, K., Lawrie, J.A., Bennett, C.M., Goff, D.V., Sarson, D.L. and Bloom, S.R. (1982b) Slow release carbohydrate improves second meal tolerance. *American Journal of Clinical Nutrition* 35, 1339–1346.

Jenkins, D.J.A., Wolever, T.M.S., Jenkins, A.L., Thorne, M.J., Lee, R., Kalmusky, J., Reichert, R. and Wong, G.S. (1983) The glycaemic index of foods tested in diabetic patients: a new basis for carbohydrate exchange favouring the use of legumes. *Diabetologia* 24, 257–264.

Jenkins, D.J.A., Wolever, T.M.S., Wong, G.S., Kenshole, A., Josse, R.G., Thompson, L.U. and Lam, K.Y. (1984) Glycemic responses to foods: possible differences between insulin-dependent and non-insulin-dependent diabetics. *American Journal of Clinical Nutrition* 40, 971–981.

Jenkins, D.J.A., Wolever, T.M.S., Collier, G.R., Ocana, A., Rao, A.V., Buckley, G., Lam, K.Y., Meyer, A. and Thompson, L.U. (1987a) The metabolic effects of a low glycemic index diet. *American Journal of Clinical Nutrition* 46, 968–795.

Jenkins, D.J.A., Mayer, A., Jenkins, A.L., Wolever, T.M.S., Collier, G.R., Wesson, V. and Cuff, D. (1987b) Simple and complex carbohydrates: lack of glycemic difference between glucose and glucose polymers. *Journal of Clinical Nutrition and Gastroenterology* 2, 113–116.

Jenkins, D.J.A., Thorne, M.J., Wolever, T.M.S., Jenkins, A.L., Rao, A.V. and Thompson, L.U. (1987c) The effect of starch–protein interaction in wheat on the glycemic response and rate of *in vitro* digestion. *American Journal of Clinical Nutrition* 45, 946–951.

Jenkins, D.J.A., Cuff, D., Wolever, T.M.S., Knowland, D., Thompson, L.U., Cohen, Z. and Prokipchuk, E. (1987d) Digestibility of carbohydrate foods in an ileostomate: relationship to dietary fiber, *in vitro* digestibility, and glycemic response. *American Journal of Gastroenterology* 82, 709–717.

Jenkins, D.J.A., Wesson, V., Wolever, T.M.S., Kalmusky, J., Giudici, S., Csima, A., Josse, R.G. and Wong, G.S. (1988) Wholemeal versus wholegrain breads: proportion of whole or cracked grain and the glycaemic response. *British Medical Journal* 297, 958–960.

Jenkins, D.J.A., Wolever, T.M.S., Vuksan, V., Brighenti, F., Cunnane, S.C., Rao, A.V., Jenkins, A., Buckley, G., Patten, R., Singer, W., Corey, P. and Josse, R.G. (1989) "Nibbling versus gorging": metabolic advantages of increased meal frequency. *New England Journal of Medicine* 321, 929–934.

Jenkins, D.J.A., Wolever, T.M.S., Ocana, A.M., Vuksan, V., Cunnane, S.C., Jenkins, M., Wong, G.S., Singer, W., Bloom, S.R., Blendis, L.M. and Josse, R.G. (1990) Metabolic effects of reducing rate of glucose ingestion by single bolus versus continuous sipping. *Diabetes* 39, 775–781.

Jenkins, D.J.A., Wolever, T.M.S., Jenkins, A., Brighenti, F., Vuksan, V., Rao, A.V., Cunnane, S.C., Ocana, A., Corey, P., Versina, C., Connelly, P., Buckley, G. and Patten, R. (1991) Specific types of colonic fermentation may raise low-density-lipoprotein–cholesterol concentrations. *American Journal of Clinical Nutrition* 54, 141–147.

Jenkins, D.J.A., Ocana, A., Jenkins, A.L., Wolever, T.M.S., Vuksan, V., Katzman, L., Hollands, M., Greenberg, G., Corey, P., Patten, R., Wong, G.S. and Josse, R.G. (1992) Metabolic advantages of spreading the nutrient load: effects of increased meal frequency in non-insulin-dependent diabetes. *American Journal of Clinical Nutrition* 55, 461–467.

Jenkins, D.J.A., Vuksan, V., Kendall, C.W., Wursch, P., Jeffcoat, R., Waring, S., Mehling, C.C., Vidgen, E., Augustin, L.S. and Wong, E. (1998) Physiological effects of resistant starches on fecal bulk, short chain fatty acids, blood lipids and glycemic index. *Journal of the American College of Nutrition* 17, 609–616.

Jenkins, D.J.A., Vuksan, V., Rao, A.V., Vidgen, E., Kendall, C.W., Tariq, N., Wursch, P., Koellreutter, B., Shiwnarain, N. and Jeffcoat, R. (1999) Colonic bacterial activity and serum lipid risk factors for cardiovascular disease. *Metabolism: Clinical and Experimental* 48, 264–268.

Jeppesen, J., Schaaf, P., Jones, C., Zhou, M.Y., Chen, Y.D. and Reaven, G.M. (1997) Effects of low-fat, high-carbohydrate diets on risk factors for ischemic heart disease in postmenopausal women. *American Journal of Clinical Nutrition* 65, 1027–1033.

Jimenez-Cruz, A., Bacardi-Gascon, M., Turnbull, W.H., Rosales-Garay, P. and Severino-Lugo, I. (2003) A flexible, low-glycemic index Mexican-style diet in overweight and obese subjects with type 2 diabetes improves metabolic parameters during a 6-week treatment period. *Diabetes Care* 26, 1967–1970.

Johnson, K.J., Anderson, K.E., Harnack, L., Hong, C.P. and Folsom, A.R. (2005) No association between dietary glycemic index or load and pancreatic cancer incidence in postmenopausal women. *Cancer Epidemiology, Biomarkers and Prevention* 14, 1574–1575.

Johnston, D.G., Alberti, K.G.M.M., Faber, O.K., Binder, C. and Wright, R. (1977) Hyperinsulinism of hepatic cirrhosis: diminished degradation or hypersecretion? *Lancet* i, 10–13.

Johnston, K.L., Clifford, M.N. and Morgan, L.M. (2003) Coffee acutely modifies gastrointestinal hormone secretion and glucose tolerance in humans: glycemic effects of chlorogenic acid and caffeine. *American Journal of Clinical Nutrition* 78, 728–733.

Jungheim, K. and Koschinsky, T. (2002) Glucose monitoring at the arm: risky delays of hypoglycemia and hyperglycemia detection. *Diabetes Care* 25, 956–960.

Juntunen, K.S., Niskanen, L.K., Liukkonen, K.H., Poutanen K.S., Holst, J.J. and Mykkänen, H.M. (2002) Post-prandial glucose, insulin, and incretin responses to grain products in healthy subjects. *American Journal of Clinical Nutrition* 75, 254–262.

Juntunen, K.S., Laaksonen, D.E., Poutanen, K.S., Niskanen, L.K. and Mykkänen, H.M. (2003) High-fiber rye bread and insulin secretion and sensitivity in healthy postmenopausal women. *American Journal of Clinical Nutrition* 77, 385–391.

Kabir, M., Rizkalla, S.W., Champ, M., Luo, J., Boillot, J., Bruzzo, F. and Slama, G. (1998a) Dietary amylase–amylopectin starch content affects glucose and lipid metabolism in adipocytes of normal and diabetic rats. *Journal of Nutrition* 128, 35–43.

Kabir, M., Rizkalla, S.W., Quignard-Boulange, A., Guerre-Millo, M., Boillot, J., Ardouin, B., Luo, J. and Slama, G. (1998b) A high glycemic index starch diet affects lipid storage-related enzymes in normal and to a lesser extent in diabetic rats. *Journal of Nutrition* 128, 1878–1883.

Kahn, S.E. (2003) The relative contributions of insulin resistance and beta-cell dysfunction to the pathophysiology of type 2 diabetes. *Diabetologia* 46, 3–19.

Kahn, S.E., Beard, J.C., Schwartz, M.W., Ward, W.K., Ding, H.L., Bergman, R.N., Taborsky, G.J. Jr and Porte, D. Jr (1989) Increased beta-cell secretory capacity as mechanism for islet adaptation to nicotinic acid-induced insulin resistance. *Diabetes* 38, 562–568.

Kahn, S.E., Larson, V.G., Beard, J.C., Cain, K.C., Fellingham, G.W., Schwartz, R.S., Veith, R.C., Stratton, J.R., Cerqueira, M.D. and Abrass, I.B. (1990) Effect of exercise on insulin action, glucose tolerance, and insulin secretion in aging. *American Journal of Physiology* 258, E937–E943.

Kahn, M.B., Gannon, M.C. and Nuttall, F.Q. (1992) Glucose appearance rate following protein ingestion in normal subjects. *Journal of the American College of Nutrition* 11, 701–706.

Kahn, S.E., Prigeon, R.L., McCulloch, D.K., Boyko, E.J., Bergman, R.N., Schwartz, M.W., Neifing, J.L., Ward, W.K., Beard, J.C., Palmer, J.P. and Porte, D. Jr (1993) Quantification of the relationship between insulin sensitivity and β-cell function in human subjects: evidence for a hyperbolic function. *Diabetes* 42, 1663–1672.

Kanarek, R. (1997) Psychological effects of smacks and altered meal frequency. *British Journal of Nutrition* 77 (Suppl. 1), S105–S120.

Kandelman, D. (1997) Sugar, alternative sweeteners and meal frequency in relation to caries prevention: new perspectives. *British Journal of Nutrition* 77 (Suppl. 1), S121–S128.

Kaplan, R.J., Greenwood, C.E., Winocur, G. and Wolever, T.M.S. (2000) Cognitive performance is associated with glucose regulation in healthy elderly persons and can be enhanced with glucose and dietary carbohydrates. *American Journal of Clinical Nutrition* 72, 825–836.

Kaplan, R.J., Greenwood, C.E., Winocur, G. and Wolever, T.M. (2001) Dietary protein, carbohydrate, and fat enhance memory performance in the healthy elderly. *American Journal of Clinical Nutrition* 74, 687–693.

Katz, A., Nambi, S.S., Mather, K., Baron, A.D., Follmann, D.A., Sullivan, G. and Quon, M.J. (2000) Quantitative insulin sensitivity check index: a simple, accurate method for assessing insulin sensitivity in humans. *Journal of Clinical Endocrinology and Metabolism* 85, 2402–2410.

Keijzers, G.B., De Galan, B.E., Tack, C.J. and Smits, P. (2002) Caffeine can decrease insulin sensitivity in humans. *Diabetes Care* 25, 364–369.

Kelly, S., Frost, G., Whittaker, V. and Summerbell, C. (2004) Low glycaemic index diets for coronary heart disease. *Cochrane Database of Systematic Reviews* (4), CD004467.

Khayat, Z.A., Patel, N. and Klip, A. (2002) Exercise- and insulin-stimulated muscle glucose transport: distinct mechanisms of regulation. *Canadian Journal of Applied Physiology* 27, 129–151.

Kiens, B. and Richter, E.A. (1996) Types of carbohydrate in an ordinary diet affect insulin action and muscle substrates in humans. *American Journal of Clinical Nutrition* 63, 47–53.

Kim, T.H., Yang, J., Darling, P.B. and O'Connor, D.L. (2004) A large pool of available folate exists in the large intestine of human infants and piglets. *Journal of Nutrition* 134, 1389–1394.

Koistinen, H.A. and Zierath, J.R. (2002) Regulation of glucose transport in human skeletal muscle. *Annal of Medicine* 34, 410–418.

Kolb, H. and Pozzilli, P. (1999) Cow's milk and type I diabetes: the gut immune system deserves attention. *Immunology Today* 20, 108–110.

Kolonel, L.N., Henderson, B.E., Hankin, J.H., Nomura, A.M., Wilkens, L.R., Pike, M.C., Stram, D.O., Monroe, K.R., Earle, M.E. and Nagamine, F.S. (2000) A multiethnic cohort in Hawaii and Los Angeles: baseline characteristics. *American Journal of Epidemiology* 151, 346–357.

Koopmans, S.J., Frolich, M., Gribnau, E.H., Westendorp, R.G.J. and DeFronzo, R.A. (1998) Effect of hyperinsulinemia on plasma leptin concentrations and food intake in rats. *American Journal of Physiology* 274, E998–E1001.

Koruda, M.J., Rolandelli, R.H., Settle, R.G., Saul, S.H. and Rombeau, J.L. (1986) The effect of a pectin-supplemented elemental diet on intestinal adaptation to massive small bowel resection. *Journal of Parenteral and Enteral Nutrition* 10, 343–350.

Kristal, A.R., Feng, Z., Coates, R.J., Oberman, A. and George V. (1997) Associations of race/ethnicity, education, and dietary intervention with the validity and reliability of a food frequency questionnaire: The Women's Health Trial Feasibility Study in Minority Populations. *American Journal of Epidemiology* 146, 856–869.

Krotkiewski, M. (1984) Effect of guar gum on body-weight, hunger ratings and metabolism in obese subjects. *British Journal of Nutrition* 52, 97–105.

Krotkiewski, M., Szelachowska, M. and Górski, J. (1987) Secretion and removal of insulin by diet. *American Journal of Clinical Nutrition* 46, 976–979.

La Coudraie, R. and Malloizel, G. (1881) *L'Oeuvre de Claude Bernard.* J.B. Baillière, Paris.

Laine, D.C., Thomas, W., Levitt, M.D. and Bantle, J.P. (1987) Comparison of predictive capabilities of diabetic exchange lists and glycemic index of foods. *Diabetes Care* 10, 387–394.

Lajous, M., Willett, W., Lazcano-Ponce, E., Sanchez-Zamorano, L.M., Hernandez-Avila, M. and Romieu, I. (2005) Glycemic load, glycemic index, and the risk of breast cancer among Mexican women. *Cancer Causes and Control* 16, 1165–1169.

Lamarche, B., Uffelman, K.D., Carpentier, A., Cohn, J.S., Steiner, G., Barrett, P.H. and Lewis, G.F. (1999) Triglyceride enrichment of HDL enhances *in vivo* metabolic clearance of HDL apo A-I in healthy men. *Journal of Clinical Investigation* 103, 1191–1199.

Lampeter, E.F., Klinghammer, A., Scherbaum, W.A., Heinze, E., Haastert, B., Giani, G. and Kolb, H. (1998) The Deutsche Nicotinamide Intervention Study: an attempt to prevent type 1 diabetes. DENIS Group. *Diabetes* 47, 980–984.

Lang, D.A., Matthews, D.R., Burnett, M. and Turner, R.C. (1981) Brief, irregular oscillations of basal plasma insulin and glucose concentrations in diabetic man. *Diabetes* 30, 435–439.

Lang, V., Bellisle, F., Alamowitch, C., Craplet, C., Bornet, F.R.J., Slama, G. and Guy-Grand, B. (1999a) Varying the protein source in mixed meals modifies glucose, insulin and glucagon kinetics in healthy men, has weak effects on subjective satiety and fails to affect food intake. *European Journal of Clinical Nutrition* 53, 959–965.

Lang, V., Vaugelade, P., Bernard, F., Darcy-Vrillon, B., Alamowitch, C., Slama, G., Duée, P.H. and Bornet, F.R. (1999b) Euglycemic hyperinsulinemic clamp to assess posthepatic glucose appearance after carbohydrate loading. 1. Validation in pigs. *American Journal of Clinical Nutrition* 69, 1174–1182.

Lang, V., Bornet, F.R., Vaugelade, P., van Ypersele de Strihou, M., Luo, J., Pacher, N., Rossi, F., La Droitte, P., Duée, P.H. and Slama, G. (1999c) Euglycemic hyperinsulinemic clamp to assess posthepatic glucose appearance after carbohydrate loading. 2. Evaluation of corn and mung bean starches in healthy men. *American Journal of Clinical Nutrition* 69, 1183–1188.

Langfort, J., Budohoski, L., Kaciuba-Uscilko, H., Nazar, K., Challiss, J.R. and Newsholme, E.A. (1991) Effect of endurance and sprint exercise on the sensitivity of glucose metabolism to insulin in the epitrochlearis muscle of sedentary and trained rats. *European Journal of Applied Physiology and Occupational Physiology* 62, 145–150.

Langkilde, A.M., Andersson, H., Schweizer, T.F. and Würsch, P. (1994) Digestion and absorption of sorbitol, maltitol and isomalt from the small bowel. A study in ileostomy subjects. *European Journal of Clinical Nutrition* 48, 768–775.

Langkilde, A.M., Champ, M. and Andersson, H. (2002) Effects of high-resistant-starch banana flour (RS(2)) on *in vitro* fermentation and the small-bowel excretion of energy, nutrients, and sterols: an ileostomy study. *American Journal of Clinical Nutrition* 75, 104–111.

Langworthy, C.F. and Deuel, H.J. Jr (1922) Digestibility of raw rice, arrowroot, canna, cassava, taro, tree-fern, and potato starches. *Journal of Biological Chemistry* 52, 251–261.

Larivière, R., Chiasson, J.-L., Schiffrin, A., Taveroff, A. and Hoffer, L.J. (1994) Effects of dietary protein restriction on glucose and insulin metabolism in normal and diabetic humans. *Metabolism: Clinical and Experimental* 43, 462–467.

Larsen, H.N., Rasmussen, O.W., Rasmussen, P.H., Alstrup, K.K., Biswas, S.K., Tetens, I., Thilsted, S.H. and Hermansen, K. (2000) Glycaemic index of parboiled rice depends on the severity of processing: study in type 2 diabetic subjects. *European Journal of Clinical Nutrition* 54, 380–385.

Lau, C., Faerch, K., Glumer, C., Tetens, I., Pedersen, O., Carstensen, B., Jorgensen, T. and Borch-Johnsen, K. (2005) Dietary glycemic index, glycemic load, fiber, simple sugars, and insulin resistance: the Inter99 study. *Diabetes Care* 28, 1397–1403.

Lavin, J.H. and Read, N.W. (1995) The effect on hunger and satiety of slowing the absorption of glucose: relationship with gastric emptying and postprandial blood glucose and insulin responses. *Appetite* 25, 89–96.

Leahy, J.L., Cooper, H.E. and Weir, G.C. (1987) Impaired insulin secretion associated with near normoglycemia. Study in normal rats with 96-h *in vivo* glucose infusions. *Diabetes* 36, 459–464.

Leahy, J.L., Bonner-Weir, S. and Weir, G.C. (1988) Minimal chronic hyperglycemia is a critical determinant of impaired insulin secretion after incomplete pancreatectomy. *Journal of Clinical Investigation* 81, 1407–1414.

Leathwood, P. and Pollet, P. (1988) Effects of slow release carbohydrates in the form of bean flakes on the evolution of hunger and satiety in man. *Appetite* 10, 1–11.

Lean, M.E.J., Han, T.S. and Seidell, J.C. (1998) Impairment of health and quality of life in people with large waist circumference. *Lancet* 351, 853–856.

Lee, B.M. and Wolever, T.M.S. (1998) Effect of glucose, sucrose and fructose on plasma glucose and insulin responses in normal humans: comparison with white bread. *European Journal of Clinical Nutrition* 52, 924–928.

Leeson, C.P., Kattenhorn, M., Morley, R., Lucas, A. and Deanfield, J.E. (2001) Impact of low birth weight and cardiovascular risk factors on endothelial function in early adult life. *Circulation* 103, 1264–1268.

Le Floch, J.-P., Escuyer, P., Baudin, E., Baudon, D. and Perlemuter, L. (1990) Blood glucose area under the curve: methodological aspects. *Diabetes Care* 13, 172–175.

Le Floch, J.P., Baudin, E., Escuyer, P., Wirquin, E., Nillus, P. and Perlemuter, L. (1992) Influence of non-carbohydrate foods on glucose and insulin responses to carbohydrates of different glycaemic index in type 2 diabetic patients. *Diabetic Medicine* 9, 44–48.

Letexier, D., Pinteur, C., Large, V., Frering, V. and Beylot, M. (2003) Comparison of the expression and activity of the lipogenic pathway in human and rat adipose tissue. *Journal of Lipid Research* 44, 2127–2134.

Levitt, M.D. and Donaldson, R.M. (1970) Use of respiratory hydrogen ($H_2$) excretion to detect carbohydrate malabsorption. *Journal of Laboratory and Clinical Medicine* 75, 937–945.

Levitt, M.D., Hirsh, P., Fetzer, C.A., Sheahan, M. and Levine, A.S. (1987) $H_2$ excretion after ingestion of complex carbohydrates. *Gastroenterology* 92, 383–389.

Lewis, C.J., Park, Y.K., Behlen Dexter, P. and Yetley, E.A. (1992) Nutrient intakes and body weights of persons consuming high and moderate levels of added sugars. *Journal of the American Dietetic Association* 92, 708–713.

Lewis, G.F., Uffleman, K.D., Szeto, L.W. and Steiner, G. (1993) Effects of acute hyperinsulinemia on VLDL triglyceride and VLDL apoβ production in normal weight and obese individuals. *Diabetes* 42, 833–842.

Lewis, G.F., Uffelman, K.D., Szeto, L.W., Weller, B. and Steiner, G. (1995) Interaction between free fatty acids and insulin in the acute control of very low density lipoprotein production in humans. *Journal of Clinical Investigation* 95, 158–166.

Lewis, G.F., Zinman, B., Groenewoud, Y., Vranic, M. and Giacca, A. (1996) Hepatic glucose production is regulated both by direct hepatic and extrahepatic effects of insulin in humans. *Diabetes* 45, 454–462.

Lewis, G.F., Vranic, M., Harley, P. and Giacca, A. (1997) Fatty acids mediate the acute extrahepatic effects of insulin on hepatic glucose production in humans. *Diabetes* 46, 1111–1119.

Lewis, G.F., Vranic, M. and Giacca, A. (1998) Role of free fatty acids and glucagon in the peripheral effect of insulin on glucose production in humans. *American Journal of Physiology* 275, E177–E186.

Lien, H.C., Chen, G.H., Chang, C.S., Kao, C.H. and Wang, S.J. (1995) The effect of coffee on gastric emptying. *Nuclear Medicine Communications* 16, 923–926.

Liljeberg, H.G. and Björck, I.M. (1996) Delayed gastric emptying rate as a potential mechanism for lowered glycemia after eating sourdough bread: studies in humans and rats using test products with added organic acids or an organic salt. *American Journal of Clinical Nutrition* 64, 886–893.

Liljeberg, H. and Björck, I. (1998) Delayed gastric emptying rate may explain improved glycaemia in healthy subjects to a starchy meal with added vinegar. *European Journal of Clinical Nutrition* 52, 368–371.

Liljeberg, H. and Björck, I. (2000) Effects of a low-glycaemic index spaghetti meal on glucose tolerance and lipaemia at a subsequent meal in healthy subjects. *European Journal of Clinical Nutrition* 54, 24–28.

Liljeberg Elmstahl, H. and Björck, I. (2001) Milk as a supplement to mixed meals may elevate postprandial insulinaemia. *European Journal of Clinical Nutrition* 55, 994–999.

Liljeberg, H., Granfeldt, Y. and Björck, I. (1992) Metabolic responses to starch in bread containing intact kernels versus milled flour. *European Journal of Clinical Nutrition* 46, 561–575.

Liljeberg, H.G.M., Åkerberg, A.K.E. and Björck I.M.E. (1999) Effect of the glycemic index and content of indigestible carbohydrates of cereal-based breakfast meals on glucose tolerance at lunch in healthy subjects. *American Journal of Clinical Nutrition* 69, 647–655.

Lingstrom, P., van Houte, J. and Kashket, S. (2000a) Food starches and dental caries. *Critical Reviews in Oral Biology and Medicine* 11, 366–380.

Lingstrom, P., Liljeberg, H., Bjorck, I. and Birkhead, D. (2000b) The relationship between plaque pH and glycemic index of various breads. *Caries Research* 34, 75–81.

Lissner, L. and Heitmann, B.L. (1995) Dietary fat and obesity: evidence from epidemiology. *European Journal of Clinical Nutrition* 49, 79–90.

Liu, G.C., Coulston, A.M. and Reaven, G.M. (1983) Effect of high-carbohydrate-low-fat diets on plasma glucose, insulin and lipid responses in hypertriglyceridemic humans. *Metabolism: Clinical and Experimental* 32, 750–753.

Liu, S., Willett, W.C., Stampfer, M.J., Hu, F.B., Franz, M., Sampson, L., Hennekens, C.H. and Manson, J.E. (2000) A prospective study of dietary glycemic load, carbohydrate intake and risk of coronary heart disease in US women. *American Journal of Clinical Nutrition* 71, 1455–1461.

Liu, S., Manson, J.E., Stampfer, M.J., Holmes, M.D., Hu, F.B., Hankinson, S.E. and Willett, W.C. (2001) Dietary glycemic load assessed by food-frequency questionnaire in relation to plasma high-density-lipoprotein cholesterol and fasting plasma triacylglycerols in postmenopausal women. *American Journal of Clinical Nutrition* 73, 560–566.

Liu, S., Manson, J.E., Buring, J.E., Stampfer, M.J., Willett, W.C. and Rikder, P.M. (2002) Relationship between a diet with a high glycemic load and plasma concentrations of high-sensitivity C-reactive protein in middle-aged women. *American Journal of Clinical Nutrition* 75, 492–498.

Liu, P., Perry, T. and Monro, J.A. (2003a) Glycaemic glucose equivalent: validation as a predictor of the relative glycaemic effect of foods. *European Journal of Clinical Nutrition* 57, 1141–1149.

Liu, S., Willett, W.C., Manson, J.E., Hu, F.B., Rosner, B. and Colditz, G. (2003b) Relation between changes in intakes of dietary fiber and grain products and changes in weight and development of obesity among middle-aged women. *American Journal of Clinical Nutrition* 78, 920–927.

Livesey, G. (1992) The energy values of dietary fibre and sugar alcohols for man. *Nutrition Research Reviews* 2, 61–84.

Livesey, G. (2003) Health potential of polyols as sugar replacers, with emphasis on low glycaemic properties. *Nutrition Research Reviews* 16, 163–191.

Livesey, G. and Elia, M. (1995) Short-chain fatty acids as an energy source in the colon: metabolism and clinical implications. In: Cummings, J.H., Rombeau, J.L. and Sakata, T. (eds) *Physiological and Clinical Aspects of Short-Chain Fatty Acids*. Cambridge University Press, Cambridge, UK, pp. 427–482.

Livesey, G., Johnson, I.T., Gee, J.M., Smith, T., Lee, W.E., Hillan, K.A., Meyer, J. and Turner, S.C. (1993) 'Determination' of sugar alcohol and polydextrose® absorption in humans by the breath hydrogen ($H_2$) technique: the stoichiometry of hydrogen production and the interaction between carbohydrates assessed *in vivo* and *in vitro*. *European Journal of Clinical Nutrition* 47, 419–430.

Livesey, G., Wilson, P.D.G., Roe, M.A., Faulks, R.M., Oram, L.M., Brown, J.C., Eagles, J., Greenwood, R.H. and Kennedy, H. (1998) Splanchnic retention of intraduodenal and intrajejunal glucose in healthy adults. *American Journal of Physiology – Endocrinology and Metabolism*, 275, E709–E716.

Logan, A.G. (2000) Sodium sensitivity, not level of salt intake, predicts salt effects. *Current Hypertension Reports* 2, 115–119.

Lonnoth, P., Jansson, P.A. and Smith, U. (1987) A microdialysis method allowing characterization of intercellular water space in humans. *American Journal of Physiology* 253, E228–E231.

Lopez-Ridaura, R., Willett, W.C., Rimm, E.B., Liu, S., Stampfer, M.J., Manson, J.E. and Hu, F.B. (2004) Magnesium intake and risk of type 2 diabetes in men and women. *Diabetes Care* 27, 134–140.

Ludvik, B., Nolan, J.J., Roberts, A., Baloga, J., Joyce, M., Bell, J.M. and Olefsky, J.M. (1995) A noninvasive method to measure splanchnic glucose uptake after oral glucose administration. *Journal of Clinical Investigation* 95, 2232–2238.

Ludvik, B., Nolan, J.J., Roberts, A., Baloga, J., Joyce, M., Bell, J.M. and Olefsky, J.M. (1997) Evidence for decreased splanchnic glucose uptake after oral glucose administration in non-insulin-dependent diabetes mellitus. *Journal of Clinical Investigation* 100, 2354–2361.

Ludwig, D.S. (2000) Dietary glycemic index and obesity. *Journal of Nutrition* 130 (Suppl. 2S), 280S–283S.

Ludwig, D.S., Pereira, M.A., Kroenke, C.H., Hilner, J.E., Van Horn, L., Slattery, M.L. and Jacobs, D.R. Jr (1999a) Dietary fiber, weight gain, and cardiovascular disease risk factors in young adults. *Journal of the American Medical Association* 282, 1539–1546.

Ludwig, D.S., Majzoub, J.A., Al-Zahrani, A., Dallal, G.E., Blanco, I. and Roberts, S.B. (1999b) High glycemic index foods, overeating, and obesity. *Pediatrics* 103, E26. Available at: http://www.pediatrics.org/cgi/content/full/103/3/e26

Ludwig, D.S., Peterson, K.E. and Gortmaker, S.L. (2001) Relation between consumption of sugar-sweetened drinks and childhood obesity: a prospective, observational analysis. *Lancet* 357, 505–508.

Lupton, J.R. and Turner, N.D. (2003) Dietary fiber and coronary disease: does the evidence support an association? *Current Atherosclerosis Reports* 5, 500–505.

Lütjens, A., Verleur, H. and Plooij, M. (1975) Glucose and insulin levels on loading with different carbohydrates. *Clinica Chimica Acta* 62, 239–243.

Lyons, T.J. (1992) Lipoprotein glycation and its metabolic consequences. *Diabetes*, 41 (Suppl. 2), 67–73.

Ma, Y., Olendzki, B., Chiriboga, D., Hebert, J.R., Li, Y., Li, W., Campbell, M.J., Gendreau, K. and Ockene, I.S. (2005) Association between dietary carbohydrates and body weight. *American Journal of Epidemiology* 161, 359–367.

Macdonald, I., Keyser, A. and Pacy, D. (1978) Some effects, in man, of varying the load of glucose, sucrose, fructose, or sorbitol on various metabolites in blood. *American Journal of Clinical Nutrition* 31, 1305–1311.

MacIntosh, C.G., Holt, S.H.A. and Brand-Miller, J.C. (2003) The degree of fat saturation does not alter glycemic, insulinemic or satiety responses to a starchy staple in healthy men. *Journal of Nutrition* 133, 2577–2580.

MacLean, H. (1922) *Modern Methods in the Diagnosis and Treatment of Glycosuria and Diabetes*. Constable & Co Ltd, London, pp. 26–27.

Maheux, P., Azhar, S., Kern, P.A., Chen, Y.-D.I. and Reaven, G.M. (1997) Relationship between insulin-mediated glucose disposal and regulation of plasma and adipose tissue lipoprotein lipase. *Diabetologia* 40, 850–858.

Malherbe, C., de Gasparo, M., de Hertogh, R. and Hoet, J.J. (1969) Circadian variations of blood sugar and plasma insulin levels in man. *Diabetologia* 5, 397–404.

Malik, V. (2003) Development and validation of a food frequency questionnaire to assess the diet glycemic index of adults in Trinidad & Tobago. MSc thesis, University of Toronto, Toronto, Ontario.

Malinow, M.R., Duell, P.B., Hess, D.L., Anderson, P.H., Kruger, W.D., Phillipson, B.E., Gluckman, R.A., Block, P.C. and Upson, M.B. (1998) Reduction of plasma homocyst(e)ine levels by breakfast cereal fortified with folic acid in patients with coronary heart disease. *New England Journal of Medicine* 338, 1009–1015.

Marks, P.A. and Bishop, J.S. (1957) The glucose metabolism of patients with malignant disease and of normal subjects as studied by means of an intravenous glucose tolerance test. *Journal of Clinical Investigation* 36, 254–264.

Martin, B.C., Warran, J.H., Krolewski, A.S., Bergman, R.N., Soeldner, J.S. and Kahn, C.R. (1992) Role of glucose and insulin resistance in development of type 2 diabetes mellitus: results of a 25-year follow-up study. *Lancet* 340, 925–929.

Martin, L.J., Su, W., Jones, P.J., Lockwood, G.A., Tritchler, D.L. and Boyd, N.F. (1996) Comparison of energy intakes determined by food records and doubly labeled water in women participating in a dietary intervention trial. *American Journal of Clinical Nutrition* 63, 483–490.

Matsuda, M. and DeFronzo, R.A. (1999) Insulin sensitivity indices obtained from oral glucose tolerance testing: comparison with the euglycemic insulin clamp. *Diabetes Care* 22, 1462–1470.

Matthews, D.R., Lang, D.A., Burnett, M. and Turner, R.C. (1983) Control of pulsatile insulin secretion in man. *Diabetologia* 24, 231–237.

Matthews, D.R., Hosker, J.P., Rudenski, A.S., Naylor, B.A., Treacher, D.F. and Turner, R.C. (1985) Homeostasis model assessment: insulin resistance and β-cell function from fasting plasma glucose and insulin concentrations in man. *Diabetologia* 28, 412–419.

Mayer-Davis, E.J., Vitolins M.Z., Carmichael, S.L., Hemphill, S., Tsaroucha, G., Rushing, J. and Levin, S. (1999) Validity and reproducibility of a food frequency interview in a multi-cultural epidemiologic study. *Annals of Epidemiology* 9, 314–324.

McBurney, M.I., Thompson, L.U. and Jenkins, D.J.A.J. (1987) Colonic fermentation of some breads and its implication for energy availability in man. *Nutrition Research* 7, 1229–1241.

McBurney, M.I., Thompson, L.U., Cuff, D.J. and Jenkins, D.J.A. (1988) Comparison of ileal effluents, dietary fibers, and whole foods in predicting the physiological importance of colonic fermentation. *American Journal of Gastroenterology* 83, 536–540.

McCleary, B.V. and Monaghan, D.A. (2002) Measurement of resistant starch. *Journal of the Association of Official Analytical Chemists International* 85, 665–675.

McKeown, N.M., Meigs, J.B., Liu, S., Saltzman, E., Wilson, P.W.F. and Jacques, P.F. (2004) Carbohydrate nutrition, insulin resistance, and the prevalence of the metabolic syndrome in the Framingham Offspring cohort. *Diabetes Care* 27, 538–546.

McKeown-Essen, G. (1994) Epidemiology of colorectal cancer revisited: are serum triglycerides and/or plasma glucose associated with risk? *Cancer Epidemiology, Biomarkers and Prevention* 3, 687–695.

McNeil, N.I. (1984) The contribution of the large intestine to energy supplies in man. *American Journal of Clinical Nutrition* 39, 338–342.

McNeil, N.I., Cummings, J.H. and James, W.P.T. (1978) Short chain fatty acid absorption by the human large intestine. *Gut* 19, 819–822.

Mehalski, K., Brand-Miller, J., Blakesmith, S., Kirby, A., Pollicino, C., Baghurst, K., Record, S., Hague, W., Simes, J., Nestel, P., Tonkin, A. and Colquhoun, D. (2003) Baseline diet glycemic load and glycemic index are determinants of HDL cholesterol levels in patients with coronary heart disease: results from the LIPID study. *Atherosclerosis Supplements* 4, 282–283.

Melanson, K.J., Westerterp, M.S., Smith, F.J., Campfield, L.A. and Saris, W.H.M. (1999a) Blood glucose patterns and appetite in time-blinded humans: carbohydrate versus fat. *American Journal of Physiology* 46, R337–R345.

Melanson, K.J., Westerterp-Plantenga, M.S., Campfield, L.A. and Saris, W.H.M. (1999b) Blood glucose and meal patterns in time-blinded males, after aspartame, carbohydrate, and fat consumption, in relation to sweetness perception. *British Journal of Nutrition* 82, 437–446.

Merier, C., Charbonnière, R., Grebaut, J. and de la Guerivière, J.F. (1980) Formation of amylose–lipid complexes by twin-screw extrusion cooking of manioc starch. *Cereal Chemistry* 57, 4–9.

Metz, G., Gassull, M.A., Leeds, A.R., Blendis, L.M. and Jenkins, D.J. (1976) A simple method of measuring breath hydrogen in carbohydrate malabsorption by end-expiratory sampling. *Clinical Science and Molecular Medicine* 50, 237–240.

Meyer, J. (1955) Regulation of energy intake and the body weight, the glucostatic theory and the lipostatic hypothesis. *Annals of the New York Academy of Sciences* 63, 15–43.

Michaud, D.S., Liu, S., Giovannucci, E., Willett, W.C., Colditz, G.A. and Fuchs, C.S. (2002) Dietary sugar, glycemic load, and pancreatic cancer risk in a prospective study. *Journal of the National Cancer Institute* 94, 1293–1300.

Mikines, K.J., Sonne, B., Farrell, P.A., Tronier, B. and Galo, H. (1988) Effect of physical exercise on sensitivity and responsiveness to insulin in humans. *American Journal of Physiology* 254, E248–E259.

Miller, C.J., Dunn, E.V. and Hashim, I.B. (2003) The glycaemic index of dates and date/yoghurt mixed meals. Are dates 'the candy that grows on trees'? *European Journal of Clinical Nutrition* 57, 427–430.

Mimura, A., Kageyama, S., Maruyama, M., Ikeda, Y. and Isogai, Y. (1994) Insulin sensitivity test using a somatostatin analogue, Octreotide (Sandostatin®). *Hormone and Metabolic Research* 26, 183–186.

Mittendorfer, B. and Sidossis, L.S. (2001) Mechanism for the increase in plasma triacylglycerol concentrations after consumption of short-term, high-carbohydrate diets. *American Journal of Clinical Nutrition* 73, 892–899.

Mohammed, N.H. and Wolever, T.M.S. (2004) Effect of carbohydrate source on postprandial blood glucose in subjects with type 1 diabetes treated with insulin lispro. *Diabetes Research and Clinical Practice* 65, 29–35.

Mokdad, A.H., Bowman, B.A., Ford, E.S., Vinicor, F., Marks, J.S. and Koplan, J.P. (2001) The continuing epidemics of obesity and diabetes in the United States. *Journal of the American Medical Association* 286, 1195–1200.

Monro, J.A. (2002) Glycaemic glucose equivalent: combining carbohydrate content, quantity and glycaemic index of foods for precision in glycaemia management. *Asia Pacific Journal of Clinical Nutrition* 11, 217–225.

Monro, J.A. (2003) Redefining glycemic index for dietary management of postprandial glycemia. *Journal of Nutrition* 133, 4256–4258.

Monro, J.A. (2005) Expressing the glycaemic potency of foods. *Proceedings of the Nutrition Society* 64, 115–122.

Montague, C.T. and O'Rahilly, S. (2000) The perils of portliness: causes and consequences of visceral adiposity. *Diabetes* 49, 883–888.

Mooradian, A.D. and Thurman, J.E. (1999) Drug therapy of postprandial hyperglycaemia. *Drugs* 57, 19–29.

Morgan, L.M., Hampton, S.M., Tredger, J.A., Cramb, R. and Marks, V. (1988a) Modifications of gastric inhibitory polypeptide (GIP) secretion in man by a high fat diet. *British Journal of Nutrition* 59, 373–380.

Morgan, L.M., Tredger, J.A., Hampton, S.M., French, A.P., Peake, J.C. and Marks, V. (1988b) The effect of dietary modification and hyperglycaemia on gastric emptying and gastric inhibitory polypeptide (GIP) secretion. *British Journal of Nutrition* 60, 29–37.

Motulsky, H. (1995) *Intuitive Biostatistics.* Oxford University Press, Oxford, UK.

Mourot, J., Thouvenout, P., Couet, C., Antoine, J.M., Krobicka, A. and Debry, G. (1988) Relationship between the rate of gastric emptying and glucose and insulin responses to starchy foods in young healthy adults. *American Journal of Clinical Nutrition* 48, 1035–1040.

Mozaffarian, D., Rimm, E.R. and Herrington, D.M. (2005) Dietary fats, carbohydrate, and progression of coronary atherosclerosis in postmenopausal women. *American Journal of Clinical Nutrition* 80, 1175–1184.

Muggeo, M., Verlato, G., Bonora, E., Zoppini, G., Corbellini, M. and de Marco, R. (1997) Long-term instability of fasting plasma glucose, a novel predictor of cardiovascular mortality in elderly patients with non-insulin-dependent diabetes mellitus. *Circulation* 96, 1750–1754.

Muggeo, M., Zoppini, G., Bonora, E., Brun, E., Bonadonna, R.C., Moghetti, P. and Verlato, G. (2000) Fasting plasma glucose variability predicts 10-year survival of type 2 diabetic patients: the Verona Diabetes Study. *Diabetes Care* 23, 45–50.

Muir, J.G., Walker, K.Z., Kaimakamis, M.A., Cameron, M.A., Govers, M.J., Lu, Z.X., Young, G.P. and O'Dea, K. (1998) Modulation of fecal markers relevant to colon cancer risk: a high-starch Chinese diet did not generate expected beneficial changes relative to a Western-type diet. *American Journal of Clinical Nutrition* 68, 372–379.

Murphy, E.L. and Calloway, D.H. (1972) The effect of antibiotic drugs on the volume and composition of intestinal gas from beans. *American Journal of Digestive Diseases* 17, 639–642.

Murphy, M.C., Isherwood, S.G., Sethi, S., Gould, B.J., Wright, J.W., Knapper, J.A. and Williams, C.M. (1995) Postprandial lipid and hormone responses to meals of varying fat contents: modulatory role of lipoprotein lipase? *European Journal of Clinical Nutrition* 49, 579–588.

Nagulesparan, M., Savage, P.J., Unger, R.H. and Bennett, P.H. (1979) A simplified method using somatostatin to assess *in vivo* insulin resistance over a range of obesity. *Diabetes* 28, 980–983.

Nakaji, S., Tokunaga, S., Sakamoto, J., Todate, M., Shimoyama, T., Umeda, T. and Sugawara, K. (2002) Relationship between lifestyle factors and defecation in a Japanese population. *European Journal of Nutrition* 41, 244–248.

Nauck, M.A., Baller, B. and Meier, J.J. (2004) Gastric inhibitory polypeptide and glucagon-like peptide-1 in the pathogenesis of type 2 diabetes. *Diabetes* 53 (Suppl. 3), S190–S196.

Nawrot, P., Jordan, S., Eastwood, J., Rotstein, J., Hugenholtz, A. and Feeley M. (2003) Effects of caffeine on human health. *Food Additives and Contaminants* 20, 1–30.

Naylor, C.D., Sermer, M., Chen, E. and Sykora, K. (1996) Cesarean delivery in relation to birth weight and gestational glucose tolerance: pathophysiology or practice style? Toronto Trihospital Gestational Diabetes Investigators. *Journal of the American Medical Association* 275, 1165–1170.

Naylor, C.D., Sermer, M., Chen, E. and Farine, D. (1997) Selective screening for gestational diabetes mellitus. Toronto Trihospital Gestational Diabetes Project Investigators. *New England Journal of Medicine* 337, 1591–1596.

Neel, J.V. (1962) Diabetes mellitus: a "thrifty" genotype rendered detrimental by "progress." *American Journal of Human Genetics* 14, 353–362.

Neel, J.V. (1982) The thrifty genotype revisited. 1982. The genetics of diabetes mellitus. In: Kobberling, J., Tattersall, J. and Tattersall, R. (eds) *The Genetics of Diabetes Mellitus.* Academic Press, London, pp. 283–293.

Nestler, J.E., Barlascini, C.O., Clore, J.N. and Blackard, W.G. (1988) Absorption characteristic of breakfast determines insulin sensitivity and carbohydrate tolerance for lunch. *Diabetes Care* 11, 755–760.

Ng, D.S. (2004) Treating low HDL – from bench to bedside. *Clinical Biochemistry* 37, 649–659.

Nielsen, P.H. and Nielsen, G.L. (1989) Preprandial blood glucose values: influence on glycemic response studies. *American Journal of Clinical Nutrition* 49, 1243–1246.

Niness, K.R. (1999) Inulin and oligofructose: what are they? *Journal of Nutrition* 129, 1402S–1406S.

Noah, L., Guillon, F., Bouchet, B., Buléon, A., Molis, C., Gratas, M. and Champ, M. (1998) Digestion of carbohydrate from white beans (*Phaseolus vulgaris*) in healthy humans. *Journal of Nutrition* 128, 977–985.

Normand, S., Pachiaudi, C., Khalfallah, Y., Guilluy, R., Mornex, R. and Riou, J.P. (1992) $^{13}C$ appearance in plasma glucose and breath $CO_2$ during feeding with naturally $^{13}C$-enriched starchy food in normal humans. *American Journal of Clinical Nutrition* 55, 430–435.

Normand, S., Khalfallah, Y., Louche-Pelissier, C., Pachiaudi, C., Antoine, J., Blanc, S., Desage, M., Riou, J. and Laville, M. (2001) Influence of dietary fat on postprandial glucose metabolism (exogenous and endogenous) using intrinsically $^{13}C$-enriched durum wheat. *British Journal of Nutrition* 86, 3–11.

Novotny, J.A., Rumpler, W.V., Riddick, H., Hebert, J.R., Rhodes, D., Judd, J.T., Baer, D.J., McDowell, M. and Briefel, R. (2003) Personality characteristics as predictors of underreporting of energy intake on 24-hour dietary recall interviews. *Journal of the American Dietetic Association* 103, 1146–1151.

Nuttall, F.Q. and Gannon, M.C. (1990) Metabolic response to egg white and cottage cheese protein in normal subjects. *Metabolism: Clinical and Experimental* 39, 749–755.

Nuttall, F.Q., Mooradian, A.D., DeMarais, R. and Parker, S. (1983) The glycemic effect of different meals approximately isocaloric and similar in protein, carbohydrate and fat content as calculated using the ADA exchange lists. *Diabetes Care* 6, 432–435.

Nuttall, F.Q., Mooradian, A.D., Gannon, M.C., Billington, C. and Krezowski, P. (1984) Effect of protein ingestion on the glucose and insulin response to a standardized oral glucose load. *Diabetes Care* 7, 465–470.

Nuttall, F.Q., Khan, M.A. and Gannon, M.C. (2000) Peripheral glucose appearance rate following fructose ingestion in normal subjects. *Metabolism: Clinical and Experimental* 49, 1565–1571.

O'Dea, K., Snow, P. and Nestel, P. (1981) Rate of starch hydrolysis *in vitro* as a predictor of metabolic responses to complex carbohydrates *in vivo*. *American Journal of Clinical Nutrition* 34, 1991–1993.

Odeleye, O.E., de Courten, M., Pettitt, D.J. and Ravussin, E. (1997) Fasting hyperinsulinemia is a predictor of increased body weight gain and obesity in Pima Indian children. *Diabetes* 46, 1341–1345.

Oh, K., Hu, F.B., Cho, E., Rexrode, K.M., Stampfer, M.J., Manson, J.E., Liu, S. and Willett, W.C. (2005) Carbohydrate intake, glycemic index, glycemic load, and dietary fiber in relation to risk of stroke in women. *American Journal of Epidemiology* 161, 161–169.

Olesen, M., Rumessen, J.J. and Gudmand-Høyer, E. (1994) Intestinal transport and fermentation of resistant starch evaluated by the hydrogen breath test. *European Journal of Clinical Nutrition* 48, 692–701.

Onning, G. and Asp, N.G. (1995) Effect of oat saponins and different types of dietary fibre on the digestion of carbohydrates. *British Journal of Nutrition* 74, 229–237.

Opperman, A.M., Venter, C.S., Oosthuizen, W., Thompson, R.L. and Vorster, H.H. (2004) Meta-analysis of the health effects of using the glycaemic index in meal-planning. *British Journal of Nutrition* 92, 367–381.

Osei, K., Rhinesmith, S., Gaillard, T. and Schuster, D. (2004) Impaired insulin sensitivity, insulin secretion, and glucose effectiveness predict future development of impaired glucose tolerance and type 2 diabetes in pre-diabetic African Americans: implications for primary diabetes prevention. *Diabetes Care* 27, 1439–1446.

Östman, E.M., Liljeberg, H.G.M. and Björck, I.M.E. (2001) Inconsistency between glycemic and insulinemic responses to regular and fermented milk products. *American Journal of Clinical Nutrition* 74, 96–100.

Östman, E.M., Liljeberg, H.G.M. and Björck, I.M.E. (2002) Barley bread containing lactic acid improves glucose tolerance at a subsequent meal in healthy men and women. *Journal of Nutrition* 132, 1173–1175.

Ostman, E.M., Frid, A.H., Groop, L.C. and Bjorck, I.M. (2005) A dietary exchange of common bread for tailored bread of low glycaemic index and rich in dietary fibre improved insulin economy in young women with impaired glucose tolerance. *European Journal of Clinical Nutrition* advance online publication, 19 October 2005; doi:10.1038/sj.ejcn.1602319.

Owen, B. and Wolever, T.M.S. (2003) Effect of fat on glycaemic responses in normal subjects: a dose–response study. *Nutrition Research* 23, 1341–1347.

Panlasigui, L.N., Thompson, L.U., Juliano, B.O., Perez, C.M., Yiu, S.H. and Greenberg, G.R. (1991) Rice varieties with similar amylose content differ in starch digestibility and glycemic response in humans. *American Journal of Clinical Nutrition* 54, 871–877.

Parillo, M., Giacco, R., Riccardi, G., Pacioni, D. and Rivellese, A. (1985) Different glycaemic responses to pasta, bread and potatoes in diabetic patients. *Diabetic Medicine* 2, 374–377.

Parsons, S.R. (1984) Effects of high fiber breakfasts on glucose metabolism in noninsulin-dependent diabetics. *American Journal of Clinical Nutrition* 40, 66–71.

Pastors, J.G., Blaisdell, P.W., Balm, T.K., Asplin, C.M. and Pohl, S.L. (1991) Psyllium fiber reduces rise in postprandial glucose and insulin concentrations in patients with non-insulin-dependent diabetes. *American Journal of Clinical Nutrition* 53, 1431–1435.

Patil, D.H., Grimble, G.K. and Silk, D.B.A. (1987) Lactitol, a new hydrogenated lactose derivative: intestinal absorption and laxative threshold in normal human subjects. *British Journal of Nutrition* 57, 195–199.

Pawlak, D.B., Bryson, J.M., Denyer, G.S. and Brand-Miller, J.C. (2001) High glycemic index starch promotes hypersecretion of insulin and higher body fat in rats without affecting insulin sensitivity. *Journal of Nutrition* 131, 99–104.

Pawlak, D.B., Kushner, J.A. and Ludwig, D.S. (2004) Effects of dietary glycaemic index on adiposity, glucose homoeostasis, and plasma lipids in animals. *Lancet* 364, 778–785.

Pelletier, X., Donazzolo, Y., Barbier-Latreille, M., Laure-Boussuge, S., Ruel, C. and Debry, G. (1998) Effect of cream cheese consumption on the glycemic response to the meal in healthy subjects. *Nutrition Research* 18, 767–774.

Perfetti, R., Zhou, J., Doyle, M.E. and Egan, J.M. (2000) Glucagon-like peptide-1 induces cell proliferation and pancreatic-duodenum homeobox-1 expression and increases endocrine cell mass in the pancreas of old, glucose-intolerant rats. *Endocrinology* 141, 4600–4605.

Peters, A.L. and Davidson, M.B. (1993) Protein and fat effects on glucose responses and insulin requirements in subjects with insulin-dependent diabetes mellitus. *American Journal of Clinical Nutrition* 58, 555–560.

Peters, U., Sinha, R., Chatterjee, N., Subar, A.F., Ziegler, R.G., Kulldorff, M., Bresalier, R., Weissfeld, J.L., Flood, A., Schatzkin, A., Hayes, R.B. for the Prostate, Lung, Colorectal, and Ovarian Cancer Screening Trial Project Team (2003) Dietary fibre and colorectal adenoma in a colorectal cancer early detection programme. *Lancet* 361, 1491–1495.

Pettitt, D.J., Forman, M.R., Hanson, R.L., Knowler, W.C. and Bennett, P.H. (1997) Breastfeeding and incidence of non-insulin-dependent diabetes mellitus in Pima Indians. *Lancet* 350, 166–168.

Phenekos, C. (2001) Influence of fetal body weight on metabolic complications in adult life: review of the evidence. *Journal of Pediatric Endocrinology* 14 (Suppl. 5), 1361–1363.

Phillips, D.I., Clark, P.M., Hales, C.N. and Osmond, C. (1995) Understanding oral glucose tolerance: comparison of glucose or insulin measurements during the oral glucose tolerance test with specific measurements of insulin resistance and insulin secretion. *Diabetic Medicine* 11, 286–292.

Pischon, T., Girman, C.J., Rifai, N., Hotamisligil, G.S. and Rimm, E.B. (2005) Association between dietary factors and plasma adiponectin concentrations in men. *American Journal of Clinical Nutrition* 81, 780–786.

Pisters, P.W., Restifo, N.P., Cersosimo, E. and Brennan, M.F. (1991) The effects of euglycemic hyperinsulinemia and amino acid infusion on regional and whole body glucose disposal in man. *Metabolism: Clinical and Experimental* 40, 59–65.

Pi-Sunyer, F.X. (2002) Glycemic index and disease. *American Journal of Clinical Nutrition* 76 (Suppl.), 290S–298S.

Poppitt, S.D., Swann, D., Black, A.E. and Prentice, A.M. (1998) Assessment of selective under-reporting of food intake by both obese and non-obese women in a metabolic facility. *International Journal of Obesity and Related Metabolic Disorders* 22, 303–311.

PowerBar Sport When To Use/FAQ. Available at: http://powerbar.ca/en/Products/PowerBar_SPORT/When_to_Use/index (accessed 12 January, 2005)

Prentki, M. and Corkey, B.E. (1996) Are the β-cell signaling molecules malonyl-CoA and cytosolic long-chain acyl-CoA implicated in multiple tissue defects of obesity and NIDDM? *Diabetes* 45, 273–283.

Prentice, A.M. (1998) Manipulation of dietary fat and energy density and subsequent effects on substrate flux and food intake. *American Journal of Clinical Nutrition* 67, 535S–541S.

Přibylová, J. and Kozlová, J. (1979) Glucose and galactose infusions in newborns of diabetic and healthy mothers. *Biology of the Neonate* 36, 193–197.

Přibylová, H., Sternová, H. and Kimlová, I. (1979) Plasma insulin, carbohydrate, and free fatty acid changes in newly born infants of diabetic and non-diabetic mothers after loading with glucose, fructose, and galactose. *Physiologia Bohemoslovenica* 28, 113–121.

Qi, L., Rimm, E., Liu, S., Rifai, N. and Hu, F.B. (2005) Dietary glycemic index, glycemic load, cereal fiber, and plasma adiponectin concentration in diabetic men. *Diabetes Care* 28, 1022–1028.

Quon, M.J., Cochran, C., Taylor, S.I. and Eastman, R.C. (1994) Non-insulin-mediated glucose disappearance in subjects with IDDM. Discordance between experimental results and minimal model analysis. *Diabetes* 43, 890–896.

Raatz, S.K., Torkelson, C.J., Redmon, J.B., Reck, K.P., Kwong, C.A., Swanson, J.E., Liu, C., Thomas, W. and Bantle, J.P. (2005) Reduced glycemic index and glycemic load diets do not increase the effects of energy restriction on weight loss and insulin sensitivity in obese men and women. *Journal of Nutrition* 135, 2387–2391.

Raben, A., Tagliabue, A., Christensen, N.J., Madsen, J., Holst, J.J. and Astrup, A. (1994) Resistant starch: the effect on postprandial glycemia, hormonal response, and satiety. *American Journal of Clinical Nutrition* 60, 544–551.

Raben, A., Vasilaras, T.H., Moller, A.C. and Astrup, A. (2002) Sucrose compared with artificial sweeteners: different effects on *ad libitum* food intake and body weight after 10 wk of supplementation in overweight subjects. *American Journal of Clinical Nutrition* 76, 721–729.

Randle, P.J., Hales, C.N., Garland, P.B. and Newsholme, E.A. (1963) The glucose fatty-acid cycle. Its role in insulin insensitivity and the metabolic disturbances of diabetes mellitus. *Lancet* i, 785–789.

Ranganath, L.R., Beety, J.M., Morgan, L.M., Wright, J.W., Howland, R. and Marks, V. (1996) Attenuated GLP-1 secretion in obesity: cause of consequence? *Gut* 38, 916–919.

Ranganath, L., Norris, F., Morgan, L., Wright, J. and Marks, V. (1999a) The effect of circulating non-esterified fatty acids on the entero-insular axis. *European Journal of Clinical Investigation* 29, 27–32.

Ranganath, L., Norris, F., Morgan, L., Wright, J. and Marks, V. (1999b) Inhibition of carbohydrate-mediated glucagon-like peptide-1 (7–36) amide secretion by circulating non-esterified fatty acids. *Clinical Science* 96, 335–342.

Ranganathan, S., Champ, M., Pechard, C., Blanchard, P., Nguyen, M., Colonna, P. and Krempf, M. (1994) Comparative study of the acute effects of resistant starch and dietary fibers on metabolic indexes in men. *American Journal of Clinical Nutrition* 59, 879–883.

Rasmussen, O. (1993a) Dose-dependency of the glycemic response to starch-rich meals in non-insulin-dependent diabetic subjects: studies with varying amounts of white rice. *Metabolism: Clinical and Experimental* 42, 214–217.

Rasmussen, O. (1993b) Dose-dependency of the glycemic response to starch-rich meals in insulin-dependent diabetic subjects: studies at constant insulinemia. *Metabolism: Clinical and Experimental* 42, 710–713.

Rasmussen, O., Gregersen, S. and Hermansen, K. (1990) The predictive capability of the glycaemic response to spaghetti in non-insulin dependent (NIDDM) and insulin dependent (IDDM) diabetic subjects. *Journal of Internal Medicine* 228, 97–101.

Rasmussen, O.W., Gregersen, S., Dørup, J. and Hermansen, K. (1992) Day-to-day variation of blood glucose and insulin responses in NIDDM subjects after starch-rich meal. *Diabetes Care* 15, 522–524.

Rasmussen, O.W., Lauszus, F.F., Christiansen, C., Thomsen, C. and Hermansen, K. (1996) Differential effects of saturated and monounsaturated fat on blood glucose and insulin responses in subjects with non-insulin-dependent diabetes mellitus. *American Journal of Clinical Nutrition* 63, 249–253.

Ravich, W.J., Bayless, T.M. and Thomas, M. (1983) Fructose: incomplete intestinal absorption in humans. *Gastroenterology* 84, 26–29.

Ravussin, E. and Swinburn, B.A. (1996) Insulin resistance is a result, not a cause of obesity: Socratic debate: the pro side. In: Angel, A., Anderson, H., Bouchard, C., Lau, D., Lieter, L. and Mendelson, R. (eds) *Progress in Obesity Research: 7.* 7th International Congress on Obesity, John Libbey & Co, London, pp. 173–178.

Rea, R.L., Thompson, L.U. and Jenkins, D.J.A. (1985) Lectins in foods and their relation to starch digestibility. *Nutrition Research* 5, 919–929.

Read, N.W., Aljancki, M.N., Bates, T.E. and Barber, D.C. (1984) Effect of gastrointestinal intubation on the passage of a solid meal through the stomach and small intestine in humans. *Gastroenterology* 83, 1568–1572.

Reaven, G.M. (1988) Role of insulin resistance in human disease. *Diabetes* 37, 1595–1607.

Reaven, G.M. (1994) Syndrome X: is one enough? *American Heart Journal* 127, 1439–1442.

Reaven, G.M. and Laws, A. (1994) Insulin resistance, *compensatory* hyperinsulinaemia and coronary heart disease. *Diabetologia* 37, 948–952.

Reaven, G.M., Lerner, R.L., Stern, M.P. and Farquhar, J.W. (1967) Role of insulin in endogenous hypertriglyceridemia. *Journal of Clinical Investigation* 46, 1756–1767.

Reaven, G.M., Bernstein, R., Davis, B. and Olefsky, J.M. (1976) Nonketotic diabetes mellitus: insulin deficiency or insulin resistance. *American Journal of Medicine* 60, 80–88.

Reidelberger, R.D. (1994) Cholecystokinin and control of food intake. *Journal of Nutrition* 124, S1327–S1333.

Reimer, R.A. and McBurney, M.I. (1996) Dietary fiber modulates intestinal proglucagon messenger ribonucleic acid and postprandial secretion of glucagon-like peptide-1 and insulin in rats. *Endocrinology* 137, 3948–3956.

Reiser, S., Powell, A.S., Yang, C.-Y. and Canary, J.J. (1987) An insulinogenic effect of oral fructose in humans during postprandial hyperglycemia. *American Journal of Clinical Nutrition* 45, 580–587.

Riby, J.E., Fujisawa, T. and Kretchmer, N. (1993) Fructose absorption. *American Journal of Clinical Nutrition* 58 (Suppl.), 748S–753S.

Richieri, G.V., Ogata, R.T., Zimmerman, A.W., Veerkamp, J.H. and Kleinfeld, A.M. (2000) Fatty acid binding proteins from different tissues show distinct patterns of fatty acid interactions. *Biochemistry* 39, 7197–7204.

Ridker, P.M., Cannon, C.P., Morrow, D., Rifai, N., Rose, L.M., McCabe, C.H., Pfeffer, M.C. and Braunwald, E. for the Pravastatin or Atorvastatin Evaluation and Infections Therapy – Thrombolysis in Myocardial Infarction

22 (PROVE IT-TIMI 22) Investigators (2005) C-reactive protein levels and outcomes after statin therapy. *New England Journal of Medicine* 352, 20–28.

Rigaud, D., Paycha, F., Meulemans, A., Merrouche, M. and Mignon, M. (1998) Effect of psyllium on gastric emptying, hunger feeling and food intake in normal volunteers: a double blind study. *European Journal of Clinical Nutrition* 52, 239–245.

Rimm, E.B., Giovannucci, E.L., Stampfer, M.J., Colditz, G.A., Litin, L.B. and Willett, W.C. (1992) Reproducibility and validity of an expanded self-administered semiquantitative food frequency questionnaire among male health professionals. *American Journal of Epidemiology* 135, 1114–1126.

Risso, A., Mercuri, F., Quagliaro, L., Damante, G. and Ceriello, A. (2001) Intermittent high glucose enhances apoptosis in human umbilical vein endothelial cells in culture. *American Journal of Physiology – Endocrinology and Metabolism* 281, E924–E930.

Ritz, P., Cloarec, D., Beylot, M., Champ, M., Charbonnel, B., Normand, S. and Krempf, M. (1993) Effects of colonic fermentation on respiratory gas exchanges following a glucose load in man. *Metabolism: Clinical and Experimental* 42, 347–352.

Rizkalla, S.W., Taghrid, L., Laromiguiere, M., Huet, D., Boillot, J., Rigoir, A., Elgrably, F. and Slama, G. (2004) Improved plasma glucose control, whole-body glucose utilization, and lipid profile on a low-glycemic index diet in type 2 diabetic men: a randomized trial. *Diabetes Care* 27, 1866–1872.

Robb, P.A., Wolever, T.M.S. and Hassanein, J. (1991) Use of breath hydrogen to quantify carbohydrate malabsorption: lack of effect of soluble fibre (guar). *Nutrition Research* 11, 1349–1356.

Roberge, J.N and Brubaker, P.L. (1991) Secretion of proglucagon-derived peptides in response to intestinal luminal nutrients. *Endocrinology* 128, 3169–3174.

Roberge, J.N and Brubaker, P.L. (1993) Regulation of intestinal proglucagon-derived peptide secretion by glucose-dependent insulinotropic peptide in a novel enteroendocrine loop. *Endocrinology* 133, 233–240.

Robertson, M.D., Livesey, G., Morgan, L.M., Hampton, S.M. and Mathers, J.C. (1999) The influence of the colon on postprandial glucagons-like peptide 1 (7–36) amide concentration in man. *Journal of Endocrinology* 161, 25–31.

Robertson, M.D., Jackson, K.G., Fielding, B.A., Williams, C.M. and Frayn, K.N. (2002) Acute effects of meal fatty acid composition on insulin sensitivity in healthy post-menopausal women. *British Journal of Nutrition* 88, 635–640.

Robertson, M.D., Currie, J.M., Morgan, L.M., Jewell, D.P. and Frayn, K.N. (2003) Prior short-term consumption of resistant starch enhances postprandial insulin sensitivity in healthy subjects. *Diabetologia* 46, 659–665.

Robinson, K.M., Heineke, E.W. and Begovic, M.E. (1990) Quantitative relationship between intestinal sucrase inhibition and reduction of the glycemic response to sucrose in rats. *Journal of Nutrition* 120, 105–111.

Robinson, K., Arheart, K., Refsum, H., Brattstrom, L., Boers, G., Ueland, P., Rubba, P., Palma-Reis, R., Meleady, R., Daly, L., Witteman, J. and Graham, I. (1998) Low circulating folate and vitamin B6 concentrations: risk factors for stroke, peripheral vascular disease and coronary heart disease. European COMAC. *Circulation* 97, 437–443.

Rocca, A.S. and Brubaker, P.L. (1995) Stereospecific effects of fatty acids on proglucagon-derived peptide secretion in fetal rat intestinal cultures. *Endocrinology* 136, 5593–5599.

Rodin, J. (1991) Effects of pure sugar vs. mixed starch fructose loads on food intake. *Appetite* 17, 213–219.

Rodin, J., Wack, J., Ferrannini, E. and DeFronzo, R.A. (1985) Effect of insulin and glucose on feeding behavior. *Metabolism: Clinical and Experimental* 34, 826–831.

Rodin, J., Reed, D. and Jamner, L. (1988) Metabolic effects of fructose and glucose: implications for food intake. *American Journal of Clinical Nutrition* 47, 683–689.

Rohdenburg, G.L., Bernhard, A. and Krehbiel, O. (1919) Sugar tolerance in cancer. *Journal of the American Medical Association* 72, 1528–1530.

Rolls, B.J. and Hammer, V.A. (1995) Fat, carbohydrate, and the regulation of energy intake. *American Journal of Clinical Nutrition* 62 (Suppl. 5), 1086S–1095S.

Rolls, B.J., Bell, E.A. and Thorwart, M.L. (1999) Water incorporated into a food but not served with a food decreases energy intake in lean women. *American Journal of Clinical Nutrition* 70, 448–455.

Rolls, B.J., Bell, E.A. and Waugh, B.A. (2000) Increasing the volume of a food by incorporating air affects satiety in men. *American Journal of Clinical Nutrition* 72, 361–368.

Romieu, I., Willett, W.C., Stampfer, M.J., Colditz, G.A., Sampson, L., Rosner, B., Hennekens, C.H. and Speizer, F.E. (1988) Energy intake and other determinants of relative weight. *American Journal of Clinical Nutrition* 47, 406–412.

Rosengren, A., Wedel, H. and Wilhelmsen, L. (1999) Body weight and weight gain during adult life in men in relation to coronary heart disease and mortality. A prospective population study. *European Heart Journal* 20, 269–277.

Rosenthal, S.M. and Ziegler, E.E. (1929) The effect of uncooked starches on the blood sugar or normal and of diabetic subjects. *Archives of Internal Medicine* 44, 344–350.

Ross, S.W., Brand, J.C., Thorburn, A.W. and Truswell, A.S. (1987) Glycemic index of processed wheat products. *American Journal of Clinical Nutrition* 46, 631–635.

Rouch, C., Meile, M.J. and Orosco, M. (2003) Extracellular hypothalamic serotonin and plasma amino acids in response to sequential carbohydrate and protein meals. *Nutritional Neuroscience* 6, 117–124.

Rowe, A.H. and Rogers, H. (1927) Carbohydrate tolerance in normal persons and in nondiabetic patients. *Archives of Internal Medicine* 39, 330–342.

Royall, D., Wolever, T.M.S. and Jeejeebhoy, K.N. (1990) Clinical significance of colonic fermentation. *American Journal of Gastroenterology* 85, 1307–1312.

Rubins, H.B., Robins, S.J., Collins, D., Fye, C.L., Anderson, J.W., Elam, M.B., Faas, F.H., Linares, E., Schaefer, E.J., Schectman, G., Wilt, T.J. and Wittes, J. (1999) Gemfibrozil for the secondary prevention of coronary heart disease in men with low levels of high-density lipoprotein cholesterol. *New England Journal of Medicine* 341, 410–418.

Rugg-Gunn, A.J., Hackett, A.F., Jenkins, G.N. and Appleton, D.R. (1991) Empty calories? Nutrient intake in relation to sugar intake in English adolescents. *Journal of Human Nutrition and Dietetics* 4, 101–111.

Rumessen, J.J. (1992) Hydrogen and methane breath tests for evaluation of resistant carbohydrates. *European Journal of Clinical Nutrition* 46, S77–S90.

Rumessen, J.J. and Gudmand-Høyer, E. (1986) Absorption capacity of fructose in healthy adults. Comparison with sucrose and its constituents monosaccharides. *Gut* 27, 1161–1168.

Rumessen, J.J. and Gudmand-Høyer, E. (1988) Functional bowel disease: malabsorption and abdominal distress after ingestion of fructose, sorbitol and fructose–sorbitol mixtures. *Gastroenterology* 95, 694–700.

Rumessen, J.J., Hamberg, O. and Gudmand-Høyer, E. (1990) Interval sampling of end-expiratory hydrogen ($H_2$) concentrations to quantify carbohydrate malabsorption by means of lactulose standards. *Gut* 31, 37–42.

Saad, M.F., Knowler, W.C., Pettitt, D.J., Nelson, R.G., Charles, M.A. and Bennett, P.H. (1991) A two-step model for development of non-insulin-dependent diabetes mellitus. *American Journal of Medicine* 90, 229–235.

Sahyoun, N.R., Anderson, A.L., Kanaya, A.M., Koh-Banerjee, P., Kritchevsky, S.B., de Rekeneire, N., Tylavsky, F.A., Schwartz, A.V., Lee, J.S. and Harris, T.B. (2005) Dietary glycemic index and load, measures of glucose metabolism, and body fat distribution in older adults. *American Journal of Clinical Nutrition* 82, 547–552.

Salmerón, J., Ascherio, A., Rimm, E.B., Colditz, G.A., Spiegelman, D., Jenkins, D.J., Stampfer, M.J., Wing, A.L. and Willett, W.C. (1997a) Dietary fiber, glycemic load, and risk of NIDDM in men. *Diabetes Care* 20, 545–550.

Salmerón, J., Manson, J.E., Stampfer, M.J., Colditz, G.A., Wing, A.L. and Willett, W.C. (1997b) Dietary fiber, glycemic load and risk of non-insulin-dependent diabetes mellitus in women. *Journal of the American Medical Association* 277, 472–477.

Samaha, F.F., Iqbal, N., Seshadri, P., Chicano, K.L., Daily, D.A., McGrory, J., Williams, T., Williams, M., Gracely, E.J. and Stern, L. (2003) A low-carbohydrate as compared with a low-fat diet in severe obesity. *New England Journal of Medicine* 348, 2074–2081.

Samra, R.A., Smirnakis, F., Anderson, G.H., Wolever, T., Geleva, D. and Woodend, D. (2004) Hyperinsulinemia in men does not impair their caloric compensation in response to a glucose drink. *FASEB Journal* 18 (Suppl. S), A1109.

Saris, W.H.M., Astrup, A., Prentice, A.M., Zunft, H.J.F., Formiguera, X., Verboeket-van de Venne, W.P.H.G., Raben, A., Poppitt, S.D., Seppelt, B., Johnston, S., Vasilaras, T.H. and Keogh, G.F. (2000) Randomized controlled trial of changes in dietary carbohydrate/fat ratio and simple vs complex carbohydrates on body weight and blood lipids: the CARMEN study. The Carbohydrate Ratio Management in European National diets. *International Journal of Obesity* 24, 1310–1318.

Särnblad, S., Kroon, M. and Åman, J. (2002) The short insulin tolerance test lacks validity in adolescents with type 1 diabetes. *Diabetic Medicine* 19, 51–56.

Sattar, N., Gaw, A., Scherbakova, O., Ford, I., O'Reilly, D.S., Haffner, S.M., Isles, C., Macfarlane, P.W., Packard, C.J., Cobbe, S.M. and Shepherd, J. (2003) Metabolic syndrome with and without C-reactive protein as a predictor of coronary heart disease and diabetes in the West of Scotland Coronary Prevention Study. *Circulation* 108, 414–419.

Sawaya, A.L., Tucker, K., Tsay, R., Willett, W., Saltzman, E., Dallal, G.E. and Roberts, S.B. (1996) Evaluation of four methods for determining energy intake in young and older women: comparison with doubly labeled water measurements of total energy expenditure. *American Journal of Clinical Nutrition* 63, 491–499.

Scaglioni, S., Stival, G. and Giovanni, M. (2004) Dietary glycemic load, overall glycemic index, and serum insulin concentrations in healthy schoolchildren. *American Journal of Clinical Nutrition* 79, 339–340.

Schäfer, G., Schenk, U., Ritzel, U., Romadori, G. and Leonhardt, U. (2003) Comparison of the effects of dried peas with those of potatoes in mixed meals on postprandial glucose and insulin concentrations in patients with type 2 diabetes. *American Journal of Clinical Nutrition* 78, 99–103.

Schauberger, G., Brinck, U.C., Guldner, G., Spaethe, R., Niklas, L. and Otto, H. (1977) Exchange of carbohydrates according to their effect on blood glucose. *Diabetes* 26 (Suppl. 1), 415 (Abstract).

Scheen, A.J. (2003) Is there a role for alpha-glucosidase inhibitors in the prevention of type 2 diabetes mellitus? *Drugs* 63, 933–951.

Scheppach, W., Fabian, C., Ahrens, F., Spengler, M. and Kasper, H. (1988a) Effect of starch malabsorption on colonic function and metabolism in humans. *Gastroenterology* 95, 1549–1555.

Scheppach, W., Richter, F., Joeres, R., Richter, E. and Kasper, H. (1988b) Systemic availability of propionate and acetate in liver cirrhosis. *American Journal of Gastroenterology* 83, 850–853.

Scheppach, W., Wiggins, H.S., Halliday, D., Self, R., Howard, J., Branch, W.J., Schrezenmeir, J. and Cummings, J.H. (1988c) Effect of gut-derived acetate on glucose turnover in man. *Clinical Science* 75, 363–370.

Scheppach, W., Pomare, W.E., Elia, M. and Cummings, J.H. (1991) The contribution of the large intestine to blood acetate in man. *Clinical Science* 80, 177–182.

Schley, P.D. and Field, C.J. (2002) The immune-enhancing effects of dietary fibres and prebiotics. *British Journal of Nutrition* 87 (Suppl. 2), S221–S230.

Schmidt, F.J., Sluiter, W.J. and Schoonen, A.J.M. (1993) Glucose concentration in subcutaneous extracellular space. *Diabetes Care* 16, 695–700.

Schneeman, B.O. (1999) Fiber, inulin and oligofructose: similarities and differences. *Journal of Nutrition* 129, 1424S–1427S.

Scholl, T.O., Hediger, M.L., Schall, J.I., Ances, I.G. and Smith, W.K. (1995) Gestational weight gain, pregnancy outcome, and postpartum weight retention. *Obstetrics and Gynecology* 86, 423–427.

Scholl, T.O., Chen, X., Khoo, C.S. and Lenders, C. (2004) The dietary glycemic index during pregnancy: influence on birth weight, fetal growth, and biomarkers of carbohydrate metabolism. *American Journal of Epidemiology* 159, 467–474.

Schrezenmeir, J. and Jagla, A. (2000) Milk and diabetes. *Journal of the American College of Nutrition* 19, 176S–190S.

Schulz, M., Liese, A.D., Mayer-Davis, E.J., D'Agostino, R.B., Fang, F., Sparks, K.C. and Wolever, T.M. (2005) Nutritional correlates of dietary glycemic index: new aspects from a population perspective. *British Journal of Nutrition* 94, 397–406.

Schulze, M.B., Liu, S., Rimm, E.B., Manson, J.E., Willett, W.C. and Hu, F.B. (2004) Glycemic index, glycemic load, and dietary fiber intake and incidence of type 2 diabetes in younger and middle-aged women. *American Journal of Clinical Nutrition* 80, 348–356.

Schwartz, M.W., Bergman, R.N., Kahn, S.E., Taborsky, G.J., Fisher, L.D., Sipols, A.J., Woods, S.C., Steil, G.M. and Porte, D. Jr (1991) Evidence for uptake of plasma insulin into cerebrospinal fluid through an intermediate compartment in dogs: quantitative aspects and implication for transport. *Journal of Clinical Investigation* 88, 1272–1281.

Schwartz, J.G., Phillips, W.T., Blumhardt, M.R. and Langer, O. (1994) Use of a more physiological oral glucose solution during screening for gestational diabetes mellitus. *American Journal of Obstetrics and Gynecology* 171, 685–691.

Schwartz, M.C., Boyko, E.J., Kahn, S.E., Ravussin, E. and Borgardus, C. (1995) Reduced insulin secretion: an independent predictor of body weight gain. *Journal of Clinical Endocrinology and Metabolism* 80, 1571–1576.

Schweizer, T.F., Andersson, H., Langkilde, A.M., Reimann, S. and Torsdottir, I. (1990) Nutrients excreted in ileostomy effluents after consumption of mixed diets with beans or potatoes. II. Starch, dietary fibre and sugars. *European Journal of Clinical Nutrition* 44, 567–575.

Secchi, A., Pontiroli, A.E., Cammelli, L., Bizzi, A., Cini, M. and Pozza, G. (1986) Effects of oral administration of maltitol on plasma glucose, plasma sorbitol, and serum insulin levels in man. *Klinische Wochen-schrift* 64, 265–269.

Segura, A.G., Josse, R.G. and Wolever, T.M.S. (1995) Acute metabolic effects of increased meal frequency in Type II diabetes: three vs six, nine and twelve meals. *Diabetes, Nutrition and Metabolism* 8, 331–338.

Seino, Y., Seino, S., Ikeda, M., Matsukura, S. and Imura, H. (1983) Beneficial effects of high protein diet in treatment of mild diabetes. *Human Nutrition: Applied Nutrition* 37A, 226–230.

Sermer, M., Naylor, C.D., Gare, D.J., Kenshole, A.B., Ritchie, J.W., Farine, D., Cohen, H.R., McArthur, K., Holzapfel, S., Biringer, A. and Chen, E. (1995) Impact of increasing carbohydrate intolerance on maternal–fetal outcomes in 3637 women without gestational diabetes. The Toronto Tri-Hospital Gestational Diabetes Project. *American Journal of Obstetrics and Gynecology* 173, 146–156

Service, F.J., Hall, L.D., Westland, R.E., O'Brien, P.C., Go, V.L.W., Haymond, M.W. and Rizza, R.A. (1983) Effects of size, time of day and sequence of meal ingestion on carbohydrate tolerance in normal subjects. *Diabetologia* 25, 316–321.

Shaheen, S.M. and Fleming, S.E. (1987) High-fiber foods at breakfast: influence on plasma glucose and insulin responses at lunch. *American Journal of Clinical Nutrition* 46, 804–811.

Shen, S.W., Reaven, G.M. and Farquhar, J.W. (1970) Comparison of impedance to insulin-mediated glucose uptake in normal subjects and in subjects with latent diabetes. *Journal of Clinical Investigation* 49, 2151–2160.

Sherlock, S. (1975) Acute (fulminant) hepatic failure. In: *Diseases of the Liver and Biliary System*, 5th edn. Blackwell Scientific Publications, Oxford, UK, p. 113.

Shetty, P.S. and Kurpad, A.V. (1986) Increasing starch intake in the human diet increases fecal bulking. *American Journal of Clinical Nutrition* 43, 210–212.

Shide, D.J. and Rolls, B.J. (1995) Information about the fat content of preloads influences energy intake in healthy women. *Journal of the American Dietetic Association* 95, 993–998.

Sievenpiper, J.L., Vuksan, V., Wong, E.Y., Mendelson, R.A. and Bruce-Thompson, C. (1998) Effect of meal dilution on the postprandial glycemic response. Implications for glycemic testing. *Diabetes Care* 21, 711–716.

Sievenpiper, J.L., Jenkins, D.J., Josse, R.G. and Vuksan, V. (2000) Dilution of 75-g oral glucose tolerance test increases postprandial glycemia: implications for diagnostic criteria. *Canadian Medical Association Journal* 162, 993–996.

Sievenpiper, J.L., Jenkins, D.J., Josse, R.G. and Vuksan, V. (2001) Dilution of 75-g oral glucose tolerance test improves overall tolerability but not reproducibility in subjects with different body compositions. *Diabetes Research and Clinical Practice* 51, 87–95.

Sigalet, D.L. and Martin, G. (1999) Lymphatic absorption of glucose and fatty acids as determined by direct measurement. *Journal of Pediatric Surgery* 34, 39–43.

Silvera, S.A.N., Jain, M., Howe, G.R., Miller, A.B. and Rohan, T.E. (2005a) Dietary carbohydrates and breast cancer risk: a prospective study of the roles of overall glycemic index and glycemic load. *International Journal of Cancer* 114, 653–658.

Silvera, S.A., Rohan, T.E., Jain, M., Terry, P.D., Howe, G.R. and Miller, A.B. (2005b) Glycemic index, glycemic load, and pancreatic cancer risk (Canada). *Cancer Causes and Control* 16, 431–436.

Silvester, K.R., Englyst, H.N. and Cummings, J.H. (1995) Ileal recovery of starch from whole diets containing resistant starch measured *in vitro* and fermentation of ileal effluent. *American Journal of Clinical Nutrition* 62, 403–411.

Simpson, R.W., McDonald, J., Wahlqvist, M.L., Atley, L. and Outch, K. (1985) Macronutrients have different metabolic effects in nondiabetics and diabetics. *American Journal of Clinical Nutrition* 42, 449–453.

Sims, E.A.H. (1996) Insulin resistance is a result, not a cause of obesity: socratic debate: the con side. In: Angel, A., Anderson, H., Bouchard, C., Lau, D., Lieter, L. and Mendelson, R. (eds) *Progress in Obesity Research: 7.* 7th International Congress on Obesity, John Libbey & Co, London, pp. 587–592.

Singh, R.B., Dubnov, G., Niaz, M.A., Ghosh, S., Singh, R., Rastogi, S.S., Manor, O., Pella, D. and Berry, E.M. (2002) Effect of an Indo-Mediterranean diet on progression of coronary artery disease in high risk patients (Indo-Mediterranean Diet Heart Study): a randomised single-blind trial. *Lancet* 360, 1455–1461.

Sisk, C.W., Burnham, C.E., Stewart, J. and McDonald, G.W. (1970) Comparison of the 50 and 100 gram oral glucose tolerance test. *Diabetes* 19, 852–862.

Skov, A.R., Toubro, S., Bülow, J., Krabbe, K., Parving, H.-H. and Astrup, A. (1999) Changes in renal function during weight loss induced by high vs low-protein low-fat diets in overweight subjects. *International Journal of Obesity* 23, 1170–1177.

Slabber, M., Barnard, H.C., Kuyl, J.M., Dannhauser, A. and Schall, R. (1994) Effects of low-insulin-response, energy-restricted diet on weight loss and plasma insulin concentrations in hyperinsulinemic obese females. *American Journal of Clinical Nutrition* 60, 48–53.

Slaughter, S.L., Ellis, P.R. and Butterworth, P.J. (2001) An investigation of the action of porcine pancreatic α-amylase on native and gelatinized starches. *Biochimica et Biophysica Acta* 1525, 29–36.

Sloth, B., Krog-Mikkelsen, I., Flint, A., Tetens, I., Björck, I., Vinoy, S., Elmståhl, H., Astrup, A., Lang, V. and Raben, A. (2004) No difference in body weight decrease between a low-glycemic-index and a high-glycemic-index diet but reduced LDL cholesterol after 10-wk *ad libitum* intake of the low-glycemic-index diet. *American Journal of Clinical Nutrition* 80, 337–347.

Slyper, A., Jurva, J., Pleuss, J., Hoffmann, R. and Gutterman, D. (2005) Influence of glycemic load on HDL cholesterol in youth. *American Journal of Clinical Nutrition* 81, 376–379.

Smith, A. (2002) Effects of caffeine on human behavior. *Food and Chemical Toxicology* 40, 1243–1255.

Sniderman, A.D., Cianflone, K., Arner, P., Summers, L.K.M. and Frayn, K.N. (1998) The adipocyte, fatty acid trapping and atherogenesis. *Arteriosclerosis Thrombosis and Vascular Biology* 18, 147–151.

Soh, N.L. and Brand-Miller, J. (1999) The glycaemic index of potatoes: the effect of variety, cooking method and maturity. *European Journal of Clinical Nutrition* 53, 249–254.

Solnica, B., Naskalski, J.W. and Sieradzki, J. (2003) Analytical performance of glucometers used for routine glucose self-monitoring of diabetic patients. *Clinica Chimica Acta* 331, 29–35.

Sørensen, N.S., Marckmann, P., Hoy, C.-E., van Duyvenvoorde, W. and Princen, H.M.G. (1998) Effect of fish-oil-enriched margarine on plasma lipids, low-density-lipoprotein particle composition, size, and susceptibility to oxidation. *American Journal of Clinical Nutrition* 68, 235–241.

Spaethe, R., Brinck, U.C., Sabin, J., Wubbens, K. and Otto, H. (1972) Échange des hydrats de carbone d'après le prencipe des équivalents biologiques dans le régime por diabétiques. *Journées annuelles de Diabétologie de l'Hôtel-Dieu* 13, 253–259.

Sparks, M.J., Selig, S.S. and Febbraio, M.A. (1998) Pre-exercise carbohydrate ingestion: effect of the glycemic index on endurance exercise performance. *Medicine and Science in Sports and Exercise* 30, 844–849.

Speechly, D.P. and Buffenstein, R. (2000) Appetite dysfunction in obese males: evidence for role of hyperinsulinaemia in passive overconsumption with a high fat diet. *European Journal of Clinical Nutrition* 54, 225–233.

Spiller, G.A., Jensen, C.D., Pattison, T.S., Chuck, C.S., Whittam, J.H. and Scala, J. (1987) Effect of protein dose on serum glucose and insulin response to sugars. *American Journal of Clinical Nutrition* 46, 474–480.

Spitzer, L. and Rodin, J. (1987) Effects of fructose and glucose preloads on subsequent food intake. *Appetite* 8, 135–145.

Staub, H. (1921) Untersuchungen über den zuckerstoffwechsel des menschen. I. Mitteilung: Ueber das verhalten des blutzuckers nach peroraler zufuhr kleiner glukosemengen. Versuch einer neuen funktionsprüfung des zuckerstoffwechsels. *Zeitschrift für Klinische Medizin* 91, 44–60.

Stephen, A.M. and Cummings, J.H. (1980) The microbial contribution to human faecal mass. *Journal of Medical Microbiology* 13, 45–56.

Stephen, A.M., Haddad, A.C. and Phillips, S.F. (1983) Passage of carbohydrate into the colon. Direct measurements in humans. *Gastroenterology* 85, 589–595.

Stern, M.P. (1994) The insulin resistance syndrome: the controversy is dead, long live the controversy! *Diabetologia* 37, 956–958.

Stern, L., Iqbal, N., Seshadri, P., Chicano, K.L., Daily, D.A., McGrory, J., Williams, M., Gracely, E.J. and Samaha, F.F. (2004) The effects of low-carbohydrate versus conventional weight loss diets in severely obese adults: one-year follow-up of a randomized trial. *Annals of Internal Medicine* 140, 778–785.

Sternberg, F., Meyerhoff, C., Mennel, F.J., Bischof, F. and Pfeiffer, E.F. (1995) Subcutaneous glucose concentration in humans: real estimation and continuous monitoring. *Diabetes Care* 18, 1266–1269.

Stevens, J., Ahn, K., Juhaeri, Houston, D., Steffan, L. and Couper, D. (2002) Dietary fiber intake and glycemic index and incidence of diabetes in African-American and white adults. *Diabetes Care* 25, 1715–1721.

Stevenson, E., Williams, C. and Biscoe, H. (2005a) The metabolic responses to high carbohydrate meals with different glycemic indices consumed during recovery from prolonged strenuous exercise. *International Journal of Sport Nutrition and Exercise Metabolism* 15, 291–307.

Stevenson, E., Williams, C. and Nute, M. (2005b) The influence of the glycaemic index of breakfast and lunch on substrate utilization during the postprandial periods and subsequent exercise. *British Journal of Nutrition* 93, 885–893.

Stevenson, E., Williams, C., Nute, M., Swaile, P. and Tsui, M. (2005c) The effect of the glycemic index of an evening meal on the metabolic responses to a standard high glycemic index breakfast and subsequent exercise in men. *International Journal of Sport Nutrition and Exercise Metabolism* 15, 308–322.

Stout, R.W. (1990) Insulin and atheroma: 20-yr perspective. *Diabetes Care* 13, 631–654.

Stram, D.O., Hankin, J.H., Wilkens, L.R., Pike, M.C., Monroe, K.R., Park, S., Henderson, B.E., Nomura, A.M., Earle, M.E., Nagamine, F.S. and Kolonel, L.N. (2000) Calibration of the dietary questionnaire for a multiethnic cohort in Hawaii and Los Angeles. *American Journal of Epidemiology* 151, 358–370.

Strandberg, T.E., Strandberg, A., Slomaa, V.V., Pitkälä, K. and Miettinen, T.A. (2003) Impact of midlife weight change on mortality and quality of life in old age. Prospective cohort study. *International Journal of Obesity* 27, 950–954.

Stubbs, R.J., Harbron, C.G., Murgatroyd, P.R. and Prentice, A.M. (1995) Covert manipulation dietary fat and energy density: effect on substrate flux and food intake in men eating *ad libitum*. *American Journal of Clinical Nutrition* 62, 316–329.

Stubbs, R.J., Harbron, C.G. and Prentice, A.M. (1996) Covert manipulation of the dietary fat to carbohydrate ratio of isoenergetically dense diets: effect on food intake in feeding men *ad libitum*. *International Journal of Obesity* 20, 651–660.

Sumiyoshi, W., Urashima, T., Nakamura, T., Arai, I., Saito, T., Tsumura, N., Wang, B., Brand-Miller, J., Watanabe, Y. and Kimura, K. (2003) Determination of each neutral oligosaccharide in the milk of Japanese women during the course of lactation. *British Journal of Nutrition* 89, 61–69.

Surwit, R.S., Schneider, M.S. and Feinglos, M.N. (1992) Stress and diabetes mellitus. *Diabetes Care* 15, 1413–1422.

Swan, D.C., Davidson, P. and Albrink, M.J. (1966) Effect of simple and complex carbohydrates on plasma non-esterified fatty acids, plasma-sugar, and plasma-insulin during oral carbohydrate tolerance tests. *Lancet* i, 60–63.

Swinburn, B.A., Nyomba, B.L., Saad, M.F., Zurlo, F., Raz, I., Knowler, W.C., Lillioja, S., Bogardus, C. and Ravussin, E. (1991a) Insulin resistance associated with lower rates of weight gain in Pima Indians. *Journal of Clinical Investigation* 88, 168–173.

Swinburn, B.A., Boyce, V.L., Bergman, R.N., Howard, B.V. and Bogardus, C. (1991b) Deterioration in carbohydrate metabolism and lipoprotein changes induced by modern, high fat diet in Pima Indians and Caucasians. *Journal of Clinical Endocrinology and Metabolism* 73, 156–165.

Tan, M.H., Baksi, A., Krahulec, B., Kubalski, P., Stankiewicz, A., Urquhart, R., Edwards, G. and Johns, D. for the GLAL Study Group (2005) Comparison of pioglitazone and gliclazide in sustaining glycemic control over 2 years in patients with type 2 diabetes. *Diabetes Care* 28, 544–550.

Tappy, L., Acheson, K., Normand, S., Schneeberger, D., Thelin, A., Pachiaudi, C., Riou, J.P. and Jequier, E. (1992) Effects of infused amino acids on glucose production and utilization in healthy human subjects. *American Journal of Physiology* 262, E826–E833.

Tasman-Jones, C. (1993) Effect of dietary fiber and fiber-rich foods on structure and function of the upper gastrointestinal tract. In: Spiller, G.A. (ed.) *CRC Handbook of Dietary Fiber in Human Nutrition*, 2nd edn. CRC Press, Boca Raton, Florida, pp. 355–357.

Tavani, A., Bosetti, C., Negri, E., Augustin, L.S., Jenkins, D.J.A. and La Vecchia, C. (2003) Carbohydrates, dietary glycaemic load and glycaemic index, and risk of acute myocardial infarction. *Heart* 89, 722–726.

Temelkova-Kurtschiev, T., Koehler, C., Henkel, E., Leonhardt, W., Fuecker, K. and Hanefeld, M. (2000) Post-challenge plasma glucose and glycemic spikes are strongly associated with atherosclerosis than fasting glucose or $HbA_{1c}$ level. *Diabetes Care* 23, 1830–1834.

Terry, P.D., Jain, M., Miller, A.B., Howe, G.R. and Rohan, T.E. (2003) Glycemic load, carbohydrate intake, and risk of colorectal cancer in women: a prospective cohort study. *Journal of the National Cancer Institute* 95, 914–916.

Tessari, P., Inchiostro, S., Biolo, G., Duner, E., Nosadini, R., Tiengo, A. and Crepaldi, G. (1985) Hyperaminoacidaemia reduces insulin-mediated glucose disposal in healthy man. *Diabetologia* 28, 870–872.

Thomas, D.E., Brotherhood, J.R. and Brand, J.C. (1991) Carbohydrate feeding before exercise: effect of glycemic index. *International Journal of Sports Medicine* 12, 180–186.

Thompson, D.G., Wingate, D.L., Thomas, M. and Harrison, D. (1982) Gastric emptying as a determinant of the oral glucose tolerance test. *Gastroenterology* 82, 51–55.

Thompson, L.U., Yoon, J.H., Jenkins, D.J.A., Wolever, T.M.S. and Jenkins, A.L. (1984) Relationship between polyphenol intake and blood glucose response of normal and diabetic individuals. *American Journal of Clinical Nutrition* 39, 745–751.

Thompson, L.U., Button, C.L. and Jenkins, D.J. (1987) Phytic acid and calcium affect the *in vitro* rate of navy bean starch digestion and blood glucose response in humans. *American Journal of Clinical Nutrition* 46, 467–473.

Thompson, W.G., Rostad Holdman, N., Janzow, D.J., Slezak, J.M., Morris, K.L. and Zemel, M.B. (2005) Effect of energy-reduced diets high in dairy products and fiber on weight loss in obese adults. *Obesity Research* 13, 1344–1353.

Thomsen, C., Rasmussen, O.W., Christiansen, C., Andreasen, F., Poulsen, P.L. and Hermansen, K. (1994) The glycaemic index of spaghetti and gastric emptying in non-insulin-dependent diabetic patients. *European Journal of Clinical Nutrition* 48, 776–780.

Thorburn, A., Muir, J. and Proietto, J. (1993) Carbohydrate fermentation decreases hepatic glucose output in healthy subjects. *Metabolism: Clinical and Experimental* 42, 780–785.

Title, L.M., Cummings, P.M., Giddens, K., Genest, J.J. and Nassar, B.A. (2000) Effect of folic acid and antioxidant vitamins on endothelial dysfunction in patients with coronary artery disease. *Journal of the American College of Cardiology* 36, 758–765.

Toeller, M. and Knußmann, R. (1973) Reproducibility of oral glucose tolerance tests with three different loads. *Diabetologia* 9, 102–107.

Toeller, M., Buyken, A.E., Heitkamp, G., Cathelineau, G., Ferriss, B., Michel, G. and the EURODIAB IDDM Complications Study Group (2001) Nutrient intakes as predictors of body weight in European people with type 1 diabetes. *International Journal of Obesity* 25, 1815–1822.

Torsdottir, I. and Andersson, H. (1989) Effect on the postprandial glycaemic level of the addition of water to a meal ingested by healthy subjects and type 2 (non-insulin-dependent) diabetic patients. *Diabetologia* 32, 231–235.

Torsdottir, I., Alpsten, M., Andersson, D., Brummer, R.J. and Andersson, H. (1984) Effect of different starchy foods in composite meals on gastric emptying rate and glucose metabolism. I. Comparisons between potatoes, rice and white beans. *Human Nutrition – Clinical Nutrition* 38, 329–338.

Torsdottir, I., Alpsten, M. and Andersson, H. (1986) Effect of different starchy foods in composite meals on gastric emptying rate and glucose metabolism. II. Comparisons between potatoes, rice and white beans in diabetic subjects. *Human Nutrition – Clinical Nutrition* 40, 397–400.

Tremblay, A., Dumesnil, J.G. and Després, J.-P. (2002) Diet, satiety and obesity treatment. *British Journal of Nutrition* 87, 213–214.

Trial to Reduce IDDM in the Genetically at Risk (TRIGR) (2004) Available at: http:www.trigr.org (accessed 5 March, 2004)

Trinidad, T.P., Wolever, T.M.S. and Thompson, L.U. (1996) The effect of acetate and propionate on calcium absorption from the rectum and distal colon of humans. *American Journal of Clinical Nutrition* 63, 574–578.

Trinidad, T.P., Wolever, T.M.S. and Thompson, L.U. (1999) Effects of calcium concentration, acetate, and propionate on calcium absorption from the human distal colon. *Nutrition* 15, 529–533.

Trougott, K. (1922) Über das verhalten des blutzuckerspiegels bei wiederholter und verschiedener art enteraler zuckerzufuhr und dessen bedeutung für die leberfunktion. *Klinische Wochenschrift* 18, 892–894.

Trowell, H.C. (1972) Ischemic heart disease and dietary fiber. *American Journal of Clinical Nutrition* 25, 926–932.

Trowell, H.C. (1973) Dietary fibre, ischaemic heart disease, and diabetes mellitus. *Proceedings of the Nutrition Society* 32, 150–157.

Trowell, H.C. (1974) Diabetes mellitus death rates in England and Wales 1920–1970 and food supplies. *Lancet* ii, 998–1002.

Trumper, A., Trumper, K., Trushein, H., Arnold, R., Goke, B. and Horsch, D. (2001) Glucose-dependent insulinotropic polypeptide is a growth factor for beta (INS-1) cells by pleiotropic signaling. *Molecular Endocrinology* 15, 1559–1570.

Truswell, A.S., Seach, J.M. and Thorburn, A.W. (1988) Incomplete absorption of pure fructose in healthy subjects and the facilitating effect of glucose. *American Journal of Clinical Nutrition* 48, 1424–1430.

Tsai, C.J., Leitzmann, M.F., Willett, W.C. and Giovannucci, E.L. (2005a) Dietary carbohydrates and glycaemic load and the incidence of symptomatic gall stone disease in men. *Gut* 54, 823–828.

Tsai, C.J., Leitzmann, M.F., Willett, W.C. and Giovannucci, E.L. (2005b) Glycemic load, glycemic index, and carbohydrate intake in relation to risk of cholecystectomy in women. *Gastroenterology* 129, 105–112.

Tsihlias, E.B., Gibbs, A.L., McBurney, M.I. and Wolever, T.M.S. (2000) Comparison of high- and low-glycemic index breakfast cereals versus monounsaturated fat in the long-term dietary management of type 2 diabetes. *American Journal of Clinical Nutrition* 72, 439–449.

University of Arizona, College of Agricultural and Life Sciences, Department of Nutritional Sciences, Cooperative Extension. Nutrient content of selected sports bars. Available at: http://ag.arizona.edu/nsc/new/sn/HPsports-bars.htm (accessed 12 January, 2005)

US Department of Agriculture Handbook 8 Database Release 17 (September 2004) Available at: http://www.hoptechno.com/nightcrew/sante4me/usda17datashape.cfm (accessed 17 January, 2005)

Vaaler, S., Hanssen, K.F. and Aagenaes, Ø. (1980) Plasma glucose and insulin responses to orally administered carbohydrate-rich foodstuffs. *Nutrition and Metabolism* 24, 168–175.

Valdez, R., Mitchell, B.D., Haffner, S.M., Hazuda, H.P., Morales, P.A., Monterrosa, A. and Stern, M.P. (1994) Predictors of weight change in a bi-ethnic population: the San Antonio Heart Study. *International Journal of Obesity* 18, 85–91.

van Amelsvoort, J.M.M. and Weststrate, J.A. (1992) Amylose–amylopectin ratio in a meal affects postprandial variables in male volunteers. *American Journal of Clinical Nutrition* 55, 712–718.

van Amelsvoort, J.J.M., van Stratum, P., Kraal, J.F., Lussenburg, R.N. and Houtsmuller, U.M.T. (1989) Effects of varying the carbohydrate:fat ratio in a hot lunch on postprandial variables in male volunteers. *British Journal of Nutrition* 61, 267–283.

van Amelsvoort, J.M.M., van Stratum, P., Dubbelman, G.P. and Lussenburg, R.N. (1990a) Effects of meal size reduction on postprandial variables in male volunteers. *Annals of Nutrition and Metabolism* 34, 163–174.

van Amelsvoort, J.M.M., van Stratum, P., Kraal, J.F., Lussenburg, R.N. and Dubbelman, G.P. (1990b) Minor difference in postprandial responses of men between starch and sugar when replacing fat in a normal meal. *British Journal of Nutrition* 63, 37–51.

van Dam, R.M., Visscher, A.W.J., Feskens, E.J.M., Verhoef, P. and Kromhout, D. (2000) Dietary glycemic index in relation to metabolic risk factors and incidence of coronary heart disease: the Zutphen Elderly Study. *European Journal of Clinical Nutrition* 54, 726–731.

Van den Heuvel, E.G., Muijs, T., Van Dokkum, W. and Schaafsma, G. (1999) Lactulose stimulates calcium absorption in postmenopausal women. *Journal of Bone and Mineral Research* 14, 1211–1216.

van der Valk, P.R., van der Schatte Olivier-Steding, I., Wientjes, K.-J.C., Schoonen, A.J. and Hoogenberg, K. (2002) Alternative-site blood glucose measurement at the abdomen. *Diabetes Care* 25, 2114–2115.

van Loo, J., Cummings, J., Delzenne, N., Englyst, H., Franck, A., Hopkins, M., Kok, N., Macfarlane, G., Newton, D., Quigley, M., Roberfroid, M., van Vliet, T. and van den Heuvel, E. (1999) Functional food properties of non-digestible oligosaccharides: a consensus report from the ENDO project (DGXII AIRII-CT94-1095). *British Journal of Nutrition* 81, 121–132.

van Loon, L.J.C., Saris, W.H.M., Verhagen, H. and Wagenmakers, A.J.M. (2000) Plasma insulin responses after ingestion of different amino acid or protein mixtures with carbohydrate. *American Journal of Clinical Nutrition* 72, 96–105.

Vaughan, C.J., Murphy, M.B. and Buckley, B.M. (1996) Statins do more than just lower cholesterol. *Lancet* 348, 1079–1082.

Velangi, A., Fernandes, G. and Wolever, T.M.S. (2005) Evaluation of a glucose meter for determining the glycemic responses of foods. *Clinical Chimica Acta* 356, 191–198.

Vichayanrat, A., Ploybutr, S., Tunlakit, M. and Watanakejorn, P. (2002) Efficacy and safety of voglibose in comparison with acarbose in type 2 diabetic patients. *Diabetes Research and Clinical Practice* 55, 99–103.

Villaume, C., Beck, B., Rohr, R., Pointel, J.-P. and Debry, G. (1986) Effect of exchange of ham for boiled egg on plasma glucose and insulin responses to breakfast in normal subjects. *Diabetes Care* 9, 46–49.

Vogel, R., Corretti, M.C. and Plotnick, G.D. (1997) Effect of a single high-fat meal on endothelial function in healthy subjects. *American Journal of Cardiology* 79, 350–354.

Vogelsang, H., Ferenci, P., Frotz, S., Meryn, S. and Gangl, A. (1988) Acidic colonic microclimate – possible reason for false negative hydrogen breath tests. *Gut* 29, 21–26.

Vogt, J.A. and Wolever, T.M.S. (2003) Fecal acetate is inversely related to acetate absorption from the human rectum and distal colon. *Journal of Nutrition* 133, 3145–3148.

Vogt, J.A., Pencharz, P.B. and Wolever, T.M.S. (2004a) L-Rhamnose raises serum propionate in humans. *American Journal of Clinical Nutrition* 80, 89–94.

Vogt, J.A., Ishii-Schrade, K.B., Pencharz, P.B. and Wolever, T.M.S. (2004b) L-Rhamnose increases serum propionate after long-term supplementation, but lactulose does not raise serum acetate. *American Journal of Clinical Nutrition* 80, 1254–1261.

Vorster, H.H., Venter, C.S. and Silvis, N. (1990) The glycaemic index of foods: a critical evaluation. *South African Journal of Food Science and Nutrition* 1(2), 13–17.

Wahlqvist, M.L., Wilmshurst, E.G. and Richardson, E.N. (1978) The effect of chain length on glucose absorption and the related metabolic response. *American Journal of Clinical Nutrition* 31, 1998–2001.

Walker, A.R.P. and Walker, B.R. (1984) Glycaemic index of South African foods determined in rural blacks – a population at low risk to diabetes. *Human Nutrition: Clinical Nutrition* 36C, 215–222.

Wang, Q. and Brubaker, P.L. (2002) Glucagon-like peptide-1 treatment delays the onset of diabetes in 8-week-old db/db mice. *Diabetologia* 45, 1263–1273.

Wang, S.R., Chase, P., Garg, S.K., Hoops, S.L. and Harris, M.A. (1991) The effect of sugar cereal with and without a mixed meal on glycemic response in children with diabetes. *Journal of Pediatric Gastroenterology and Nutrition* 13, 155–160.

Warren, J.M., Henry, C.J.K. and Simonite, V. (2003) Low glycemic index breakfasts and reduced food intake in preadolescent children. *Pediatrics* 112, e414. Available at: http://www.pediatrics.org/cgi/content/full/112/5/e414

Wee, S.L., Williams, C., Tsintzas, K. and Boobis, L. (2005) Ingestion of a high-glycaemic index meal increases muscle glycogen storage at rest but augments its utilization during subsequent exercise. *Journal of Applied Physiology* 99, 707–714.

Weisenfeld, S., Heght, A. and Goldner, M.G. (1962) Tests of carbohydrate metabolism in carcinomatosis. *Cancer* 15, 18–27.

Welch, I.M., Bruce, C., Hill, S.E. and Read, N.W. (1987) Duodenal and ileal lipid suppresses postprandial blood glucose and insulin responses in man: possible implications for the dietary management of diabetes mellitus. *Clinical Science* 72, 209–216.

Welch, S., Gebhart, S.S., Bergman, R.N. and Phillips, L.S. (1990) Minimal model analysis of intravenous glucose tolerance test-derived insulin sensitivity in diabetic subjects. *Journal of Clinical Endocrinology and Metabolism* 71, 1508–1518.

Westphal, S.A., Gannon, M.C. and Nuttall, F.Q. (1990) Metabolic response to glucose ingested with various amounts of protein. *American Journal of Clinical Nutrition* 52, 267–272.

Weyer, C., Bogardus, C., Mott, D.M. and Pratley, R.E. (1999) The natural history of insulin secretory dysfunction and insulin resistance in the pathogenesis of type 2 diabetes mellitus. *Journal of Clinical Investigation* 104, 787–794.

Whitley, H.A., Humphreys, S.M., Samra, J.S., Campbell, I.T., Maclaren, D.P.M., Reilly, T. and Frayn, K.N. (1997) Metabolic responses to isoenergetic meals containing different proportions of carbohydrate and fat. *British Journal of Nutrition* 78, 15–26.

Widjaja, A., Morris, R.J., Levy, J.C., Frayn, K.N., Manley, S.E. and Turner, R.C. (1999) Within- and between-subject variation in commonly measured anthropometric and biochemical variables. *Clinical Chemistry* 45, 561–566.

Wientjes, K.J., Vonk, P., Vonk-van Klei, Y., Schoonen, A.J.M. and Kossen, N.W. (1998) Microdialysis of glucose in subcutaneous adipose tissue up to 3 weeks in healthy volunteers. *Diabetes Care* 21, 1481–1488.

Wilkinson, I.B. and McEniery, C.M. (2004) Arterial stiffness, endothelial function and novel pharmacological approaches. *Clinical and Experimental Pharmacology and Physiology* 31, 795–799.

Willett, W.C. (1998) Is dietary fat a major determinant of body fat? *American Journal of Clinical Nutrition* 67 (Suppl.), 556S–562S.

Willett, W.C. and Lenart, E. (1998) Reproducibility and validity of food-frequency questionnaires. In: Willett, W.C. (ed.) *Nutritional Epidemiology*, 2nd edn. Oxford University Press, Oxford, UK, 101 pp.

Willett, W.C., Howe, G.R. and Kushi, L.H. (1997) Adjustment for total energy intake in epidemiologic studies. *American Journal of Clinical Nutrition* 65, 1220S–1228S.

Williams, C.M. and Jackson, K.G. (2002) Inulin and oligofructose: effects on lipid metabolism from human studies. *British Journal of Nutrition* 87 (Suppl. 2), S261–S264.

Witztum, J.L. (1994) The oxidation hypothesis of atherosclerosis. *Lancet* 344, 793–795.

Wolever, T.M.S. (1985) Application of glycaemic index to mixed meals. *Lancet* ii, 944.

Wolever, T.M.S. (1986) The glycaemic index: a physiological basis for carbohydrate exchange. PhD thesis, University of Toronto, Toronto, Ontario.

Wolever, T.M.S. (1989) How important is prediction of glycemic responses? *Diabetes Care* 12, 591–593.

Wolever, T.M.S. (1990a) Metabolic effects of continuous feeding. *Metabolism: Clinical and Experimental* 39, 947–951.

Wolever, T.M.S. (1990b) The glycemic index. In: Bourne, G.H. (ed.) *World Review of Nutrition and Dietetics, Vol. 62. Aspects of Some Vitamins, Minerals and Enzymes in Health and Disease.* Karger, Basel, pp. 120–185.

Wolever, T.M.S. (1990c) Glycemic index and mixed meals. *American Journal of Clinical Nutrition* 51, 1113.

Wolever, T.M.S. (1992) Glycemic index versus glycemic response: nonsynonymous terms. *Diabetes Care* 15, 1436–1437.

Wolever, T.M.S. (2002) Low carbohydrate does not mean low glycaemic index! *British Journal of Nutrition* 87, 211–212.

Wolever, T.M.S. (2003) Carbohydrate and the regulation of blood glucose and metabolism. *Nutrition Reviews* 61, S40–S48.

Wolever, T.M.S. (2004a) Effect of blood sampling schedule and method of calculating the area under the curve on validity and precision of glycaemic index values. *British Journal of Nutrition* 91, 295–301.

Wolever, T.M.S. (2004b) Comment on validity of glycaemic glucose equivalent. *European Journal of Clinical Nutrition* 58, 1672–1673.

Wolever, T.M.S. and Bolognesi, C. (1996a) Source and amount of carbohydrate affect postprandial glucose and insulin in normal subjects. *Journal of Nutrition* 126, 2798–2806.

Wolever, T.M.S. and Bolognesi, C. (1996b) Prediction of glucose and insulin responses of normal subjects after consuming mixed meals varying in energy, protein, fat, carbohydrate and glycemic index. *Journal of Nutrition* 126, 2807–2812.

Wolever, T.M.S. and Bolognesi, C. (1996c) Time of day influences relative glycaemic effect of foods. *Nutrition Research* 16, 381–384.

Wolever, T.M.S. and Chiasson, J.L. (2000) Acarbose raises serum butyrate in subjects with impaired glucose tolerance. *British Journal of Nutrition* 84, 57–61.

Wolever, T.M.S. and Jenkins, D.J.A. (1986) The use of the glycemic index in predicting the blood glucose response to mixed meals. *American Journal of Clinical Nutrition* 43, 167–172.

Wolever, T.M.S. and Jenkins, D.J.A. (1993) Effect of dietary fiber and foods on carbohydrate metabolism. In: Spiller, G.A. (ed.) *CRC Handbook of Dietary Fiber in Human Nutrition*, 2nd Edn. CRC Press, Boca Raton, Florida, pp. 111–152.

Wolever, T.M.S. and Mehling, C. (2002) High-carbohydrate/low-glycaemic index dietary advice improves glucose disposition index in subjects with impaired glucose tolerance. *British Journal of Nutrition* 87, 477–487.

Wolever, T.M.S. and Mehling, C. (2003) Long-term effect of varying source or amount of dietary carbohydrate on postprandial plasma glucose, insulin, triacylglycerol and free fatty acid concentrations in subjects with impaired glucose tolerance. *American Journal of Clinical Nutrition* 77, 612–621.

Wolver, T.M.S. and Robb, P.A. (1992) Effect of guar, pectin, psyllium, soy polysaccharide and cellulose on breath hydrogen and methane in healthy subjects. *American Journal of Gastroenterology* 87, 305–310.

Wolever, T.M.S., Taylor, R.H. and Goff, D.V. (1978) Guar: viscosity and efficacy. *Lancet* 2, 1381.

Wolever, T.M.S., Jenkins, D.J.A., Nineham, R. and Alberti, K.G.M.M. (1979) Guar gum and reduction of post-prandial glycaemia: effect of incorporation into solid food, liquid food and both. *British Journal of Nutrition* 41, 505–510.

Wolever, T.M.S., Nuttall, F.Q., Lee, R., Wong, G.S., Josse, R.G., Csima, A. and Jenkins, D.J.A. (1985) Prediction of the relative blood glucose response of mixed meals using the white bread glycemic index. *Diabetes Care* 8, 418–428.

Wolever, T.M.S., Jenkins, D.J.A., Kalmusky, J., Jenkins, A., Giordano, C., Giudici, S., Josse, R.G. and Wong, G.S. (1986a) Comparison of regular and parboiled rices: explanation of discrepancies between reported glycemic responses to rice. *Nutrition Research* 6, 349–357.

Wolever, T.M.S., Cohen, Z., Thompson, L.U., Thorne, M.J., Jenkins, M.J.A., Prokipchuk, E.J. and Jenkins, D.J.A. (1986b) Ileal loss of available carbohydrate in man: comparison of a breath hydrogen method with direct measurement using a human ileostomy model. *American Journal of Gastroenterology* 81, 115–122.

Wolever, T.M.S., Jenkins, D.J.A., Josse, R.G., Wong, G.S. and Lee, R. (1987) The glycemic index: similarity of values derived in insulin-dependent and non-insulin-dependent diabetic patients. *Journal of the American College of Nutrition* 6, 295–305.

Wolever, T.M.S., Jenkins, D.J.A., Ocana, A.M., Rao, A.V. and Collier, G.R. (1988a) Second meal effect: low glycemic index foods eaten at dinner improve subsequent breakfast glycemic response. *American Journal of Clinical Nutrition* 48, 1041–1047.

Wolever, T.M.S., Jenkins, D.J.A., Collier, G.R., Lee, R., Wong, G.S. and Josse, R.G. (1988b) Metabolic response to test meals containing different carbohydrate foods. 1. Relationship between rate of digestion and plasma insulin response. *Nutrition Research* 8, 573–581.

Wolever, T.M.S., Jenkins, D.J.A., Jenkins, A.L., Vuksan, V., Wong, G.S. and Josse, R.G. (1988c) Effect of ripeness on the glycaemic response to banana. *Journal of Clinical Nutrition and Gastroenterology* 3, 85–88.

Wolever, T.M.S., Csima, A., Jenkins, D.J.A., Wong, G.S. and Josse, R.G. (1989) The glycemic index: variation between subjects and predictive difference. *Journal of the American College of Nutrition* 8, 235–247.

Wolever, T.M.S., Jenkins, D.J.A., Vuksan, V., Josse, R.G., Wong, G.S. and Jenkins, A.L. (1990) Glycemic index of foods in individual subjects. *Diabetes Care* 13, 126–132.

Wolever, T.M.S., Jenkins, D.J.A., Jenkins, A.L. and Josse, R.G. (1991a) The glycemic index: methodology and clinical implications. *American Journal of Clinical Nutrition* 54, 846–854.

Wolever, T.M.S., Spadafora, P. and Eshuis, H. (1991b) Interaction between colonic acetate and propionate in man. *American Journal of Clinical Nutrition* 53, 681–687.

Wolever, T.M.S., Jenkins, D.J.A., Vuksan, V., Katzman, L., Jenkins, A.L. and Josse, R.G. (1992a) Variation in meal fat content does not affect the relative glycaemic response of spaghetti in subjects with type II diabetes. *Diabetes Nutrition and Metabolism* 5, 191–197.

Wolever, T.M.S., Jenkins, D.J.A., Vuksan, V., Jenkins, A.L., Buckley, G.C., Wong, G.S. and Josse, R.G. (1992b) Beneficial effect of a low-glycaemic index diet in type 2 diabetes. *Diabetic Medicine* 9, 451–458.

Wolever, T.M.S., ter Wal, P., Spadafora, P. and Robb, P. (1992c) Guar, but not psyllium, increases breath methane and serum acetate concentrations in human subjects. *American Journal of Clinical Nutrition* 55, 719–722.

Wolever, T.M.S., Jenkins, D.J.A., Vuksan, V., Jenkins, A.L., Wong, G.S. and Josse, R.G. (1992d) Beneficial effect of low-glycemic index diet in overweight NIDDM subjects. *Diabetes Care* 15, 562–566.

Wolever, T.M.S., Vuksan, V., Katzman-Relle, L., Jenkins, A.L., Josse, R.G., Wong, G.S. and Jenkins, D.J.A. (1993) Glycaemic index of some fruits and fruit products in patients with diabetes. *International Journal of Food Science and Nutrition* 43, 205–212.

Wolever, T.M.S., Katzman-Relle, L., Jenkins, A.L., Vuksan, V., Josse, R.G. and Jenkins, D.J.A. (1994a) Glycaemic index of 102 complex carbohydrate foods in patients with diabetes. *Nutrition Research* 14, 651–669.

Wolever, T.M.S., Nguyen, P.M., Chiasson, J.-L., Hunt, J.A., Josse, R.G., Palmason, C., Rodger, N.W., Ross, S.A., Ryan, E.A. and Tan, M.H. (1994b) Determinants of diet glycemic index calculated retrospectively from diet records of 342 individuals with non-insulin-dependent diabetes mellitus. *American Journal of Clinical Nutrition* 59, 1265–1269.

Wolever, T.M.S., Bentum-Williams, A. and Jenkins, D.J.A. (1995a) Physiologic modulation of plasma FFA concentrations by diet: metabolic implications in non-diabetic subjects. *Diabetes Care* 18, 962–970.

Wolever, T.M.S., Nguyen, P.-M., Chiasson, J.-L., Hunt, J.A., Josse, R.G., Palmason, C., Rodger, N.W., Ross, S.A., Ryan, E.A. and Tan, M.H. (1995b) Relationship between habitual diet and blood glucose and lipids in non-insulin dependent diabetes (NIDDM). *Nutrition Research* 15, 843–857.

Wolever, T.M.S., Spadafora, P.J., Cunnane, S.C. and Pencharz, P.B. (1995c) Propionate inhibits incorporation of colonic [1,2–13C] acetate into plasma lipids in humans. *American Journal of Clinical Nutrition* 61, 1241–1247.

Wolever, T.M.S., Hamad, S., Gittelsohn, J., Gao, J., Hanley, A.J.G., Harris, S.B. and Zinman, B. (1997a) Low dietary fiber and high protein intakes associated with newly discovered diabetes in a remote aboriginal community. *American Journal of Clinical Nutrition* 66, 1470–1474.

Wolever, T.M.S., Hamad, S., Gittelsohn, J., Hanley, A.J.G., Logan, A., Harris, S.B. and Zinman, B. (1997b) Nutrient intake and food use in an Ojibwa-Cree community in Northern Ontario assessed by 24 h dietary recall. *Nutrition Research* 17, 603–618.

Wolever, T.M.S., Chiasson, J.-L., Csima, A., Hunt, J.A., Palmason, C., Ross, S.A. and Ryan, E.A. (1998a) Variation of postprandial plasma glucose, palatability and symptoms after a standardized mixed test meal compared to 75 g oral glucose. *Diabetes Care* 21, 336–340.

Wolever, T.M.S., Chiasson, J.-L., Hunt, J.A., Palmason, C., Ross, S.A. and Ryan, E.A. (1998b) Similarity of relative glycaemic but not relative insulinaemic responses in normal, IGT and diabetic subjects. *Nutrition Research* 18, 1667–1676.

Wolever, T.M.S., Hamad, S., Chiasson, J.-L., Josse, R.G., Leiter, L.A., Rodger, N.W., Ross, S.A. and Ryan, E.A. (1999) Day-to-day consistency in amount and source of carbohydrate intake associated with improved blood glucose control in type 1 diabetes. *Journal of the American College of Nutrition* 18, 242–247.

Wolever, T.M.S., Assiff, L., Basu, T., Chiasson, J.-L., Boctor, M., Gerstein, H.C., Hunt, J.A., Josse, R.G., Lau, D., Leiter, L.A., Maheux, P., Murphy, L., Rodger, N.W., Ross, S.A., Ryan, E., Tildesley, H.D. and Yale, J.-F. (2000) Miglitol, an α-glucosidase inhibitor, prevents the metformin-induced fall in serum folate and vitamin $B_{12}$ in subjects with type 2 diabetes. *Nutrition Research* 20, 1447–1456.

Wolever, T.M.S., Isaacs, R.L. and Ramdath, D.D. (2002a) Lower diet glycaemic index in African than South Asian men in Trinidad and Tobago. *International Journal of Food Science and Nutrition* 53, 297–303.

Wolever, T.M.S., Schrade, K.B., Vogt, J.A., Tsihlias, E.B. and McBurney, M.I. (2002b) Could colonic short chain fatty acids contribute to long-term adaptation of blood lipids on a high fiber diet in subjects with type 2 diabetes? *American Journal of Clinical Nutrition* 75, 1023–1030.

Wolever, T.M.S., Vorster, H.H., Björk, I., Brand-Miller, J., Brighenti, F., Mann, J.I., Ramdath, D.D., Granfeldt, Y., Holt, S., Perry, T.L., Venter, C. and Wu, X. (2003a) Determination of the glycaemic index of foods: interlaboratory study. *European Journal of Clinical Nutrition* 57, 475–482.

Wolever, T.M.S., Tsihlias, E.B., McBurney, M.I. and Le, N.-A. (2003b) Long-term effect of reduced carbohydrate or increased fiber intake on LDL particle size and HDL composition in subjects with type 2 diabetes. *Nutrition Research* 23, 15–26.

Wolever, T.M.S., Campbell, J.E., Geleva, D. and Anderson, G.H. (2004) High-fiber cereal reduces postprandial insulin responses in hyperinsulinemic but not normoinsulinemic subjects. *Diabetes Care* 27, 1281–1285.

Wolf, B.W., Wolever, T.M.S., Bolognesi, C., Zinker, B.A., Garleb, K.A. and Firkins, J.L. (2001a) Glycemic response of a food starch esterified by 1-octenyl succinic anhydride in humans. *Journal of Agricultural and Food Chemistry* 49, 2674–2678.

Wolf, B.W., Wolever, T.M.S., Bolognesi, C., Zinker, B.A. and Garleb, K.A. (2001b) Glycemic response to a rapidly digested starch is not affected by the addition of an indigestible dextrin in humans. *Nutrition Research* 21, 1099–1106.

Wong, M.L., Wee, S., Pin, C.H., Gan, G.L. and Ye, H.C. (1999) Sociodemographic and lifestyle factors associated with constipation in an elderly Asian community. *American Journal of Gastroenterology* 94, 1283–1291.

Woo, R., Kissileff, H.R. and Pi-Sunyer, F.X. (1984) Elevated postprandial insulin levels do not induce satiety in normal-weight humans. *American Journal of Physiology* 16, R745–R749.

Wood, I.S. and Trayhurn, P. (2003) Glucose transporters (GLUT and SGLT): expanded families of sugar transport proteins. *British Journal of Nutrition* 89, 3–9.

Woodend, D.M. and Anderson, G.H. (2001) Effect of sucrose and safflower oil preloads on short term appetite and food intake of young men. *Appetite* 37, 185–195.

Woods, S.C., Stein, L.J., McKay, L.D. and Porte, D. Jr (1984) Suppression of food intake by intravenous nutrients and insulin in the baboon. *American Journal of Physiology* 247, R393–R401.

Woods, S.C., Chavez, M., Park, C.R., Riedy, C., Kaiyala, K., Richardson, R.D., Figlewicz, D.P., Schwartz, M.W., Porte, D. Jr and Seeley, R.J. (1996) The evaluation of insulin as a metabolic signal influencing behaviour via the brain. *Neuroscience and Biobehaviour Reviews* 20, 139–144.

World Health Organization (1998) Obesity: preventing and managing the global epidemic. Report of a WHO Consultation on Obesity, Geneva.

World Health Organization (1999) *Definition, Diagnosis and Classification of Diabetes Mellitus and its Complications. Part 1: Diagnosis and Classification of Diabetes Mellitus.* World Health Organization, Geneva.

Wren, A.M., Seal, L.J., Cohen, M.A., Brynes, A.E., Frost, G.S., Murphy, K.G., Dhillo, W.S., Ghatei, M.A. and Bloom, S.R. (2001) Ghrelin enhances appetite and increases food intake in humans. *Journal of Clinical Endocrinology and Metabolism* 86, 5992–5995.

Wright, E.M., Martin, M.G. and Turk, E. (2003) Intestinal absorption in health and disease-sugars. *Best Practice and Research in Clinical Gastroenterology* 17, 943–956.

Würsch, P. (1989) Starch in human nutrition. *World Review of Nutrition and Dietetics* 60, 199–256.

Würsch, P., Koellreutter, B. and Schweizer, T.F. (1989) Hydrogen excretion after ingestion of five different sugar alcohols and lactulose. *European Journal of Clinical Nutrition* 43, 819–825.

Xavier, R.J. and Podolsky, D.K. (2000) How to get along – friendly microbes in a hostile world. *Science* 289, 1483–1484.

Yancy, W.S. Jr, Olsen, M.K., Guyton, J.R., Bakst, R.P. and Westman, E.C. (2004) A low-carbohydrate, ketogenic diet versus a low-fat diet to treat obesity and hyperlipidemia: a randomized, controlled trial. *Annals of Internal Medicine* 140, 769–777.

Yarnell, J.W., Patterson, C.C., Thomas, H.F. and Sweetnam, P.M. (2000) Comparison of weight in middle age, weight at 18 years, and weight change between, in predicting subsequent 14 year mortality and coronary events: Caerphilly Prospective Study. *Journal of Epidemiology and Community Health* 54, 344–348.

Yoon, J.H., Thompson, L.U. and Jenkins, D.J. (1983) The effect of phytic acid on *in vitro* rate of starch digestibility and blood glucose response. *American Journal of Clinical Nutrition* 38, 835–842.

Young, G.P. and Gibson, P.R. (1995) Butyrate and the human cancer cell. In: Cummings, J.H., Rombeau, J.L. and Sakata, T. (eds) *Physiological and Clinical Aspects of Short-Chain Fatty Acids.* Cambridge University Press, Cambridge, UK, pp. 319–335.

Young, K.W.H. and Wolever, T.M.S. (1998) Effect of volume and type of beverage consumed with a standard test meal on postprandial blood glucose responses. *Nutrition Research* 18, 1857–1863.

Zemel, M.B. (2004) Role of calcium and dairy products in energy partitioning and weight management. *American Journal of Clinical Nutrition* 79 (Suppl.), 907S–912S.

Zeymer, U., Schwarzmaier-D'assie, A., Petzinna, D., Chiasson, J.-L. and the STOP-NIDDM Trial Research Group (2004) Effect of acarbose treatment on the risk of silent myocardial infarctions in patients with impaired glucose tolerance: results of the randomized STOP-NIDDM trial electrocardiography study. *European Journal of Cardiovascular Prevention and Rehabilitation* 11, 412–415.

Zhou, Y.-P. and Grill, V.E. (1994) Long-term exposure of rat pancreatic islets to fatty acids inhibits glucose-induced insulin secretion and biosynthesis through a glucose fatty acid cycle. *Journal of Clinical Investigation* 93, 870–876.

Zimmet, P.Z. (1995) The pathogenesis and prevention of diabetes in adults. Genes, autoimmunity, and demography. *Diabetes Care* 18, 1050–1064.

Zumbé, A., Lee, A. and Storey, D. (2001) Polyols in confectionery: the route to sugar-free, reduced sugar and reduced calorie confectionery. *British Journal of Nutrition* 85 (Suppl. 1), S31–S45.

# Index

Page numbers in *italic* represent figures; page numbers in **bold** represent tables